A Short Textbook of Preventive Medicine for the Tropics

University Medical Texts

General Editor
SELWYN TAYLOR D.M., M.CH.(OXON), F.R.C.S.

A Short Textbook of Medicine Fourth Edition
J. C. HOUSTON M.D., F.R.C.P.
C. L. JOINER M.D., F.R.C.P.
J. R. TROUNCE M.D., F.R.C.P.

A Short Textbook of Surgery Third edition
SELWYN TAYLOR D.M., M.CH., F.R.C.S.
L. T. COTTON M.CH., F.R.C.S.

A Short Textbook: Ear, Nose and Throat
R. PRACY F.R.C.S.
J. SIEGLER M.B., B.S., F.R.C.S., D.L.O.
P. M. STELL M.B., F.R.C.S.

A Short Textbook of Chemical Pathology Third edition
D. N. BARON M.D., D.SC., F.R.C.P., F.R.C.PATH.

A Short Textbook of Orthopaedics and Traumatology
J. N. ASTON M.B., F.R.C.S.

A Short Textbook of Psychiatry
W. L. LINFORD REES B.SC., M.D., F.R.C.P., D.P.M.

A Short Textbook of Venereology Second edition
R. D. CATTERALL F.R.C.P.(EDIN.)

A Short Textbook of Medical Microbiology Third edition
D. C. TURK D.M., M.R.C.P., F.R.C.PATH.
I. A. PORTER M.D., F.R.C.PATH.

A Short Textbook of Gynaecology and Obstetrics
G. D. PINKER M.D., F.R.C.S., F.R.C.O.G.
D. W. T. ROBERTS M.CHIR., F.R.C.S., F.R.C.O.G.

A Short Textbook of
Preventive Medicine
for the Tropics

Adetokunbo O. Lucas

B.Sc.(Durh.), M.D.(Newcastle), D.P.H.(Belf.), D.T.M. & H.(Eng.),
F.R.C.P.(Lond.), S.M.Hyg.(Harv.), F.M.C.P.H.(Nig.)
Professor of Preventive and Social Medicine, University of Ibadan

Herbert M. Gilles

B.Sc., M.D.(Malta), B.Sc.(Oxon), F.R.C.P.(Lond.), F.F.C.M.(U.K.),
F.M.C.P.H.(Nig.), D.T.M. & H. Professor of Tropical Medicine,
Liverpool School of Tropical Medicine
Formerly Professor of Preventive and Social Medicine,
University of Ibadan

The English Universities Press Limited

To Kofo and Mina

ISBN 0 340 05347 x Boards
ISBN 0 340 05348 8 Paperback

First published 1973

The English Universities Press Ltd
St Paul's House, Warwick Lane, London EC4P 4AH

Printed and bound in England by
T. and A. Constable Ltd, Edinburgh

Editor's Foreword

I look on this book as quite the most important of the 'University Medical Texts' since it is concerned with far greater numbers of potential patients and far bigger disease risks than is to be found in any of the other books in the series. The developing countries have enormous problems in preventive and social medicine and it is obviously right that all the resources and help that can be mobilised should be directed to this end in the first place rather than to the relatively less important subject of curing diseases already established.

Clearly the authors are right when they say that it is impossible to cover the whole of the tropical countries in one brief text, but I believe that by having the general principles right and by having painted on a broad canvas, they have achieved very good coverage.

I know that too many medical students face too many examinations in too many places at the present time, but if this book should lighten the burden for a few of them and at the same time encourage them to think along broad preventive and social medical lines then it will have succeeded. I am delighted to be in some small way responsible for its publication.

Selwyn Taylor

Authors' Preface

In many of the new universities of the developing countries, the teaching of preventive and social medicine spans the whole five years of the medical curriculum. Students seem to find it very difficult to pick out the important aspects of this diffuse subject and are often dependent on stencilled notes as their only source of study and revision.

In this textbook we have attempted to emphasise basic concepts of the epidemiology and control of disease as well as other aspects of social medicine and public health relevant to the tropics. We are only too conscious of the error of lumping the 'tropics' as a homogenous whole, since we are very aware that places such as Singapore, Lagos and Buenaventura have only a hot humid climate in common. Nevertheless, we have attempted to bring the whole subject of preventive and social medicine in one compact volume drawing on our basic experience in West Africa, supplemented by relatively short but instructive visits in many other parts of the tropical world. We have aimed at producing a textbook suitable for most places where the socio-economic environment is similar to that of West Africa, but which also lends itself to essential modifications to suit local differences in pattern of disease and development. It is in this area especially that we would expect individual academic teachers to forge their own stamp on the basic general concepts we have covered emphasising or watering down various sections at will.

The Singaporean student, for example, will find the section on communicable disease unduly long, while that on occupational health dismally short. In instances such as this we have given recommendations for further reading that we knew to be available. In other cases we would expect local experience to supplement or even correct our views in the light of indigenous conditions or customs.

For the over-examined medical student in the tropics we have sometimes provided a short summary at the end of some sections for quick revision, and we sincerely hope that this textbook will help to lighten his burden in the final examination.

A. O. LUCAS
H. M. GILLES

vi

Contents

* by Dr F. T. Sai, formerly Director of Medical Services, Ministry of Health, Accra and Professor of Preventive Medicine, University of Ghana Medical School, Accra.

† by Dr A. Adeniyi-Jones, Professor of Community Care, University of Ife, Nigeria.

‡ by Dr O. Adeniyi-Jones, Director of Health Services, W H O, A F R O, Brazzaville, People's Republic of the Congo.

Chapter One

The Tropical Environment

Man's total environment includes all the living and non-living elements in his surroundings. It consists basically of three major components: physical, biological and social. Man's relationship to his environment is reciprocal in that the environment has a profound influence on man whilst, at the same time, man extensively alters his environment to suit his needs and desires.

(a) *Physical Environment*

This refers to the non-living part of the environment—the air, soil, water, minerals; the temperature, humidity and other physical characteristics. The physical environment is extremely variable in the tropics covering arid deserts, savannahs, upland jungle, cold dry or humid plateaux, marshlands, high mountain steppes or tropical rain forest.

Climatic factors such as temperature and humidity have a direct effect on man, his comfort and his physical performance. The influence of the physical environment on the biological environment has an indirect effect on man. It determines the distribution of plants and animals which provide him with materials for food, clothing and shelter; it determines the natural distribution of the predators which prey on him and other animals which compete with him for food; and it determines the prevalence and distribution of parasites and their vectors.

Man alters the natural characteristics of his physical environment sometimes on a small scale but often on a very large scale. He may clear a small patch of bush, build a hut and dig a small canal to irrigate his vegetable garden; or he may build large cities, drain swamps, irrigate arid zones, dam rivers and create large artificial lakes. Many such changes have proved beneficial to man but some aspects of these changes have created new hazards.

(b) *Biological Environment*

All the living things in an area—the plants, animals and micro-organisms—constitute the biological environment. All these living things are interdependent on each other and they are ultimately dependent on their physical environment. Thus, the photosynthetic plants trap energy from the sun and circulate it among the living things in the area.

Nitrogen-fixing organisms convert atmospheric nitrogen into the nitrates which are essential for plant life. A mammal may obtain its nourishment by feeding on plants (herbivore) or on other animals (carnivore) or both (omnivore). Under natural conditions, there is a balanced relationship between the growth and the size of the population of a particular species, on the one hand, and its sources of food and prevalence of competitors and predators, on the other hand.

Man deliberately manipulates the biological environment. He cultivates useful plants to provide food, clothing and shelter, and he raises farm animals for their meat, milk, leather, wool and other useful products. He hunts and kills wild animals and other predators, and he destroys insects which transmit disease or which compete with him for food.

In many parts of the tropics, insects, snails and other vectors of disease abound and thrive. This is partly because the natural environment favours their survival but also because, in some of these areas, relatively little has been done to control these agents.

(c) *Social Environment*

This represents the part of the environment which is entirely man-made. In essence it represents the situation of man as a member of society: his family group, his village or urban community, his culture including beliefs and attitudes, the organisation of society, politics and government, laws and the judicial system, the educational system, transport and communication, and social services including the health services.

There is much variation in the extent of technical development in the various countries in the tropics. Some of these countries are now highly developed whilst others are still in the early stages of technical development. Some of the developing countries show certain common features —limited central organisation of services, scattered populations living in small self-contained units, low level of economic development, limited educational facilities, and inadequate control of common agents of disease. Some of these communities are still held tightly in the vicious cycle of ignorance, poverty and disease.

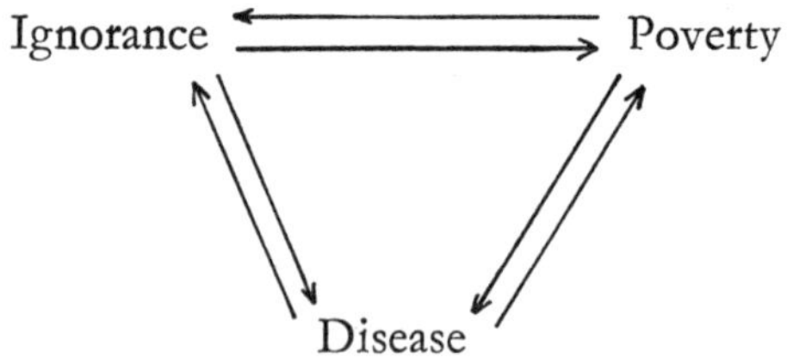

Many areas in the tropics are in transition. Rapid economic development and the growth of modern industries is causing mass migrations from rural to urban areas. Faster means of transportation, progress in education, the control and eradication of major endemic diseases, and other developments are effectively breaking the chains of disease, poverty and ignorance. At the same time new problems are emerging, including those resulting from the social and psychological stresses imposed by these bewildering changes and their destructive effects on traditional family life and communal relationships.

In these transitional societies there have been marked changes in the pattern of diseases. Communicable diseases which were formerly the predominant causes of disability, disease and death are now being replaced by non-communicable diseases and conditions. Malnutrition in the form of the deficiency of specific nutrients is being succeeded by problems resulting from over-indulgence, thus obesity is replacing marasmus as the predominant nutritional problem. Alcoholism and drug abuse are emerging as manifestations of social stresses and tensions.

The Ecological Approach to Preventive Medicine

In preventive medicine, it is useful to consider the reciprocal relationship between man and his total environment. In the search of the causes of diseases, it is not sufficient merely to identify the specific agent of disease such as a virus or a parasite, but it is desirable to identify the influence of environmental factors on the interaction between man and the specific agent. For example, the typhoid bacillus (*Salmonella typhi*) is known to be the causative agent of disease but the occurrence of outbreaks of typhoid disease is determined by various environmental factors; water supply, methods of sewage disposal, prevalence of typhoid carriers, personal habits of the people (cleanliness), use of raw water, etc., attitude to and use of medical services, including vaccination. Similarly, a specific nutritional deficiency such as ariboflavinosis should not be viewed merely as a discrete metabolic defect but it should be seen in the context of the food habits of the community including food taboos, level of education and income of the population and local agriculture.

From this ecological approach, one can derive a rational basis for the control of diseases within the population. The control of typhoid is then seen not solely in terms of treating the individual patient with an antibiotic but also in terms of water supply, sewage disposal, food hygiene and vaccination. Malnutrition is managed not only by giving pills containing concentrated nutrients but also by giving suitable advice about diet and promoting the cultivation of nutritional foods both commercially by farmers and privately in home gardens; in more complex situations it may extend to promotion of welfare services such as unemployment benefits and food supplements for the needy.

Chapter Two

Health Statistics

The assessment of the health of the individual is made on clinical grounds by medical history, physical examination, laboratory tests and other special investigations. Theoretically, the health of a whole community can be assessed by conducting repeatedly a detailed clinical assessment of each individual. In practice, the health of the community is assessed less directly by the collection, analysis and interpretation of data about important events which serve as indicators of the health of the community—deaths (mortality data), sickness (morbidity data) and data about the utilisation of medical services.

Vital Statistics
These are records of certain vital events, births, deaths, marriages and divorces.

Health Statistics
These include vital statistics, and other data pertinent to health. Health statistics are derived from a variety of sources:

(a) *Notification* of diseases—infectious, industrial and other notifiable diseases.

(b) *Institutions*—records from hospitals, health centres, dispensaries, etc.

(c) *Special programmes*—school health service; control and eradication programmes of specific diseases, e.g. tuberculosis, yaws, smallpox, measles.

(d) *Epidemiological Surveys*—information is obtained from the whole community or from a sample by:
    (i) questionnaire—e.g. sickness survey
    (ii) physical examination—e.g. nutrition survey
    (iii) special investigation—e.g. mass miniature radiography (MMR), sputum, immunological tests.

(e) *Utilisation of medical services*—useful data can be obtained from:

(i) Attendance at out-patient clinics—apart from the records of general out-patient clinics where sick patients are treated, pertinent statistical data can be obtained from special clinics such as antenatal clinics, child welfare, family planning.

(ii) The distribution and sales of drugs and vaccines can also yield valuable information.

(f) *Data initially collected for other purposes*—a variety of such data can give useful indication of some aspects of the health of the community:

(i) Routine medical inspection, e.g. pre-employment, insurance, army recruits.

(ii) Sickness absence records from schools, industry and other institutions may for example indicate an acute epidemic such as influenza.

Collection of Data

A variety of mechanisms are used for the collection of the data which form the basis of health statistics. In order that health statistics from various communities can be compared, standardisation is essential nationally and desirable internationally:

A. *Census of the Population*

This is required to provide the essential population base for calculating various rates. The census usually includes not only a total count of the population but also a record of the age and sex distribution, and also some other personal data.

National censuses

In most countries, censuses are held periodically, usually every ten years.

Local censuses

The public health worker may need to conduct a census on a small scale in a local area where census data are unobtainable or not sufficiently accurate for a proposed epidemiological survey. For some studies, the census is conducted on the basis of the number of persons who are actually present on the census date in the defined area; this *de facto* population may include temporary residents and visitors but may exclude permanent residents who happen to be away. For other studies, especially where a longitudinal survey is planned, the census enumerates all persons who are normally resident in an area, i.e. this *de jure* population would exclude temporary residents and visitors but will include permanent residents who are temporarily away.

Population pyramid

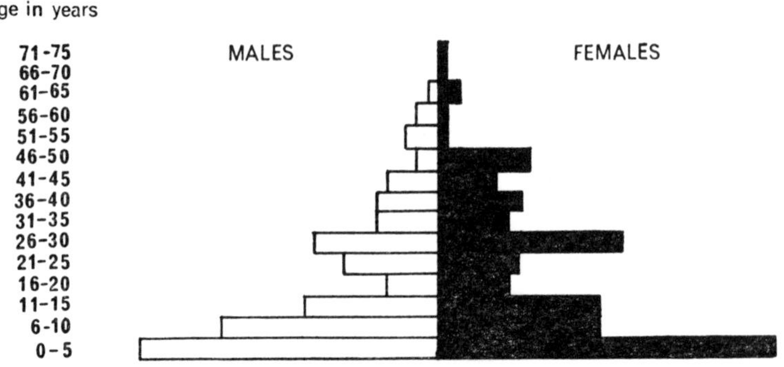

FIG. 2.1   Population pyramid of a developing country.

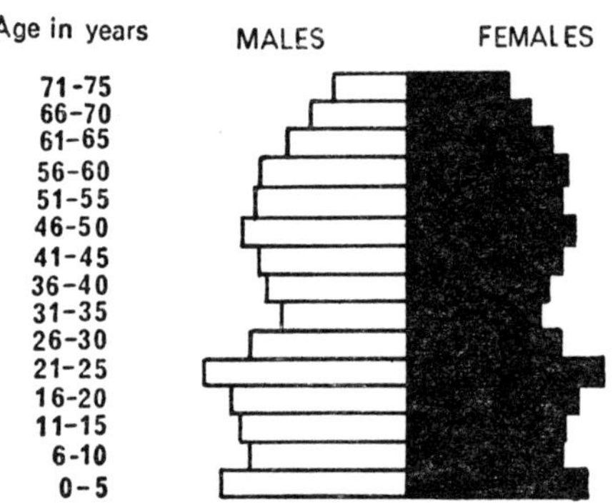

FIG. 2.2   Population pyramid of a more developed country.

The age and sex structure of the population is often displayed in the form of a histogram showing the percentage distribution of each sex at 5-year-age intervals. The shape is roughly pyramidal; the base representing the younger age-group, tapers to a narrow peak in the old age-group. In most developing countries the pyramid is typically broad, with a rapid tapering off in the older age-groups. This represents the characteristic feature of a relatively young population. The shape of the pyramid is determined by the high birth rate and high child death rate in these communities (Fig. 2.1). In the more developed countries, the population pyramid shows more gradual decline, indicating the relatively older population with a low death rate in childhood (Fig. 2.2).

B. *Registration of Births and Deaths*
The registration of births and deaths is compulsory in the developed countries but only in some of the developing countries. Births and deaths are two important events which can be clearly recognised by lay

persons and as such the data can be collected by literate laymen. In addition to recording the fact of death, it is useful to establish the cause of death. The certification of the cause of death is done at various levels of sophistication, ranging from simple diagnoses that can be made by auxiliaries to more difficult diagnoses that can only be obtained from elaborate investigations of the patients by highly trained personnel and post-mortem examination by competent pathologists. In many developing countries there is difficulty in obtaining a complete registration of births and deaths. Even where the local laws make such registrations compulsory, the enforcement of these regulations is difficult and unpopular. Various devices have been tried to improve the quality of the data:

(a) *Registration centres*
These should be conveniently sited so that each person has reasonable access to the registration centre in his district. The registration centre should be adapted to the local social structure, using such persons as village heads, compound heads, religious scribes, or any other institutions that are appropriate in the particular area.

(b) *Rewards and penalties*
In some countries the population is induced to register births by attaching rewards to the possession of birth certificates. For example, the government free primary school may be available only to children whose births have been registered. By and large, unduly harsh penalties against defaulters are not to be recommended because such actions may antagonise the public and alienate them from other public health programmes and personnel.

(c) *Education*
Regardless of the method of registration that is adopted, the success of the scheme will depend on being able to get appropriate and sufficient information to the general public about the programme. They must know why the procedure is considered necessary and they must know of the benefits to them as individuals and communities.

C. Notification of Diseases
In every country there is a list of certain diseases, cases of which must be reported to the appropriate health authority. These notifiable diseases (or reportable diseases) include the list of six diseases which are notifiable internationally, the 'Convention Diseases' which are covered by the International Sanitary Regulations. Thus, cases of plague, cholera, smallpox and yellow fever must be reported to the World Health Organisation by the national health authority.

The national reporting of diseases primarily includes communicable diseases, but in addition there are specific regulations about the reporting of certain industrial diseases. The notification of acute epidemic diseases is designed to provide the health authorities with information at an early stage so that they can take urgent action to control outbreaks of these infections. For example, the early notification of a case of smallpox would enable the health authorities to confine the epidemic to the smallest possible area in the shortest possible time. The notification of chronic and non-epidemic infections provides information which can be used in the long term planning of health services and also in the assessment and monitoring of control programmes. Various factors limit the usefulness of notification of diseases in the control of diseases:

(a) *Incomplete reporting* of diagnosed cases. This may be from the ignorance or negligence on the part of the health worker.

(b) *Missed diagnoses*—these would include atypical cases, mild and sub-clinical infections. In certain diseases a high proportion of infected persons who harbour the agent do not feel or appear ill, and yet they may transmit infection, i.e. they are 'carriers'.

(c) *Concealment of cases*—this may result from fear of consequences such as forcible confinement in an institution in an isolation hospital or ostracism in diseases which carry a social stigma in the community, e.g. leprosy, venereal diseases.

(d) *Over diagnosis*—because of mistaken diagnosis, some of the reported cases may prove not to be due to the particular disease.

Improvement of Notifications

1 *Simple forms*
The notification form should be as simple as possible. In some communities with low levels of literacy, the notification has been achieved by the use of appropriate colour coded cards which already contain the address of the health office and the particular village. The village head can therefore notify a case of an infectious disease merely by dropping one card of the appropriate colour in the post box.

2 *Education*
As in other aspects of public health, the cooperation of the public depends on providing them with sufficient information, in this case telling them how notification of diseases can help the individual and the community.

3 *Feed-back*
The data that are compiled should be made available to all those who contributed information. They can thereby see how the information is being used.

D. *Data from Medical Institutions*

Hospitals, health centres, clinical laboratories and other medical institutions provide easily accessible sources of health statistics, but such institutional data must be used and interpreted most cautiously. The pattern of disease as seen in hospitals and in other medical institutions is distorted by many factors of selection which operate from the patient's home to the point at which he is seen and his condition diagnosed in an institution. With regard to the patient, his action depends on his awareness that he is sick and his knowledge that relief is available at a particular institution. He then makes his choice of treatment, from various alternatives which are available to him:

(*a*) self-treatment
(*b*) home medication with traditional drugs or patent medicine
(*c*) treatment by traditional healers
(*d*) treatment by quack or other unqualified persons
(*e*) modern medical treatment by a private medical practitioner or at the dispensary, health centre or hospital.

Factors in the institutions which influence the pattern of disease include the following:

(*a*) the types of services offered by the institution
(*b*) accessibility of the institution including such factors as the distance from the patient's home and the fees charged
(*c*) the special interests and reputation of the personnel.

Thus, for example, the establishment of a bacteriological laboratory in a hospital might lead to an increase in the frequency with which certain diseases such as typhoid is being diagnosed. The appointment of a specialist obstetrician in a hospital may lead to a concentration of difficult obstetric problems in the hospital as a result of referrals from other doctors and self-selection by patients who have heard of the specialist's reputation. A free clinic may attract large numbers of patients, including relatively large numbers of the poor, whereas an expensive private clinic will be used mainly by the rich and those who have financial provision through insurance.

Another defect of institutional data is that although the numerator (i.e. number of cases) is known, the denominator (i.e. the population at risk) is not easy to define. Comparisons from community to community on the basis of institutional data are difficult and fraught with the danger that erroneous conclusions may be based on the distorted pattern of hospital data.

In spite of these limitations and dangers, the information that is derived from medical institutions can supplement data from other sources. Useful data can be obtained from the following sources:

(a) *General out-patient clinics*—dispensaries, health centres, hospitals.

(b) *Special clinics*—infant and child welfare, school health, ante-natal, industrial, specific diseases—tuberculosis, leprosy.
(c) *Hospitals*—records of in-patients and deaths, autopsy records, laboratory reports.

Analysis and Presentation of Data

Health statistics may be presented as absolute numbers but they are often expressed as rates, i.e. the number of events are related to the population involved, and in order to simplify comparisons, rates are usually expressed in relation to an arbitrary total e.g. 1000, 100 000 or 1 000 000.

$$\text{RATE} = \frac{\text{Number of persons affected or number of events}}{\text{Population at risk}} \times 1000$$

Rates which are calculated with the total population in an area as the denominator are known as *crude* rates.

The rates which are calculated with the particular segments of the population at risk as the denominator, are called *specific* rates.

Some Commonly Used Rates in Public Health
Crude rates

$$\text{CRUDE BIRTH RATE} = \frac{\text{Number of live births reported during the year}}{\text{Mid-year population}} \times 1000$$

$$\text{CRUDE DEATH RATE} = \frac{\text{Number of deaths reported during the year}}{\text{Mid-year population}} \times 1000$$

$$\text{NATURAL INCREASE RATE} = \frac{\text{Number of live births minus number of deaths}}{\text{Mid-year population}} \times 1000$$

Crude rates from different populations cannot be easily compared, especially where there are striking differences in the age and sex structure of the population. Thus, the crude death rate may be relatively high in a population which has a high proportion of elderly persons compared with the rate in a younger population. Thus, if the death rate is to be used as an indicator of the health status of a population, adjustment of the crude rate is required. This adjustment may be in the form of:

(a) *Standardised rates*—there are rates which have been adjusted to correct for the age and sex structure or other peculiarities of the population. The adjustment is made to a standard population.
(b) *Specific rates*—these rates are calculated using data from specified segments of the population.

AGE-SPECIFIC AND SEX-SPECIFIC DEATH RATES =

$$\frac{\text{Number of deaths in persons in a specified age and sex group}}{\text{Number of persons in the specified age and sex group}} \times 1000$$

The death rate in a total population may be analysed separately for each sex in one-year age-groups, or more conveniently in 5- or 10-year age-groups.

Some Commonly Used Specific Rates
(a) *Specific rates* relating to infants and children:

INFANT MORTALITY RATE =

$$\frac{\text{Number of deaths in infants under 1 year}}{\text{Number of live births during the year}} \times 1000$$

NEONATAL MORTALITY RATE =

$$\frac{\text{Number of deaths in infants under 1 month of age}}{\text{Number of live births during the year}} \times 1000$$

POST-NEONATAL MORTALITY RATE =

$$\frac{\text{Number of deaths in infants between 1 month and 1 year}}{\text{Number of live births during the year}} \times 1000$$

(b) *Specific rates* relating to pregnancy and the puerperium:

STILL BIRTH RATE =

$$\frac{\text{Number of foetal deaths of 28 or more completed weeks of gestation}}{\text{Number of live births and still births}} \times 1000$$

PERINATAL MORTALITY RATE =

$$\frac{\text{Number of still births and deaths under 1 week}}{\text{Number of live births and still births}} \times 1000$$

MATERNAL MORTALITY RATE =

$$\frac{\text{Number of maternal deaths due to pregnancy, child birth and puerperal conditions}}{\text{Total number of live births and still births}} \times 1000$$

FERTILITY RATE =

$$\frac{\text{Number of births in a year}}{\text{Number of women between the ages of 15 and 49 years in the population}} \times 1000$$

The Use of Vital Statistics
These various rates are used to reflect the health status of a community; some relate to the community as a whole but others deal more specific-

ally with special groups. Thus, the standardised death rate gives an indication of the overall health condition of the community, but the specific mortality rates in the most susceptible age-groups have in practice proved to be more sensitive indicators. Thus, the infant mortality rate is widely acepted as one of the most useful single measures of the health status of community. The infant mortality rate may be very high (200-300/1000 live births) in communities where health and social services are poorly developed. Experience has shown that it can respond dramatically to relatively simple measures. Thus, with the establishment of maternal and child health services, the infant mortality rate may fall from being very high (200-300/1000 live births) to a moderate level (50-100/1000 live births). In the most advanced nations the rate is low (below 20/1000 live births). Even in these developed communities, the infant mortality rate shows striking differences in the different socio-economic groups; it may be as low as 10 deaths/1000 live births in the upper socio-economic group whilst it is 40 deaths/1000 live births in the lower socio-economic group of the same country.

The infant mortality rate is usually subdivided into two segments: the neonatal and the post-neonatal death rates. The neonatal death rate is related to factors operating on the foetus *in utero*, and also during and immediately after delivery. Thus, neonatal mortality rate is related to maternal and obstetric factors. On the other hand the post-neonatal mortality rate is related to a variety of environmental factors and especially to the level of child care. Improvement in maternal and child health services brings about a fall in both the neonatal and the post-neonatal death rates, but the fall occurs more dramatically in the latter rate. Thus, at high infant mortality rates (200 deaths/1000 live births), most of the deaths occur in the post-neonatal period but at very low levels (20 deaths/1000 live births), a high proportion of the deaths are neonatal and are mainly due to such problems as congenital abnormalities and immaturity.

In developed countries, the first year of life represents the period of highest risk in childhood and the death rate is very low in the older children. In many tropical developing countries, although the first year does represent the period of highest risk, a high mortality rate persists in the older children. Thus, the infant mortality rate taken by itself underestimates the loss of child life. The child death rate, which measures deaths in the 1-4 year age-group, is used to complete the picture.

Vital statistics can be used to study specific health problems and aspects of the health services. Thus, the maternal death, the still birth and the perinatal mortality rates are of value in studying obstetric problems and obstetric services.

The Presentation of Data
Statistical data can be summarised and presented in graphic form or

non-graphically. In each case the aim is to produce a precise and accurate demonstration of the data, summarised to simplify and accented to draw attention to the most important features.

Numerical presentation may at its simplest be no more than an arrangement of the figures in order of magnitude, so that the range of the data from the smallest to the largest is clearly displayed. Simple statistical calculations can indicate salient features of the data. For example, a series of values can be summarised by calculating statistics such as:

(a) *Mean, median or mode*—each is a single value which is representative of the series of figures, i.e. an average.

(b) *Range or standard deviation*—these are measures of dispersion which show the degree of variability within the series of values.

Data can be presented in tabular form. Often the raw data are classified, compressed and grouped into a frequency distribution. For example, rather than showing the individual ages of persons, data may be classified into 5-year or 10-year age-groups, with a record of the number of persons in each group. For tabular presentation, data are sorted, arranged, condensed and set out in such a way as to bring out the essential points. For effective presentation, a few simple rules must be observed:

(*a*) The title of the table should clearly describe the material contained within the text. Three elements commonly feature in the title:
   (i) What? The material contained in the table.
   (ii) Where? Location of the study.
   (iii) When? Time of the study.

(*b*) Each *column* and each *row* should be clearly labelled; the units of measurement must be stated. If a rate is used, the base of measurement and the number of observations must be stated.

(*c*) The *totals* for columns and *rows* should be shown where appropriate.

(*d*) *Abbreviations* and *symbols* should be explained in footnotes except when they are well known and universally familiar (e.g. £, $, etc.).

Graphic Representation of Data

Statistical data can be summarised and displayed in the form of graphs, geometric figures or pictures. The aim of the graphic representation is to provide a simple, visual aid such that the reader will rapidly appreciate the important features of the data. The following examples will be described:

(*a*) Bar diagram   (*b*) Histogram   (*c*) Pie diagram   (*d*) Graph.

(a) *Bar diagram*

In a bar diagram, the data are represented by a series of bars (i.e. slender rectangles). Each item in the group is represented by a bar, the *length* of the bar is proportional to the value of the item. It is particularly useful in representing discrete variables (Fig. 2.3).

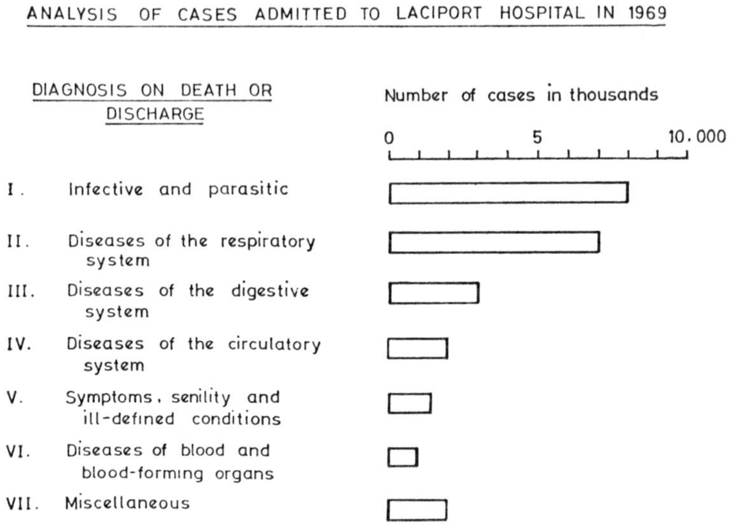

ANALYSIS OF CASES ADMITTED TO LACIPORT HOSPITAL IN 1969

FIG. 2.3   Bar diagram.

(b) *Histogram*
A histogram represents a frequency distribution in the form of adjoining rectangles which represent the frequency of each variable. The class intervals of the frequency distribution are shown on the horizontal axis, the frequencies are shown on the vertical axis (Fig. 2.4).

(c) *Pie diagram*
This consists of a circle which is divided into sectors which are proportional to the value of each variable (Fig. 2.5).

(d) *Graphs*
The simplest graph shows two variables: one on the horizontal axis and the other on the vertical axis (Fig. 2.6).

Morbidity Statistics
In addition to vital statistics, data about the occurrence of sickness within the community can provide more detailed assessment of the health of the community. Morbidity data are, however, more difficult to collect and interpret than the records of births and deaths (Fig. 2.7).

   (i) Births and deaths are easily recognisable events which can be recorded by lay persons. Success in the collection of morbidity statistics

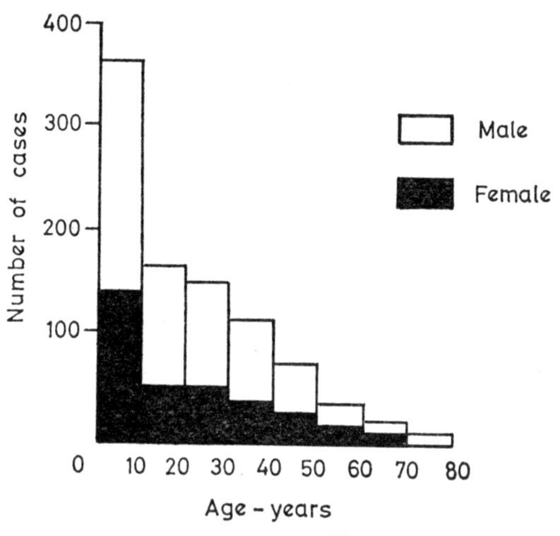

FIG. 2.4   Histogram.

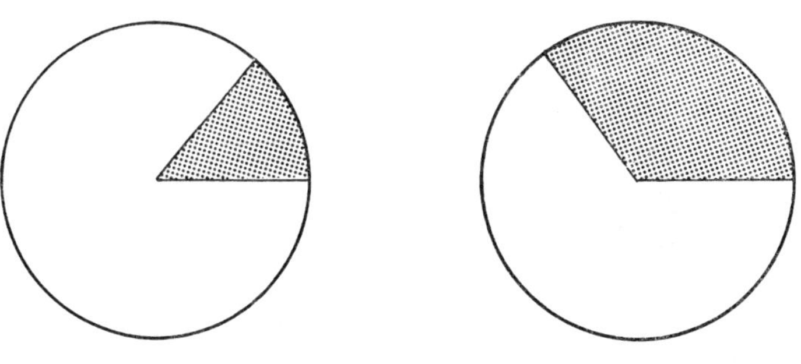

FIG. 2.5   Pie diagram. (Dotted area indicates proportion infected.)

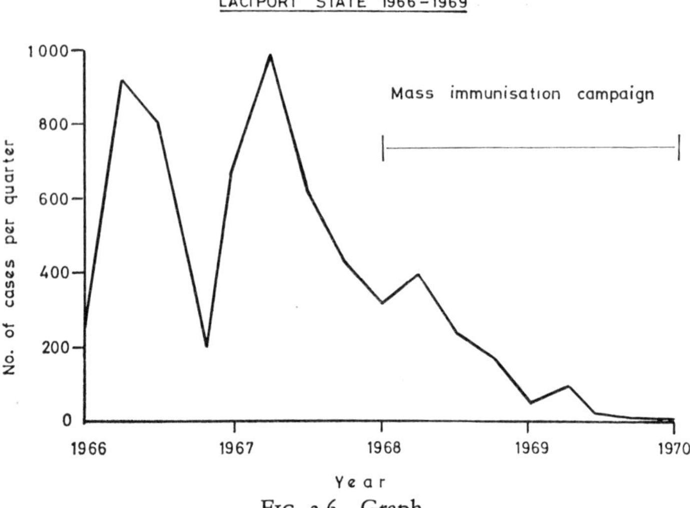

FIG. 2.6   Graph.

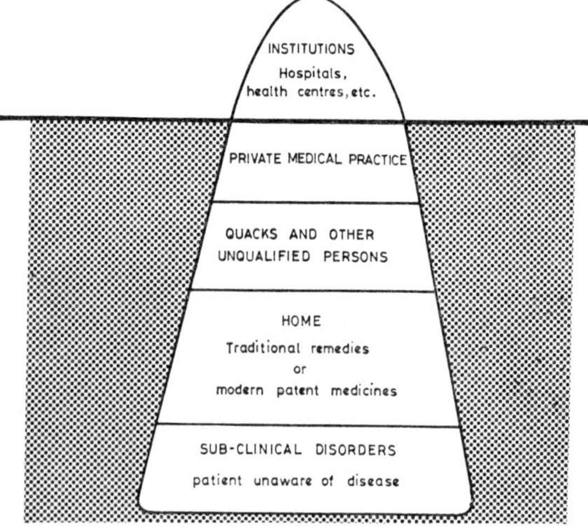

FIG. 2.7   The iceberg phenomenon. Data from institutions such as hospitals represent an unknown proportion and in some conditions, a very small proportion of the cases in the community. Institutional cases are often no more than the tip of the iceberg; the nature and extent of the larger mass beneath the surface can be discovered by well-designed epidemiological studies.

depends on the extent to which individuals recognise departures from health and also on the availability of facilities for the diagnosis of the illnesses. Thus, the quality of morbidity statistics depend on the extent of coverage and the degree of sophistication of the medical services.

(ii) Whereas each vital event of birth and death can occur only on one occasion in the lifetime of any persons, sickness may occur repeatedly in the same person. In addition one person may, at one and the same time, suffer from several disease processes.

The various sources of morbidity data have been listed in the introductory section of this chapter.

Statistical Analysis of Morbidity Data

In describing the pattern of sickness in a community, various morbidity rates are calculated. These fall into four major groups:

1 Incidence rates

These describe the frequency of occurrence of new cases of a disease or spells of illness. The incidence rate may be defined in terms of *numbers of persons* who start a spell of sickness in the defined period, or alternatively, in terms of the spells of illness during the period:

$$\text{INCIDENCE RATE (PERSONS)} = \frac{\text{Number of persons who start a spell of illness during the defined period}}{\text{Average number of persons exposed to risk during the period}} \times 1000$$

$$\text{INCIDENCE RATE (SPELLS)} = \frac{\text{Number of spells of illness which start during the defined period}}{\text{Average number of persons exposed to risk during the period}} \times 1000$$

2 Prevalence rates

The prevalence rate of illness can be defined as the number of persons who are currently sick at a specific point in time.

$$\text{POINT PREVALENCE RATE (PERSONS)} = \frac{\text{The number of persons who are sick at a given time}}{\text{Average number of persons exposed to risk}} \times 1000$$

3 Duration of illness

The average duration of illness can be measured per completed spell of illness, per sick person, or per person.

4 Fatality rate

The fourth element is the number of deaths in relation to the number of new cases of a particular disease.

THE CASE FATALITY RATE =

$$\frac{\text{Number of deaths ascribed to a specified disease}}{\text{Number of reported cases of the specified disease}} \times 1000$$

This is in part a measure of the severity of the illness.

Statistical Classification of Diseases and Causes of Death

The use of standard classification of diseases and injuries has greatly aided the statistical analysis of morbidity and mortality data. Through the United Nations and the World Health Organisation, an internationally recommended classification has been evolved, and it is periodically revised. Although this classification may be extended or modified to suit local and national conditions, the essential structure for international comparisons must be preserved.

The cause of death can be defined as 'the morbid condition or disease process, abnormality injury or poisoning leading directly or indirectly to death. Symptoms or modes of dying such as heart failure, asthenia, etc., are not considered to be the causes of death for statistical purposes'.

These causes of death are classified broadly under seventeen main sections:

    I Infective and Parasitic Diseases
    II Neoplasms
    III Allergic, Endocrine System, Metabolic and Nutritional Diseases
    IV Diseases of the Blood and Blood-forming Organs
    V Mental, Psychoneurotic and Personality Disorders
    VI Diseases of the Nervous System and Sense Organs
    VII Diseases of the Circulatory System
    VIII Diseases of the Respiratory System
    IX Diseases of the Digestive System
    X Diseases of the Genito-urinary System
    XI Deliveries and Complications of Pregnancy, Childbirth and the Puerperium
    XII Diseases of the Skin and Cellular Tissue
    XIII Diseases of the Bones and Organs of Movement
    XIV Congenital Malformations
    XV Certain Diseases of Early Infancy
    XVI Symptoms, Senility and Ill-defined Conditions
    XVII Accidents, Poisonings and Violence

Two alternative classifications of items included in Group XVII have been provided:

    E XVII Alternative Classification of Accidents, Poisonings and Violence (External Cause)
    N XVII Alternative Classification of Accidents, Poisonings and Violence (Nature of Injury)

FIG. 2.8   International form of medical certificate of cause of death

CAUSE OF DEATH		Approximate interval between onset and death
I Disease or condition directly leading to death	(a) .... due to (or as a consequence of)	....
Antecedent causes Morbid conditions, if any, giving rise to the above cause, stating the under-lying condition last	(b) .... due to (or as a consequence of) (c)	....
II Other significant conditions contributing to the death, but not related to the disease or condition causing it	....	....

I   This does not mean the mode of dying, e.g. heart failure, asthenia, etc. It means the disease, injury, or complication which caused death.

The E and N classifications are independent and either or both can be used.

The more detailed classification includes over 600 categories of diseases, 153 external causes of injury and 189 categories showing the nature of the injury. Shorter lists are available: an Intermediate list of 150 cause groups A (list) and two Abbreviated lists of 50 causes each (list B and C).

In the rural areas of the tropics where facilities are limited and autopsies infrequent, e.g. in many provincial hospitals, the use of individual headings gives an impression of precision to diagnoses which is often not justified. The use of cause groups (A list) in these circumstances permits a more valid estimate of the size of the problem, e.g. diarrhoeal diseases; it focuses on the necessity for corrective action and makes it easier to detect change over a period of time.

Certification of the Cause of Death

This is usually provided by the physician who was in attendance on a sick patient during his last illness. The certificate is made out on a form which is usually based on the International form of medical certificate of cause of death. This form is in two parts (Fig. 2.8).

In many developing countries, only a small proportion of deaths occur under the supervision of trained doctors. In the other cases, a certificate of death may be provided by other categories of staff including health auxiliaries. Attempts have been made to evolve for the use of such staff simple classifications of causes of death, based mainly on symptoms and broad descriptions. Such methods of recording crude causes of death can be of great value if the data are interpreted with care. Such statistics should, however, be tabulated separately from certifications from qualified physicians.

Chapter Three

Epidemiology

Originally, the term 'epidemiology' meant 'the study of epidemics', but the techniques which were originally used in the study and control of epidemics have also been usefully applied in the study of non-communicable diseases. In its modern usage, the term epidemiology refers to the study of the distribution of disease in human populations against the background of their total environment. It includes a study of the patterns of diseases as well as a search for the determinants of diseases.

The modern definition of epidemiology includes three important elements:

(a) *All Diseases Included*
The term is no longer restricted to the study of infections but it includes cancer, malnutrition, road accidents, mental illness and other non-communicable diseases. Epidemiological techniques are also being applied to the study of the operation of health services.

(b) *Populations*
Whereas clinical medicine is concerned with the features of disease in the individual, epidemiology deals with the distribution of disease in populations, communities or groups.

(c) *Ecological Approach*
The frequency and distribution of disease are examined against the background of various circumstances in man's total environment—physical, biological and social. This is an ecological approach; the occurrence of disease is examined in terms of the interrelationship between man and his total environment.

The Distribution of Disease
Three major questions are usually asked in epidemiology:
WHO? What is the distribution of the disease in terms of *persons*?
WHERE? What is the distribution of the disease in terms of *place*?
WHEN? What is the distribution of the disease in terms of *time*?

Answers to these questions provide clues to the factors which determine the occurrence of the disease.

The Epidemiological Tool—the Rate

The basic tool of epidemiology is the rate—it relates the number of cases to the population at risk. In order to compare populations of different sizes easily, the rate is usually expressed as the number of events in an arbitrary total, e.g. 1000 or 100 000.

Two main types of rates are calculated:

(1) *Incidence rate*
This indicates the occurrence of new cases within a stated period:

$$\text{INCIDENCE RATE} = \frac{\text{Number of new cases in a stated period}}{\text{Population at risk}} \times 1000$$

(2) *Prevalence rate* (Point Prevalence Rate)
This is the number of cases which are present within the population at a particular point in time.

$$\text{PREVALENCE RATE} = \frac{\text{Number of current cases at a specified time}}{\text{Population at risk}} \times 1000$$

Incidence, Prevalence and Duration

There is obviously some relationship between the rate at which new cases occur and the number of cases present at any particular point in time. The third factor to be considered is the *duration* of the illness. The prevalence rate would rise:

(*a*) if the incidence of illness increases but the average duration remains unchanged.
(*b*) if the incidence rate remains unchanged but the average duration of the illness increases.

Thus, the prevalence rate is dependent on the combination of these two factors, incidence rate and duration of illness. Under certain conditions where no marked changes are occurring in these factors, there is a simple mathematical relationship:

$$\text{Prevalence rate} = \text{Incidence rate} \times \text{Average duration}$$

This relationship becomes altered if the incidence rate is rapidly altering as during an acute epidemic or if the average duration of the illness is changing perhaps in response to treatment.

Epidemiological Methods

There are three main types of epidemiological studies:

1. *Descriptive Epidemiology*

The distribution of disease is described in terms of the three major variables: Person, Place and Time. This is the first phase of epidemiological studies in which one answers the questions:

'Who is affected? In what place? And at what time?'

The answers to these questions together with knowledge of the clinical and pathological features of the disease and information about the population and its environment, assist in developing hypotheses about the determinants of the disease. These hypotheses can be tested by analytical studies.

Various characteristics of persons, place and time are used in descriptive epidemiology:

Persons
> Age, sex, marital status;
> Race, ethnic group, religion;
> Occupation, education, socio-economic status;
> Personal habits—use of alcohol and tobacco.

Place
> Climatic zones;
> Country, region, state, district;
> Urban or rural;
> Local community, city wards;
> Precise location in an institution.

Time
> Year, season, day;
> Secular trends, periodic changes;
> Seasonal variations and other cyclical fluctuations.

Some of these and other variables may be used to describe the distribution of the disease.

2. *Analytical Epidemiology*

Two types of study are employed:

(a) *Case history studies ('retrospective studies')*
For case history studies, a group of affected persons are compared with suitably matched control groups of non-affected persons.

For example, in a study designed to test the hypothesis that cigarette smoking is an important factor in the causation of cancer of the lung, a number of patients with this disease ('cases') were questioned about their smoking habits. Similar questions were asked from a group of patients who had cancer at other sites (controls). This enquiry showed significant differences in the smoking habits of cases compared with controls. This was a case history study in that the subjects were selected on the basis of being *affected* or *non-affected persons*.

(b) *Cohort studies*
For cohort studies, a group of persons who are exposed to the suspected aetiological agent are compared with matched control subjects who have not been similarly exposed. For example, in a further study on cancer of the lung, a large group of persons were questioned about their smoking habits. The incidence rate of cancer of the lung among the smokers (exposed) was compared with the rate among non-smokers (non-exposed). Thus in this cohort study the subjects were selected on the basis of *exposure* or *non-exposure*.

Compared with cohort studies, case history studies have the advantage of being relatively quick, easy and cheap. A significant number of cases can be assembled for the case history study and a variety of hypotheses can be rapidly screened. The more promising ones can be further examined by the more laborious, time-consuming and expensive cohort studies. The latter have the advantage of giving a more direct estimation of the risk from exposure to each factor.

3. *Experimental Epidemiology*
This involves studies in which one group which is deliberately subjected to an experience is compared with a control group which has not had a similar experience. Field trials of vaccines and of chemoprophylactic agents are examples of experimental epidemiology. In such trials, one group receives the vaccine or drug, whilst the control group is given a placebo; alternatively, a new vaccine or drug may be compared with a well-established agent of known potency. The opportunities for experimental epidemiology in man are not numerous; often it is not feasible to carry out such controlled trials especially on things that are related to personal behaviour.

Epidemiological Data
As in clinical medicine, epidemiological data may be obtained in the form of answers to questions, physical examination of persons and results of laboratory and special investigations. In assessing the value of a particular method the following qualities should be considered:

(a) *Sensitivity*—ability of the test to detect the condition when it is present. A highly sensitive test will be positive whenever the condition is present; a less sensitive test will be positive in a proportion of cases, but will give a *false negative* case in others.

(b) *Specificity*—ability of the test to differentiate cases in which the condition is present from those in which it is absent. A highly specific test will be positive only when the relevant condition is present but a less specific test will give *false positive* results.

(c) *Repeatability*—the extent to which the same result is obtained when the test is repeated on the same subject or material. The variation which occurs on repeating the test may be due to the following:
   (i) Variation in the thing being measured
   (ii) Limitation in the accuracy of the instrument
   (iii) Observer error or variation.

There may be variations in the findings of one observer when he measures or classifies the same object on repeated occasions, i.e. *intra-observer variation or error*. There may be differences between the findings of two observers when they measure or classify the same object, i.e. *inter-observer variation or error*.

   Observer variation and error can be minimised by:
   (i) Carefully standardising the procedures for obtaining the measurements and classifications.
   (ii) Defining the criteria in clear objective terms.
   (iii) Training all the participants in the methods to be adopted to ensure uniform standard techniques.
   (iv) Providing standard reference material such as photographs or standard X-ray films for direct comparison.
   (v) Taking measurements and making the classifications without knowledge of the status of the patient, whether he is a 'case' or a control subject. In the double-blind technique, subjects are randomly allocated to treatment and control groups; neither the subjects nor the observers know to which groups each subject is assigned. Thus, there is 'blind' assignment of subjects as well as 'blind' assessment of the results.

Epidemiology of Communicable Diseases
Communicable diseases are characterised by the existence of a living infectious agent which are transmissible. Apart from the infectious agent, two other factors, the host and the environment, affect the epidemiology of the infection:

   Agent: The Seed
   Host: The Soil
   Route of transmission: The Climate.

Infectious Agents
These may be viruses, rickettsiae, bacteria, protozoa, fungi or helminths. The biological properties of the agent may play a major role in its epidemiology.

In order to survive a parasite must be able to do the following:
  (*a*) Multiply
  (*b*) Emerge from the host
  (*c*) Reach a new host
  (*d*) Infect the new host.
The ability of the infective agent to survive in man's environment is an important factor in the epidemiology of the infection. Each infective agent has its precise habitat on which it depends for its survival. The term *reservoir of infection* is used to describe this natural habitat of the infective agent. The term 'reservoir' implies the following:
 (i) *Habitat*—the infective agent lives and multiplies there.
(ii) *Survival*—the infective agent primarily depends on the reservoir for its survival. The reservoir may be man, animal or non-living material.

A. Reservoir in Man

This includes a number of important pathogens which are specifically adapted to man—the infective agents of measles, smallpox, typhoid, meningococcal meningitis, gonorrhoea and syphilis. The human reservoir includes both active cases and carriers.

Carriers

A carrier is a person who harbours the infective agents without showing signs of disease but is capable of transmitting the agent to other persons. Convalescent carriers are persons who continue to harbour the infective agent after recovering from the illness. They may excrete the agent for only a short period; or they may become chronic carriers, excreting the organism continuously or intermittently over a period of years. A healthy carrier is a person who remains well throughout the infection. In some cases, the infected person excretes the pathogens during the incubation period, before the onset of symptoms or before the characteristic features of the disease (e.g. the measles rash or glandular swelling in mumps) are manifested; these are known as *incubatory carriers* or precocious carriers.

Carriers play an important role in the epidemiology of certain infections: poliomyelitis, meningococcal meningitis, typhoid and amoebiasis:

(*a*) The number of carriers may far outnumber the sick patients.
(*b*) The carrier and his contacts do not know that he is infected, hence neither of them will take precautions to avoid transmission of the infection.
(*c*) The carrier is not debilitated by his infection and he can continue with his normal daily routine, moving freely from place to place, making contacts over a wide area. On the contrary, the sick patient's contacts may be restricted to close family contacts, friends and visitors.

(*d*) Chronic carriers may serve as a source of infection over a very long period and as a means of repeatedly re-introducing the disease into an area which is otherwise free of infection.

B. *Reservoir in Animals*
Some infective agents which affect man have their reservoir in animals. The term *zoonosis* is applied to those infectious diseases of vertebrate animals which are transmissible to man under natural conditions:

(*a*) Where man uses the animal for food, e.g. taeniasis.
(*b*) Where there is a vector transmitting the infection from animals to man, e.g. plague (flea), viral encephalitis (mosquito).
(*c*) Where the animal bites man, e.g. rabies.
(*d*) Where the animal contaminates man's environment including his food, e.g. salmonellosis.

C. *Reservoir in Non-living Things*
Many of these agents are basically saprophytes living in soil, and fully adapted to living free in nature. Biologically, they are usually equipped to withstand marked environmental changes in temperature and humidity. Apart from the vegetative forms, some develop resistant forms such as spores which can withstand adverse environmental conditions, e.g. Clostridial organisms, the infective agents of tetanus (*Clostridium tetani*), gas gangrene (*C. welchii*) and botulism (*C. botulinum*).

The Source of Infection
This term refers to the immediate source of infection, i.e. person or object from which the infectious agent passes to a host. This source of infection may or may not be a portion of the reservoir. For example, man is the reservoir of typhoid infection; a cook who is a carrier may infect food that is served at a party; that item of food is the source of infection in that particular outbreak.

Mode of Transmission
This refers to the mechanism by which an infectious agent is transferred from one person to the other or from the reservoir to a new host. Transmission may occur by:

(a) *Contact*, either directly, person to person, or indirectly through contaminated objects. Contact infections are more likely to occur where there is crowding, since this increases the likelihood of contact with infected persons. Hence they tend to be more marked in urban than in rural areas, and they are associated with overcrowding in household.

(b) *Inhalation*—through airborne infection. Poor ventilation, overcrowding in sleeping quarters and in public places are important factors in the epidemiology of airborne infections.

(c) *Infection*—through the contamination of hands, food or water.

(d) *Penetration of skin*—directly by the organism itself (e.g. hookworm larvae, schistosomiasis) by the bite of a vector (e.g. malaria, plague) or through wounds (e.g. tetanus).

(e) *Transplacental infection*—congenital infection, e.g. syphilis, toxoplasmosis.

Host Factors
The occurrence of infection and its outcome are in part determined by host factors. The term immunity is used to describe the ability of the host to resist infection. Apart from determining the occurrence of infection, the host's immune responses also modify the nature of the pathological reaction to infection. Allergic reactions in response to infection may significantly contribute to the clinical and pathological reactions.

Resistance to infection is determined by non-specific and by specific factors:

(i) *Non-specific Resistance*
This depends on the protective covering of skin which resists penetration by most infective agents, and the mucous membranes, some of which include ciliated epithelium which mechanically scavenges particulate matter. Certain secretions—mucus, tears and gastric secretions—contain lysozymes which have anti-bacterial activity; in addition, the acid content of gastric secretion also has some anti-microbial action. Reflex responses such as coughing and sneezing also assist in keeping susceptible parts of the respiratory tract free of foreign matter.

(ii) *Specific Immunity*
Specific immunity may be due to genetic or acquired factors.

(a) *Genetic*
Certain infective agents which infect other animals do not infect man, and vice versa. This species-specificity is, however, not always absolute and there are some infective agents which regularly pass from animals to man.

There are also variations in the susceptibility of various races and ethnic groups, e.g. Negroes tend to have a high level of resistance to vivax malaria infection.

Specific genetic factors have been associated with resistance to infection, e.g. persons who have haemoglobin S are more resistant to infection with *Plasmodium falciparum* than those with normal haemoglobin AA.

(b) *Acquired immunity*
Acquired immunity may be active or passive. In active immunity the host manufactures antibodies in response to an antigenic stimulus. In passive immunity, the host receives pre-formed antibodies. Acquired immunity may be acquired naturally or it may be induced artificially. Active immunity may be naturally acquired following clinical or sub-clinical infection; or it may be induced artificially by administering living or killed organisms or their products. The newborn baby acquires passive immunity by the transplacental transmission of antibodies; in this way the newborn babies of immune mothers are protected against such infections as measles, malaria and tetanus in the first few months of life. Passive immunity is artificially induced by the administration of antibodies from the sera of immune human beings (homologous) or animals (heterologous). Protection from passive immunity tends to be of short duration, especially when heterologous serum is used.

Factors affecting Host Immunity
The resistance of the host to infection is affected by such factors as age, sex, pregnancy, nutrition, trauma and fatigue.

(i) Age
For some infections, persons at both extremes of age tend to be most severely affected, i.e. children and the elderly. Some infections predominate in childhood; this usually occurs in situations in which most children become infected and thereby acquire lifelong immunity. Other infections predominate in adults; this may be determined by exposure, e.g. industrial (e.g. anthrax), sexual (e.g. gonorrhoea). Age may also influence the clinical pathological form of an infection, e.g. miliary tuberculosis is more likely in children whilst cavitating lung lesions are more likely in adults.

(ii) Sex
Some infective diseases show marked differences in their sex incidence; this is apart from infections which specifically affect the genital and other sex organs. Such infections as poliomyelitis and diphtheria often show a preponderance in females.

(iii) Pregnancy
Pregnancy increases susceptibility to certain infections; these occur more frequently, show more severe manifestations and have a worse prognosis than in non-pregnant women of a similar age-group, e.g. viral infections such as smallpox and poliomyelitis; bacterial infections such as pneumococcal infection; and protozoal infection such as malaria and amoebiasis. It does not appear that there is uniform depression of

resistance to all infections. Certain infections, e.g. typhoid and meningococcal infection, do not occur more frequently or show greater clinical severity in pregnant women.

(iv) *Nutrition*
Good nutrition is generally accepted as an important measure in enhancing resistance to infection. Severe specific deficiency of vitamin A renders the cornea and the skin more liable to infection. In addition to such specific effects it has been noted that poorly nourished children are more liable to succumb to gastro-enteritis and measles. The relationship has not been definitely established in the case of some other infections; it seems likely that some of the infections are not adversely affected by nutrition.

(v) *Trauma and fatigue*
Stress in the form of trauma and fatigue may render the host more susceptible to infections. One classical example is the effect of trauma and fatigue on poliomyelitis. The paralytic form of the disease may be precipitated by violent exercise during the prodromal period or by trauma in the form of injections of adjuvanted vaccine; paralysis tends to be most severe in the limb into which the vaccine was injected or which was subjected to most fatigue.

Herd Immunity
The level of immunity in the community as a whole is termed 'herd immunity'. When herd immunity is low, introduction of the infection is likely to lead to severe epidemics. For example, the introduction of measles into an island population which had no previous experience of the infection resulted in massive epidemics. On the other hand, when herd immunity is high, the introduction of infection may not lead to a propagated spread. A disease may be brought under complete control when a high proportion of the population has been immunised; even though a small proportion remains non-immune the transmission of infection may virtually cease.

Incubation Period
This is the interval of time from the infection of the host to the first appearance of symptoms and signs of the disease. In practice, it is not easy to determine precisely the time of infection and hence incubation period is measured from the time of first exposure to the onset of the first symptoms. Each infection has its characteristic range, varying from a few hours to several years.

Knowledge of the incubation period of an infection can be used in the control of infections as well as in the clinical assessment of patients.

(a) *Tracing the source of infection*

Investigation of likely sources can concentrate on the relevant period in relation to the onset of symptoms. For example, in tracing the likely source of a case of smallpox, one would want to know of the patient's movements and his contacts with sick persons 7-21 days before the onset of symptoms. In a case of syphilis, the suspects would include all his sexual partners in the three-month period preceding the appearance of the chancre.

(b) *Period of surveillance or quarantine of contacts*

The surveillance or quarantine of contacts is maintained for the period of time equal to the usual maximal incubation period of the infection.

(c) *Immunisation*

Certain infections can be prevented by immunisation of the host during the incubation period, e.g. (i) *Passive immunisation* with immune globulin can prevent or modify an attack of measles in a child who has been in contact with the infection; (ii) *Active immunisation* with smallpox vaccine early in the incubation period can protect a contact from smallpox infection.

(d) *Identifying point source epidemics*

An outbreak resulting from a simple common exposure (a point source epidemic) will give rise to cases which will all be present within the incubation period of the infection. Propagation of the epidemic apart from this single exposure would be indicated by the occurrence of cases later than the known extreme length of the incubation period.

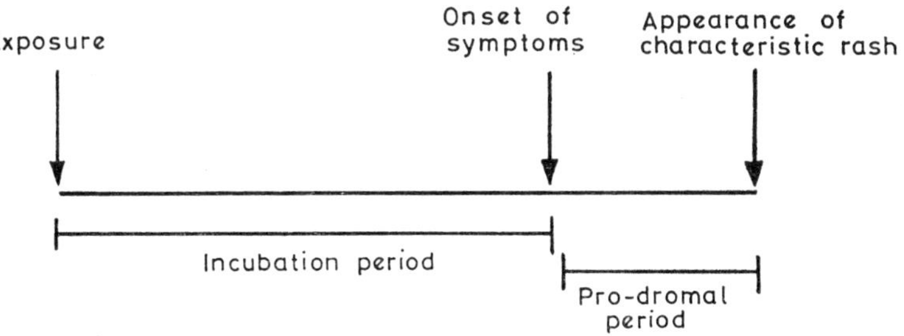

FIG. 3.1   Point source epidemic.

(e) *Prognosis*

In some infections, the prognosis is related to the incubation period. For example, the shorter the incubation period, the worse the prognosis of tetanus.

Prodromal Period

The prodromal period is the interval between the onset of symptoms of an infectious disease and the appearance of the characteristic manifestation such as a skin rash. For example, in measles, the infection presents with fever and coryza, but the characteristic rash appears about four days later.

Control of Communicable Diseases

A programme for the control of a communicable disease should be based on a detailed knowledge of the epidemiology of the infection and on effective public health organisation to plan, execute and evaluate the programme. The epidemiological information should include knowledge of the distribution of the infection in the local area, of the major foci of infection and of the overall effect of the infection on the population.

The programme must include some mechanism for

(*a*) recognising the infection and the confirmation of the diagnosis
(*b*) notifying the disease to the appropriate authority
(*c*) finding the source of infection and
(*d*) assessing the extent of the outbreak by finding other cases and the other exposed persons.

(a) *Recognition of the infection*

This is in the first instance the responsibility of the physicians and auxiliary personnel who are treating the patients. For the early recognition of communicable diseases, it is necessary that physicians and medical auxiliaries should be able to recognise the clinical manifestations of the major infective diseases in the area. This is particularly important in the case of acute epidemic diseases such as smallpox, where prompt action is required to prevent the disastrous spread of infection. Thus, the medical auxiliary at the most peripheral unit should be able to initiate appropriate action which would lead to the early recognition of the outbreak of an epidemic. Laboratory services should be used to support clinical diagnosis. Ideally there should be a Public Health Laboratory system which can process specimens from patients and from the environment.

(b) *Notification of diseases*

A notifiable disease is one the occurrence of which must be reported to the appropriate health authority. The group includes the major epidemic diseases and other communicable diseases about which the health authorities require information. Some diseases are also notifiable internationally. Formerly by the international agreement, contained in the International Sanitary Regulations, the following diseases were notifiable to the World Health Organisation:

Cholera
Plague
Smallpox
Yellow fever

(c) *Identification of the source of infection*
Epidemiological investigations are directed to finding the source of infection. This involves analysis of the information about the time sequence of the occurrence of cases and the history of the movements of the patients. Knowledge of the incubation period of the infection is of great value in interpreting the data.

(d) *Assessment of the extent of the outbreak*
This involves finding other infected persons in addition to those who have been notified, and identifying others who also have been exposed to the risk of infection: the contacts of known patients and others who have been exposed to a common source such as a polluted stream.

Methods of controlling Communicable Diseases
Basically, there are three main methods of controlling a communicable disease:
- (1) eliminate reservoir of infection
- (2) interrupt the pathway of transmission
- (3) protect the susceptible hosts.

1. *Elimination of the Reservoir*
Where the reservoir is in man, the objective would be to find and treat all infected persons, both patients and carriers, thereby eliminating sources of infection. For some infections, segregation of infected persons through isolation or quarantine may be required.

(a) *Isolation of patients*
Isolation is indicated in the control of acute epidemic diseases such as smallpox, or for chronic infections such as lepromatous leprosy. Isolation of patients is indicated for infections which have the following epidemiological features:
- (i) High morbidity and mortality
- (ii) High infectivity
- (iii) No significant extra-human reservoir
- (iv) Infectious cases easily recognisable
- (v) No significant reservoir or carriers.

(b) *Quarantine*
This refers to the limitation of movement of persons who have been

exposed to infection. The restriction continues for a period of time equal to the usual longest duration of the incubation period of the disease.

Where the reservoir of infection is in animals, the appropriate action will be determined by the usefulness of the animals, how intimately they are associated with man and the feasibility of protecting susceptible animals. Where, as in the case of the plague rat, the animal is regarded as a pest, the objective would be to destroy the animals and exclude them from human habitations. Where, as in the case of rabies in an urban area, pet dogs are susceptible, the approach would be to protect them with rabies vaccine whilst destroying stray dogs. Animals that are used as food should be examined and the infected ones eliminaated. This examination may take place in life, e.g. tuberculin testing of cattle; or it may take place after slaughter during meat inspection.

Where the reservoir is in soil, elimination of the reservoir is not feasible but it may be possible to limit man's exposure to the affected area, e.g. in some areas, infection with *Histoplasma capsulatum* occurs in persons who go into bat-infested caves. Such exposure can be avoided.

2. *Interruption of Transmission*
This mostly involves improvement of environmental sanitation and personal hygiene. The control of vectors also depends largely on alterations in the environment and in addition the use of pesticidal agents.

3. *Protection of the Susceptible Host*
This may be achieved by active or passive immunisation. Protection may also be obtained by the use of anti-microbial drugs, e.g. chemoprophylaxis is used for the prevention of malaria, meningococcal meningitis and bacillary dysentery.

Mass campaigns are sometimes indicated for dealing with acute epidemics or as a method of controlling or eradicating endemic diseases. Any vaccine or drug for a mass campaign must be effective, safe, cheap and simple to apply. Following the emergency operation of a mass campaign, the programme should be integrated into the basic health services of the community.

Surveillance of Diseases
Surveillance of diseases means the exercise of continuous scrutiny of and watchfulness over the distribution and spread of infections and the related factors, with sufficient accuracy and completeness to provide the basis for effective control. This modern concept includes three main features:

(*a*) The systematic collection of all relevant data

(*b*) The orderly consolidation and evaluation of these data
(*c*) The prompt dissemination of the results to those who need to know, particularly those who are in a position to take action.

The surveillance of communicable diseases has two main objectives. The first objective is the recognition of acute problems which demand immediate action. For example, the recognition of an outbreak of a major epidemic infection such as smallpox or the fresh introduction of it into a previously uninfected area, must be recognised promptly so that infection may be confined to the smallest possible area in the shortest possible time. Secondly, surveillance is used to provide a broad assessment of specific problems in order to discern long term trends and epidemiological patterns. Thus surveillance provides the scientific basis for ascertaining the major public health problems in an area, thereby serving as a guide for planning, implementation and assessment of programmes for the control of communicable diseases. Surveillance is essential for the proper assessment of priorities in public health programmes.

Surveillance involves the collection, evaluation and correlation of epidemiological information which is kept in separate elements by different administrative and professional groups. The sources of data include the following:

(*a*) Registration of deaths
(*b*) Notification of diseases and the reporting of epidemics
(*c*) Laboratory investigations
(*d*) Investigation of individual cases and epidemics
(*e*) Epidemiological surveys
(*f*) Distribution of the animal reservoir and the vector
(*g*) Production, distribution and care of vaccines, sera and drugs
(*h*) Demographic and environmental data.

Effective surveillance depends on the synthesis of all the data derived from the sources which are relevant to the particular problem. The detailed organisation of surveillance varies from country to country, but the basic feature is the mechanism by which pertinent epidemiological data are brought together, to be evaluated, correlated and interpreted by competent epidemiologists, thereby providing the logical basis for effective action. Most major control and eradication programmes now place considerable emphasis on surveillance in making the initial assessment and in evaluating the progress of the programme.

The techniques of surveillance are now being applied to such problems as the environmental hazards associated with atmospheric pollution, ionising radiation and road traffic accidents; to non-communicable diseases such as cancer, atheroma and other degenerative diseases; and to social problems such as drug addiction, juvenile deliquency and prostitution.

Epidemiology of Non-infectious Diseases

Epidemiological methods have been widely applied in the study of non-infectious diseases. Such studies have yielded many fruitful results, especially in providing the basis for taking effective preventive action long before the specific aetiological agent is identified and long before the mechanism of the pathogenesis of the disease are understood. For example, Lind in the eighteenth century demonstrated that the occurrence of scurvy is associated with lack of fresh fruits in the diet of sailors. He was able to take effective action in preventing scurvy by the use of lime juice more than 150 years before the recognition of vitamin C as the specific factor involved. Epidemiological studies have made important contributions to knowledge of the aetiology of various diseases including the following examples:

(a) *Nutritional disorders*—scurvy, beri-beri, pellagra, dental caries, goitre.

(b) *Cancer at various sites*—skin, lungs, penis, cervix uteri, breast, bladder, leukaemia.

(c) *Congenital abnormalities*—Down's syndrome, thalidomide poisoning.

(d) *Intoxications*—chronic beryllium poisoning, alcoholic cirrhosis.

(e) *Mental illness*—puerperal insanity, neuroses, suicide.

(f) *Accidents*—home, road and industrial accidents.

(g) *Degenerative diseases*—tropical neuropathy, coronary artery disease, hypertension, arthritis.

Epidemiological Investigation of Non-infectious Diseases

For the study of infectious diseases, it is convenient to use the simple model of 'Agent', 'Mode of transmission' and 'Host'. This model needs to be modified in dealing with non-infectious diseases. Firstly, instead of a specific aetiological agent, the non-infectious disease may result from multiple factors. Secondly, since there is no infective agent being transmitted, it is more appropriate to replace this with 'environmental factors'. Thirdly, host factors cannot be analysed in terms of active or passive immunity but rather in terms of various host factors—genetic, social, behavioural, psychological, etc.—which modify the risk of developing these various diseases.

In spite of these apparent differences, the basic epidemiological approach is identical; the epidemiological investigation of non-communicable disease involves a study of the distribution of the disease (descriptive), a search for the determinants of the distribution (analytical), and deliberate experiments designed to test hypotheses (experimental). The basic strategy is to discover populations or groups in which the disease is relatively rare; these groups can then be compared and contrasted in the hope of discovering the probable causes of the disease. The effects of making alterations in these supposed factors can be examined by controlled trials.

Chapter Four

Infections through the Gastro-intestinal Tract

A number of important pathogens gain entry through the gastro-intestinal tract. Some of these cause diarrhoeal diseases (e.g. *Salmonella*, *Shigella*) whilst others pass through the intestinal tract to cause disease in other organs (e.g. poliomyelitis, infective hepatitis).

The Infective Agents
The pathogens include viruses, bacteria, protozoa and helminths (Table 4.1).

TABLE 4.1

Examples of pathogens which are acquired through the gastro-intestinal tract

VIRUSES	BACTERIA	PROTOZOA	HELMINTHS
Poliomyelitis	*Salmonella typhi*	*Entamoeba histolytica*	*Ascaris lumbricoides*
Coxsackie	*Salmonella paratyphi* Cholera	*Giardia lamblia*	*Enterobius vermicularis*
Infective hepatitis	*Brucella* species Pathogenic *Escherichia coli*		*Dracunculus medinensis* *Taenia solium* *Taenia saginata*

Physical and Biological Characteristics

In considering the epidemiology of these infections, it is useful to note some of the physical and biological properties of each infective agent. The organisms vary in their ability to withstand physical conditions such as high or low temperatures and drying; and they also differ in their susceptibility to chemical agents including chlorine. The vegetative form of *Entamoeba histolytica* is rapidly destroyed in the stomach but the cyst form survives digestion by gastric juices. Differences in the sizes of the organisms are also of epidemiological importance. Thus, simple filtration through a clay filter will eliminate most of the large organisms—bacteria, protozoa, and the eggs or larvae of helminths—from polluted water, but the filtrate will contain the smaller organisms such as viruses.

Mode of Transmission

Viruses, bacteria and cysts of protozoa are directly infectious for man as they are passed in the faeces, but in the case of helminths, the egg may become infectious only after maturation in the soil (e.g. *Ascaris*) or after passing through an intermediate host (e.g. *Taenia saginata*). The most important pattern of transmission is the passage of infective material from human faeces into the mouth of a new host and this is known as 'Faeco-oral' or 'Intestino-oral' transmission. It should be noted, however, that not all the pathogens which infect through the mouth are excreted in the faeces; for example, guinea-worm infection is acquired by mouth but the larvae escape through the skin. On the other hand, the ova of hookworm are passed in faeces but the route of infection is by direct penetration of the skin by the infective larvae.

The Faeco-oral Route of Transmission

The direct ingestion of gross amounts of faeces is uncommon, except in young children and mentally disturbed persons. Faeco-oral transmission occurs mostly through inapparent faecal contamination of food, water and hands—the three main items which regularly make contact with the mouth (Fig. 4.1). It should be noted that minute quantities of

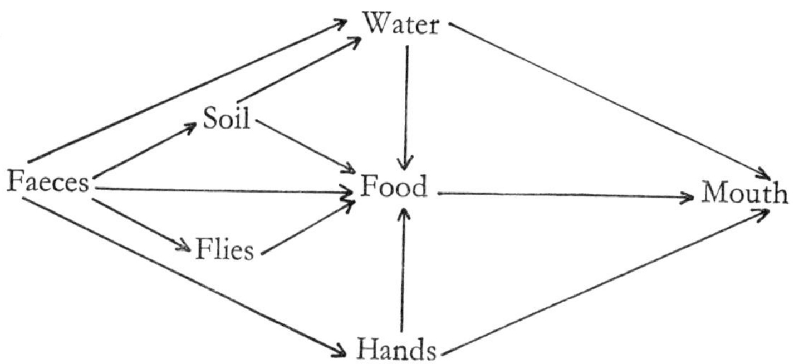

FIG. 4.1   Pathways of faeco-oral transmission.

faeces can carry the infective dose of various pathogens. Thus, dangerously polluted water may appear sparkling clear, contaminated food may be free of objectionable odour or taste, and apparently clean hands may carry and transmit disease.

As shown in the diagram, food occupies a central and important position. Not only can it be contaminated directly by faeces but also indirectly through polluted water, dirty hands, contaminated soil and filth flies. Water may be polluted directly by faeces; faecal material may be washed in from the polluted soil on the river bank. There are many opportunities for the contamination of hands: the person may contaminate his hands on cleaning after defaecation or in touching or handling contaminated objects including soil. Contamination of the soil with faeces plays an essential role in the transmission of certain helminths which must undergo a period of maturation before becoming infectious (e.g. *Ascaris*). Filth flies, in particular, the common housefly, spread faecal material and play a role in the transmission of gastro-intestinal infections. The housefly mechanically transfers faecal pollution:

(*a*) By carrying faeces on its hairy limbs
(*b*) By regurgitating the contents of its stomach on to solid food as a means of liquefying it ('Vomit drop')
(*c*) By defaecating on the food; its faeces may contain surviving organisms derived from human faeces.

Although flies are physically capable of transmitting these infections, it is not easy to determine how important they are in particular epidemiological situation and it is likely that their importance has been exaggerated in relation to the other mechanisms of transmission.

Epidemic Patterns in relation to the Mode of Transmission

Some of the infections which are acquired through the gastro-intestinal tract, characteristically occur in epidemic form, e.g. typhoid. The vehicle of infection may be water. The water-borne epidemic is typically explosive; it may affect people over a wide area who have no other traceable connection but the use of the same source of water supply. Food-borne outbreaks may be more localised, affecting persons from the same household or boarding institution, those who feed communally at a hotel, restaurant, aeroplane or staff canteen, or those who have taken part in a festive dinner or picnic.

Host Factors

Certain non-specific factors in the host play some part in preventing infection through the gastro-intestinal tract. Thus, the high acid content and the anti-bacterial lysozyme in the stomach, and the digestive juices in the upper part of the intestinal tract destroy potentially infective organisms but do not constitute an impenetrable barrier to infection. More significant is the specific immunity which can be derived from previous infections or from artificial immunisation. This immunity is in part related to specific antibodies in the sera of convalescent patients or artificially immunised persons. It has also been demonstrated that the intestinal mucosa may acquire resistance to certain pathogens such as cholera or poliomyelitis; this local resistance is mediated through fractions of immunoglobulins which are secreted by the mucosa.

Control of the Infections acquired through the Gastro-intestinal Tract

The most effective method of controlling these diseases can best be determined from a knowledge of the epidemiology of the infection with particular reference to the local community. The basic principles involved in the choice of method can be conveniently discussed with reference to Fig. 4.1. Control can operate at various levels:

1. *The infective agent*
    (*a*) Sanitary disposal of faeces
    (*b*) Elimination of human and animal reservoirs.
2. *The route of transmission*
    (*a*) Provision of safe water supply
    (*b*) Protection of food from contamination
    (*c*) Control of flies
    (*d*) Improvement of personal hygiene.
3. *The host*
    (*a*) Specific immunisation
    (*b*) Chemoprophylaxis
    (*c*) Specific treatment.

The measures listed in sections 1 and 2 relate to the improvement of environmental sanitation, and are mostly not specifically related to any particular infection.

I. Viral Infections

The most common viral infections transmitted through the gastro-intestinal tract are: (i) Poliomyelitis and other enteroviruses and (ii) Infective hepatitis.

Poliomyelitis and Other Enteroviruses

The enteroviruses, in addition to poliovirus, mainly include the *Coxsackie* and *Echo* (enteric cytopathogenic human orphan) viruses. These viruses were first isolated from the faeces of patients during poliomyelitis investigations. Healthy persons may excrete enteroviruses for short periods, and in areas where standards of environmental sanitation are low, they are prevalent among infants and young children. *Coxsackie viruses* are classified into two groups, A and B, and although frequently isolated from healthy persons they may cause a variety of human illnesses, e.g. herpangina; summer grippe; vesicular stomatitis; virus meningitis, etc. The presence of Coxsackie Group B virus can interfere with poliomyelitis virus multiplication, while a mixed Coxsackie Group A and poliomyelitis virus infection might result in a more severe paralysis.

Echo viruses are also excreted by healthy persons, particularly children, but may cause illnesses such as diarrhoea and virus meningitis. *Reo viruses* were first isolated from the faeces of healthy children but have been also found in children with diarrhoea and steatorrhoeic enteritis. By far the most important enterovirus in the tropics is poliomyelitis. *It should be noted that the enteroviruses (Coxsackie and Echo) may interfere with oral poliomyelitis vaccination campaigns in the tropics.*

Poliomyelitis is an acute febrile illness classically resulting in a flaccid paralysis 'infantile paralysis'. The *incubation period* varies from 4 to 35 days with an average of about 10 days.

Medical geography

The disease has a world-wide distribution; it is endemic in many areas of the tropics and subtropics but appears periodically in the form of epidemics.

Virology

There are three distinct types of polio virus, type I (Brunhilde), type II (Lansing) and type III (Leon), which invade the central nervous system. The viruses grow well in tissue culture, they resist desiccation but are killed in half an hour by heat (60°C).

Epidemiology

Man is the reservoir of infection, the polio virus is excreted in the stools of infected cases, convalescent and healthy carriers. The virus is transmitted by food, water, or by droplet infection of flies. The incidence rates in males and females are similar. Trauma, excessive fatigue and pregnancy during the period of acute febrile illness and intramuscular injections some time before the acute episode all seem to be provoking factors leading to paralysis. Tonsillectomy increases the risk of bulbar poliomyelitis. The mechanism of these various stresses is not clear.

In many areas of the tropics infection is hyperendemic and all of the known types of poliomyelitis virus (I, II and III) are prevalent. Within such communities the disease smoulders but epidemic outbreaks undoubtedly occur. The virus strains responsible for paralytic illness in any area may vary, and at different periods in the same area one type or other may predominate.

Poliomyelitis is a highly infectious disease and the alimentary tract is of prime importance as a portal of entry and exit of the virus, as it is with other enteroviruses. The factor of greatest importance in determining the incidence of paralytic poliomyelitis is the state of immunity of the affected population. In many tropical countries where sanitation is primitive and living conditions are crowded and poor, facilities for the spread of polio virus are good, consequently infants have the opportunity of coming into contact with all three types of poliomyelitis virus early in life, and few of them reach pre-school age without having been infected with at least one strain, although, clinically, the infection is in most cases inapparent. Immunity is acquired early. In countries where the sanitary arrangements are good, the risk of contact with the virus at an early age is diminished and older persons are affected. Thus the most significant difference between the occurrence of poliomyelitis in the well-developed countries of the temperate zone and the less-developed areas of the tropics is in the distribution of cases in the various age-groups. Serum antibody surveys carried out among children in many parts of the tropics have shown that by the time they are 3 years old 90 per cent have developed antibodies against at least one type of poliomyelitis. Passive immunity is transmitted from mother to offspring and lasts for about 3-6 months.

Laboratory diagnosis
The virus is isolated from specimens of faeces, throat swabs or from throat and nasopharyngeal washings.

Control
High standards of hygiene and mass immunisation are the two most important measures of control.

(a) *The individual*
The disease is notifiable and isolation of individual cases is highly desirable. This measure by itself is not enough to control an epidemic because of the large numbers of asymptomatic carriers. All pharyngeal and faecal discharges of patients should be treated with disinfectants and disposed of as safely as possible. Contacts should be protected with oral polio vaccine and kept under observation for a period of three weeks from the date of their last known contact. Tonsillectomy and dental extractions should be deferred when a poliomyelitis epidemic is present in the community and injections of any kind reduced to a minimum. Individuals should avoid over-exertion such as games, swimming, etc.

(b) *The community*
Crowds should be avoided during epidemics. Food should be protected from flies and sanitary disposal of faeces encouraged. Health education aimed at raising the standards of personal hygiene should be rigorously carried out. Rehabilitation for paralysed persons is essential.

(c) *Immunisation*
Immunisation provides the most reliable method for the prevention of poliomyelitis and for controlling rapid spread during an epidemic. Two types of poliomyelitis vaccine are currently available: (i) the killed (Salk) vaccine which is given by injection and (ii) the attenuated (Sabin)

vaccine which is given by mouth and through a mild infection induces protection against the disease. Unfortunately, evidence has accumulated that in many tropical countries the oral vaccine fails to provoke a satisfactory antibody response in a high percentage of recipients, probably because of interference by other enteroviruses (see pp. 41-2). Despite this, however, the Sabin vaccine does in practice appear to afford protection against the disease, especially when used in *mass immunisation* campaigns in the tropics. It is the most practical and economical method of rapidly immunising a large susceptible population and bringing an epidemic of poliomyelitis to an end. The simplest scheme for immunisation is to give 3 doses of the trivalent oral poliomyelitis vaccine at intervals of 4 weeks. For immunising small groups attending hospitals and clinics in the tropics the killed Salk vaccine might be preferable. Preparations are now available which incorporate killed poliomyelitis vaccine with triple antigen. A course of 3 injections given at 4-week intervals will thus provoke satisfactory immunity against tetanus, diphtheria, whooping cough and poliomyelitis. Children in the tropics should all be immunised against these diseases and expatriates irrespective of age should be protected against poliomyelitis before going out to the tropics.

Poliomyelitis—Summary

(1) *Occurrence*—World-wide
(2) *Organisms*—Polio virus I, II, III
(3) *Reservoir of infection*—Man
(4) *Modes of transmission*—Food, water, droplet
(5) *Control*— (i) Isolation
         (ii) Sanitary disposal of faeces
         (iii) Health education
         (iv) Immunisation

Infective Hepatitis

The disease is characterised by loss of appetite, jaundice and enlargement of the liver. The *incubation period* varies from 15 to 40 days with an average around 20 days.

Medical geography

The disease is widespread but is probably more common in the tropics.

Virology

Virus A is identified with infective hepatitis (short-incubation hepatitis), while serum hepatitis (long-incubation hepatitis) is associated with virus B. Virus-like particles, termed the hepatitis-B antigen (HbAg) have been detected in the serum of many patients with hepatitis-B, and also in patients with infective hepatitis. Several recent studies have shown that the incidence of HbAg ('Australia antigen' or 'hepatitis-associated antigen') carriers is higher in the tropics than in Europe and this antigen has been detected in wild-caught mosquitoes in Africa.

Epidemiology
Man is the reservoir of infection, excreting the organism in the faeces and possibly urine. A viraemia also occurs. Faecal-oral spread is the most important mode of transmission by direct or indirect contact. Sporadic cases are probably caused by person-to-person contact, but explosive epidemics from water and food have also occurred. Food handlers can disseminate the infection. Although in most parts of the tropics infective hepatitis is essentially a childhood disease, many adult patients are also seen and the disease is particularly severe in pregnancy. In many countries the incidence of infective hepatitis is rising. Hepatitis has many epidemiological similarities to poliomyelitis and is a sensitive indicator of poor community hygiene. Violent exercise during the early stages of the disease seem to result in severe clinical attacks of hepatitis. In general, children tolerate hepatitis well and recover more rapidly than adults. A high frequency of Glucose-6-phosphate dehydrogenase deficiency has been found among patients with hepatitis, and patients with the enzyme defect have a longer and more severe course. A high incidence of acute coma and an increased death rate was associated in Accra, Ghana, with immigration, shanty town residency, lower socio-economic status and pregnancy. In this study, men required a longer time to recover from equivalent degrees of liver damage than women.

Laboratory diagnosis
   No specific test exists for the identification of the virus and diagnosis
   is made on clinical, epidemiological, and biochemical grounds, e.g.
   liver function tests.

Control
If patients are in hospital they should if possible be barrier nursed as for any faeces-carried infection. Food handlers should not resume work until three weeks after recovery. All measures of personal and community hygiene useful in reducing the spread of infection should be encouraged.

Immunisation
Human immune serum globulin (ISG) is useful for persons going to the tropics where the disease is endemic. Even when it does not prevent infective hepatitis, it does modify the severity in those persons who

contract the disease. It is also extremely useful in protecting family contacts during epidemics (0·05 ml per kg, intramuscularly). The dose for those going to the tropics is 0·02 ml per kg of a 16 g per 100 ml solution and passive protection lasts for about 6 months. Recovery from a clinical attack creates a lasting active immunity.

Infective Hepatitis—Summary

(1) *Occurrence*—World-wide
(2) *Organism*—Virus A
(3) *Reservoir of infection*—Man
(4) *Modes of transmission*—Person to person, food, water
(5) *Control*— (i) Personal and community hygiene
          (ii) Immunisation

II. Bacterial Infections

The most important bacterial infections that gain entry through the gastro-intestinal tract are: (i) The enteric fevers, (ii) Infant gastro-enteritis, (iii) The bacillary dysenteries, (iv) Cholera, (v) Brucellosis (vi) Food poisoning.

Enteric Fevers

These infections are caused by members of the *Salmonella* group, *Salmonella typhi* and *S. paratyphi* A, B or C. They are one of the most common causes of a pyrexia of unknown origin. The *incubation period* is usually from 10 to 14 days.

Medical geography

The enteric fevers have a world-wide distribution although they are endemic only in communities where the standards of sanitation and personal hygiene are low.

Typhoid Fever
Bacteriology

S. *typhi* is a Gram-negative, aerobic, non-sporing, rod-like organism. The organism can survive in water for 7 days, in sewage for 14 days and in ice-cream for 1 month. In warm dry conditions most of the bacilli die in a few hours. Boiling of water or milk destroys the organism. There are many phage types of S. *typhi* and these have proved of great value in tracing the source of an epidemic.

Epidemiology

Typhoid fever presents one of the classical examples of a water-borne infection. All ages and both sexes are susceptible. Man is the only reservoir of infection. This may be an overt case of the disease, an ambulatory 'missed' case or a symptomless carrier. About 2-4 per cent of typhoid patients become chronic carriers of the infection. The majority are faecal carriers. Urinary carriers also occur and seem more common in association with some abnormality of the urinary tract and in patients with *Schistosoma haematobium* infection. Although in most patients the focus of persistent typhoid infection in carriers is in the gall bladder, in some, the deep biliary passages of the liver have also been incriminated. This seems particularly so in Hong Kong, where an association between *Clonorchis sinesis* and *S. typhi* carriers has been demonstrated. Food handlers, especially if they are intermittent carriers, are particularly dangerous and have been responsible for many outbreaks of the disease. Close contact with a patient whether family or otherwise, e.g. nurse, may result in infection being transmitted by soiled hands or through fomites such as handkerchiefs, towels, etc.

Contamination of water—the cause of major outbreaks—can occur through cross-connection of a main with a polluted water supply, faecal contamination of wells, or faulty purification. Typhoid can also be spread by shell-fish, particularly oysters which mature in tidal estuaries and are thus exposed to contaminated waters. Milk-borne outbreaks occur either by direct contamination from a carrier or indirectly from utensils. Ice-cream, other milk products, ice, fruit, vegetables and salads may be infected directly from a carrier or indirectly. Flies or infected dust may be sources of infection. Food (e.g. tinned meat, vegetables infected from human faeces used as manure) can also cause epidemics of typhoid fever.

Laboratory diagnosis

A leucopenia with a relative lymphocytosis is often seen. Blood or 'clot' culture during the first two weeks of the disease usually yields *S. typhi*. After about the tenth day the Widal test (O and H agglutinations) becomes positive and rises progressively—a rising titre rather than absolute values is necessary for diagnosis. The diazo test is a red coloration given by the froth of the urine of typhoid patients when mixed with the diazo reagents, despite its definite limitations it is a simple and useful diagnostic test in areas where laboratory facilities are minimal. It becomes positive during the second and third weeks. The Vi reaction is of help in the detection of the carrier state.

Control

The ultimate control of typhoid fever from a community depends on the sanitary disposal of excreta which will stop the dissemination of faecal matter from one person to another, the introduction of a permanent method of purification of water, and raising the standards of personal hygiene. In any outbreak of typhoid fever every attempt should be made to trace it to its ultimate source by the use of phage-typing, and serological tests, particularly for the presence of Vi antibody, to detect the chronic carrier.

(a) *The individual*

All typhoid patients should be barrier nursed in a general hospital or removed to an infectious diseases hospital. Cases should be immediately notified or if possible the room from where they came should be cleansed and disinfected. All fomites should be likewise disinfected. The treatment of choice is still chloramphenicol 2 g daily for 14 days while trimethoprim-sulphamethoxazole is a valuable substitute. The patients should remain in hospital until, following treatment, stools and urine are bacteriologically negative on three occasions at intervals of not less than 48 hours. The above measures are not all feasible in many parts of the tropics and a compromise has often to be arrived at.

(b) *The community*

The chronic carrier is a difficult problem especially in the tropics, each one should be assessed in relation to his occupation and kept under as much surveillance as possible. In patients in whom the gall bladder is the definite site of infection, surgery (cholecystectomy) should be carried out. The prolonged administraion of ampicillin (4 g daily for 1-3 months) has also been used successfully to treat *Salmonella* carriers; while a trimethoprim-sulphamethoxazole combination (Septrin) has given encouraging results.

If the water supply is suspect, e.g. by the simultaneous occurrence of a large number of cases in a limited area, boiling or hyperchlorination is required. If food is suspected, it should be traced back to its source and enquiries made as to any recent illness among persons handling the food, samples of the food should be taken for medical examination. Milk should be pasturised or boiled. The use of fresh human manure as fertiliser should be actively discouraged and vegetables boiled or cooked before consumption. Food should be protected from flies, the numbers of which should be reduced to a minimum.

(c) *Immunisation*

One attack of typhoid fever confers permanent immunity. Field trials in Yugoslavia, Poland, the USSR and Guyana have proved the value of typhoid vaccines, which have been shown to have a protective effect of nearly 90 per cent. Vaccines with a high content of Vi antigen are the most successful, and acetone-inactivated vaccines are superior to those killed by heat and phenol. One subcutaneous infection of 500 million killed *S. typhi* gives adequate protection. Typhoid-Paratyphoid A and B vaccine (TAB) has no advantage over typhoid vaccines as the protection it gives from paratyphoid fever is uncertain. A recent innovation is a TAB vaccine (0·2 ml) for intradermal injection. In countries where typhoid vaccine alone is easily available, this monovalent vaccine should be used as a matter of choice.

The Paratyphoid fevers are food borne rather than waterborne. Infections and fatality is much lower than for typhoid fever. In other respects the diseases are very similar and the same preventive measures are generally applicable as for typhoid fever.

Enteric Fevers—Summary

(1) *Occurrence*—World-wide
(2) *Organisms*—*S. typhi*: *S. paratyphi* A, B, C
(3) *Reservoir of infection*—Sick patient, convalescent, carrier (faecal, urinary)
(4) *Modes of transmission*—Water, food, flies
(5) *Control*— (i) Isolation, notification, search for source of infection
      (ii) Supervision of carriers
      (iii) Sanitary disposal of excreta
      (iv) Purification of water, control of flies, food hygiene
      (v) Immunisation
      (vi) Health education

Gastro-enteritis

Gastro-enteritis is one of the commonest causes of childhood mortality in the tropics. Severe vomiting and diarrhoea leading to dehydration are the cardinal features. The *incubation period* is usually from 1 to 5 days.

Medical geography
Infant gastro-enteritis has a world-wide distribution but is especially common in the tropics.

Bacteriology
Although gastro-enteritis in children can be due to a variety of causes, the bulk of infections in infants have been attributed to certain serotypes of the coliform group of bacteria or to viruses. About 2 per cent of healthy young children excrete *E. coli* organisms, the serotypes which have been identified with specific epidemics have been $O_{111}, O_{55}, O_{26}, O_{229}, O_{125}, O_{126}$ and O_{128}. Echo and Coxsackie viruses cause diarrhoea in children (see p. 41).

Epidemiology
Gastro-enteritis is much less common among infants who are breast fed. Poverty, diet, fly infestation and ignorance of elementary hygiene are responsible for the maintenance and spread of the disease. The unfortunate newly acquired habit of early cessation of breast feeding now gaining ground in the tropics and its substitution by bottle feeding

has contributed to an increased incidence of the disease among infants and is a retrograde step in more ways than one. Man is the only reservoir of infection, usually a sick child or a symptomless carrier.

Laboratory diagnosis
    This is based on isolating the organism usually an *E. coli* serotype or an enterovirus from the faeces.

Control
(a) *The individual*
The child should be treated with the appropriate antibiotic whenever possible. Scrupulous attention to personal and general cleanliness is necessary for the prevention of gastro-enteritis. Breast feeding should be encouraged to be continued for as long as possible. If artificial feeding must be used, rigorous attention to the sterilisation of all utensils used for the preparation of the feed and of the bottles should be maintained. It is wiser in these instances to teach mothers how to feed their infants using a cup and spoon, since these are easier to keep clean than bottles. Personal cleanliness, e.g. hands and nails, must be enforced in all households containing infants and young children.

(b) *The community*
Control of flies is imperative; all food, feeding utensils especially bottles and teats must be stored in fly-proof surroundings. The sanitary disposal of faeces and constant health education is necessary.

Gastro-enteritis—Summary

(1) *Occurrence*—World-wide
(2) *Organisms*— (i) *E. coli* serotypes
                 (ii) Enteroviruses
(3) *Reservoir of infection*—Man
(4) *Modes of transmission*— (i) Milk
                             (ii) Flies
(5) *Control*— (i) Personal hygiene
               (ii) Sanitary disposal of faeces
               (iii) Encouraging breast feeding
               (iv) Sterilisation of milk bottles and other utensils
               (v) Control of flies
               (vi) Health education

Bacillary Dysentery
Bacillary dysentery is characterised by diarrhoea, fever and a sudden onset of abdominal pain. The *incubation period* is 1 to 7 days.

Medical geography
The infection has a world-wide distribution but it is commoner in tropical than in temperate climates.

Bacteriology
Species and varieties of the genus *Shigella* are numerous and they can be conveniently classified into four main subgroups:

(1) *Subgroup A* contains 10 antigenically distinct serotypes, including *Sh. Shigae* and *Sh. schmitzii*

(2) *Subgroup B* contains 6 main serotypes all antigenically interrelated, including *Sh. flexneri*

(3) *Subgroup C* contains 15 antigenically distinct serotypes, including *Sh. boydii*

(4) *Subgroup D* includes *Sh. sonnei*

The proportion of infections due to individual serotypes varies from country to country, and in the same country at different times. The organisms of greatest clinical importance are *Sh. shigae* (the most severe); *Sh. flexneri*; *Sh. boydii, Sh. schmitzii* and *Sh. sonnei* (the least severe). Strains that are typeable are often sulphonamide resistant while untypeable strains are usually sensitive. The dysentery bacilli are non-motile, Gram-negative organisms.

Epidemiology
Infection is derived from cases of the disease, from healthy convalescents (who can excrete organisms for up to 2 months or more); and from symptomless carriers who keep up infection in the community.

The organisms, which are excreted in the faeces, may gain access to food through the soiled fingers of patients or carriers. They may also pass from person to person by contact with inanimate articles, e.g. lavatory seats, door handles, crockery, bedding and clothes. Fly-borne infection is important in some parts of the tropics where these insects are numerous, e.g. the Middle East. Epidemics may occasionally result from the contamination of milk, ice-cream or water. Occupation (e.g. food handlers who are carriers) is an important factor in the social epidemiology of bacillary dysentery as well as of other faeces-transmitted diseases.

Young children are more liable than older persons to acquire *Shigella* infections, and when infected to suffer from clinical disease. Diarrhoeal diseases surveys carried out in Mauritius, Sudan, United Arab Republic, Ceylon, Iran, Bangladesh and Venezuela showed that morbidity and mortality was highest among children under the age of 3. Diarrhoea was commonest during the weaning period and greater in bottle-fed than breast-fed infants. *Shigellae* were isolated both from children suffering from diarrhoea and from those having no diarrhoea.

Laboratory diagnosis
Direct microscopical examination of the faeces will reveal pus cells and sometimes red blood cells. The isolation of the specific organism from the faeces cultured as early as possible in the disease provides

the best means of diagnosis. Fluorescent antibody techniques have recently been used for more rapid identification of the organisms.

Control
(a) *The individual*
The patient should be treated at home or in hospital and barrier nursed if possible. Strict personal hygiene should be encouraged among the family contacts or nursing personnel looking after the case and the stools should be treated with a disinfectant before disposal, clothing and bed linen should be similarly treated. If the disease is notifiable, the Medical Office of Health should be informed.

(b) *The community*
The most valuable community measures are provision for the sanitary disposal of faeces, a pure water supply, food hygiene and control of flies. Health education to increase the standards of personal hygiene and stop the transmission of the disease within a family and from food handlers is essential. Hands *must* be washed before food is handled and facilities for this must be made available.

Bacillary Dysentery—Summary
(1) *Occurrence*—World-wide

(2) *Organisms*—Shigella shiga, S. flexneri, S. boydii, S. schmitzii and S. sonnei

(3) *Sources of infection*—Sick patient, convalescent, carrier (especially food handler)

(4) *Modes of transmission*— (i) Faecal contamination of food, water or fomites
(ii) Flies

(5) *Control*— (i) Sanitary disposal of faeces
(ii) Pure water supply
(iii) Food hygiene
(iv) Control of flies
(v) Health education
(vi) Adequate treatment of patient

Cholera
This is a disease of rapid onset caused by *Vibrio cholerae* and characterised by vomiting; profuse dehydrating diarrhoea with 'rice water stools' and marked toxaemia. Muscular cramps, suppression of urine and shock occur later. The *incubation period* is 1 to 7 days. Cholera is a notifiable and internationally quarantinable disease.

Medical geography
Classical cholera, caused by *Vibrio cholerae*, classical biotype is now virtually limited to the Indo-Pakistan subcontinent and notably in the

deltas of the Ganges and Brahmaputra rivers. Cholera El Tor, caused by *Vibrio cholerae,* El Tor biotype was originally confined to a limited geographical area in the Celebes in Indonesia but has been spreading in a pandemic form since 1961 to Indonesia, Sarawak, the Philippines, Sabah, Taiwan, Korea, Hong Kong, the Chinese mainland, West New Guinea, Malaysia, Singapore, Burma, Thailand, India, Pakistan, Afghanistan, Iran, Bahrein, Nepal, Turkey and Iraq. Recently it has been reported from Egypt, Libya, Tunisia, the Southern USSR, Czechoslovakia and for the first time has now entered Africa, south of the Sahara, with cases in Guinea, Ghana, Nigeria and East Africa. It has also occurred in Ethiopia, Sudan and Spain and has recently been imported to Australia and New Zealand (Fig. 4.2).

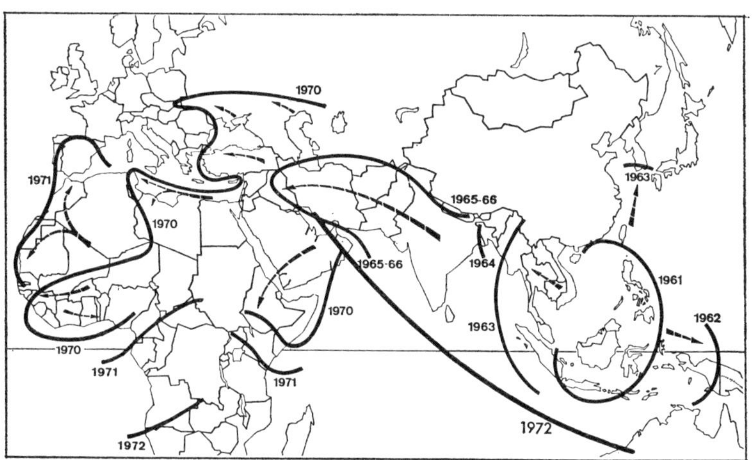

FIG. 4.2   The path of *El Tor* Cholera from 1961 to the end of 1972.

Bacteriology

V. cholerae was discovered by Koch in 1883 and is a delicate Gram-negative organism. There are two biotypes, classical and El Tor. Each biotype contains three serotypes—Inaba, Ogawa and Hikojima. The El Tor biotype is named after the El Tor quarantine station in Egypt, where it was first isolated in 1920; it is distinguished from the other three strains by being able to produce a soluble haemolysin which is active against sheep and goat erythrocytes and by other characteristics.

Epidemiology

The reservoir of infection is a sick person, a convalescent patient or a carrier through the faeces or vomit. For every typical case of the disease there may be 10-100 other symptomless persons excreting the vibrio.

Cholera may begin suddenly as a water-borne disease. In Calcutta, where cholera is endemic, the supply of filtered water falls short in summer and the people are found to use both unfiltered and tank water. Cholera also spreads by close personal contact, by contaminated food (e.g. dates in the Egyptian epidemic of 1947), infected inanimate objects and by flies. Intrafamilial spread also occurs. In order to flourish, cholera requires a combination of dense population and poor sanitation. For many years there was a tendency to overlook the role of symptomless carriers in the transmission of cholera, until it was shown that the carrier state in cholera El Tor may last for more than 7 years ('Cholera Dolores' in the Philippines) and that the vibrio can establish itself in the gall bladder.

Cholera El Tor has been proved capable of speedy and extensive spread over much wider areas than classical cholera, and in several such areas cases due to cholera El Tor have displaced those of classical cholera. In Calcutta, for instance, by the end of 1964 there was only one case of classical cholera for every ten or more cases of cholera El Tor. This epidemiological phenomenon is explained by the demonstration that the El Tor biotype eliminates the classical biotype in a few hours both *in vitro* and *in vivo*. Cholera has a seasonal pattern but the season varies from locality to locality—thus in Dacca, Bangladesh, the cholera season follows the monsoon rains and slowly disappears during the hot, dry months; while in Calcutta, India, the disease rises to a peak during the hot, dry season and ends with the onset of the rains.

The major changes in the epidemiology of cholera have been (i) recognition of the increasing importance of carriers, (ii) the frequency of personal contact infection (case to case spread) rather than water-borne epidemics and (iii) the predominance and alarming spread of the El Tor biotype.

Laboratory diagnosis

A definite diagnosis of cholera can be made only after isolation of *V. cholerae* from the faeces of patients. The faeces should be transported to the laboratory as rapidly as possible in alkaline peptone water (pH 9·0). Three methods are available for the rapid recognition of cholera vibrios: (i) the selective enrichment/fluorescent-antibody technique, (ii) the oblique-light technique and (iii) the gelatin-agar method. Microscopic examination of a stool specimen may show large numbers of vibrios.

Control

During epidemics the recognition of cases clinically is relatively easy, sporadic cases however can easily be missed and hence in endemic areas any case of severe gastro-enteritis must be considered as cholera until the contrary is proved.

(a) *The individual*
Early diagnosis, isolation and notification of cases is very important.
A search for the source of infection should be made and steps taken to
deal with that source when found. Concurrent disinfection of stools,
fomites, house, linen, clothing, etc., should be carried out. The
administration of antibiotics reduces the carrier rate. Before the patient
is discharged from hospital, two negative stool cultures are required
and terminal disinfection of bedding, etc., must be carried out.

Contacts must be traced, immunised (1 ml, 8000 million vibrios)
and watched for 5 days, or if carriers until two negative stools are
obtained. Attendants of patients must be also immunised (1 ml),
instructed to observe scrupulous cleanliness and disinfection of their
hands and should be forbidden to consume food or drink in the patient's
room or to go into the kitchen. Detailed surveillance of every person
who might have the disease is desirable but rarely feasible in most of
the cholera-prone countries.

(b) *The community*
Immediate steps must be taken to raise the existing standards of environmental sanitation and in particular to check all water supplies.
Chlorination should be stepped up to 1·3 parts per million. Excreta
and refuse disposal must be rigorously controlled and all other fly-
breeding sources eliminated; if possible, houses should be sprayed with
DDT. Bacteriological examination of pooled night-soil has been used
to detect infections in Hong Kong, and from this source the infection
can be traced backwards to its origin. The same method applied to
latrines in Calcutta was not as successful. Food sanitation should be
enforced and all public swimming-pools closed. People should be
instructed to boil water, to eat only cooked foods and raise their
standards of personal hygiene. Camps and hospitals for isolation cases
should be improvised. Congregations of persons, e.g. in markets,
places of prayer, etc., should be discouraged during epidemics. Control
of travellers and pilgrims especially from endemic areas of cholera
should be rigidly and continuously enforced. The establishment of
treatment centres for diarrhoeal diseases is advocated. Countries must
show a greater willingness to provide the WHO and their neighbours
with a regular flow of information on their current states of cholera.

(c) *Immunisation*
All people at risk or travellers entering an endemic area must be
vaccinated. Two injections given subcutaneously of 0·5 ml and 1·0 ml
respectively at weekly intervals provide some protection. During
epidemics, however, one injection of 1·0 ml is considered sufficient for
mass immunisation and for contacts.

The efficiency of cholera vaccines in preventing disease has ranged from 0-80 per cent, averaging about 50 per cent. This level of induced immunity is of relatively little public health value. The highest level of protection is generally in the first three months and may continue for an additional three months. The available evidence suggests that both classical and El Tor vaccines will protect against either biotype.

The WHO epidemiological model of cholera indicates that the improvement of sanitation is the optimal means of controlling cholera and that vaccination is beneficial when applied together with sanitation. Cholera vaccine does not however prevent the development of the carrier state in household contacts.

Under International Sanitary Regulations, the validity of a cholera vaccination certificate extends for a period of 6 months, beginning 6 days after the first injection of the vaccine, or, in the event of a re-vaccination on the date of that re-vaccination.

Cholera—Summary

(1) *Occurrence*—India/Pakistan subcontinent, S.E. Asia, the Near East, East Africa, Southern and Central Europe
(2) *Organisms*—*Vibrio cholerae*, classical and El Tor biotypes
(3) *Reservoir of infection*—Man
(4) *Modes of transmission*—Water, personal contact (case-to-case), food, flies
(5) *Control*— (i) Diagnosis, isolation, notification and antibiotics
      (ii) Search for source of infection
      (iii) Concurrent and terminal disinfection
      (iv) Environmental sanitation
      (v) Immunisation
      (vi) Health education, personal hygiene

Brucellosis

Brucellosis is one of the most important infections of animals which can affect man and which are referred to as Zoonoses. The human disease is characterised by fever, heavy night sweats, splenomegaly and weakness. The *incubation period* varies from 6 days to as long as 3 months.

Medical geography

The infection is widely distributed but is particular prevalent in the countries around the Mediterranean Sea. Brucellosis is more prevalent in the tropics than is generally supposed and has been widely reported from Africa, South America and India.

Bacteriology

Human disease is attributed to *Brucella abortus, Br. suis* and *Br. melitensis* from cattle, swine and goat exposure respectively. *Brucella* are small, non-motile, non-sporing, Gram-negative coccobacilli.

Apart from their different CO_2 requirements, the members of this group resemble each other closely in their cultural characters.

Epidemiology

Many animals can serve as sources of infection for man, among which the most important are cattle, swine, goats and sheep.

The modes of transmission are ingestion, contact, inhalation and inoculation from animals which are discharging *Brucella*. Infection by ingestion may occur by the gastro-intestinal route and by penetration of the mucous membrane of the oral cavity and throat. The transmission of *Brucella* by ingestion of contaminated milk, milk products, meat and meat products is well recorded. Viable *Brucella* may be present in the viscera and muscles of infected carcasses for periods of over 1 month. Camel meat and water are also vehicles of infection. Contact with infected material, e.g. placentae, urine, carcasses, etc., is a common mode of infection and brucellosis is an occupational disease of veterinarians, farmers, etc. Air-borne infection through the mucous membranes of the eye and respiratory tract can occur, while accidental inoculation has been recorded among veterinarians and laboratory workers. Brucellosis results in economic loss to animal husbandry. There is loss of protein food from animal abortion, premature births, infertility and reduced production of milk.

Laboratory diagnosis

The laboratory diagnosis of brucellosis includes bacteriological and serological methods as well as allergic tests. *Brucella* organisms can be cultured from the blood, bone marrow, synovial fluid, lymph nodes and other sources. A progressive rise of antibody titre occurs in acute brucellosis and the serum agglutination test nearly always gives significantly positive results in the presence of active infection. The interpretation of the agglutination test is not always easy since, owing to the occurrence of latent and past infections, a certain number of persons in countries where the disease is endemic have very high titres. The complement fixation test can also be used in the diagnosis of chronic brucellosis, while the intradermal test when positive only indicates a state of specific allergy and must be interpreted with great caution. It is a useful adjunct to other methods of diagnosis especially in epidemiological surveys.

Control

The main control of human brucellosis rests in the pasteurisation of milk and environmental sanitation of farms.

(a) *The individual*

Persons having contact with herds should observe high standards of personal hygiene. Exposed areas of skin should be washed and soiled

C

clothing renewed. Employees in the slaughter houses should wear protective clothing when handling carcasses and these should be removed and disinfected after use. The antibiotic of choice for the specific treatment of brucellosis is tetracycline.

(b) *The community*
Pasteurisation of milk is the most important method of prevention of human brucellosis; when this is not possible all milk should be boiled before use. Health education and propaganda should be carried out. Infected animals should be segregated and possibly slaughtered. High standards of animal husbandry must be encouraged and, when possible, animals should be vaccinated.

(c) *Immunisation*
Vaccination in man is dangerous, a living vaccine 19-BA (a derivative of *Br. abortus* strain 19) has been used, however, in the USSR in persons at high risk of *Brucella* infection.

Vaccination of animals can result in control and even eradication of brucellosis among them. Living attenuated vaccines of *Br. melitensis*, and 19 *Br. abortus* have been widely and successfully used. Killed vaccines are also available.

Brucellosis—Summary
(1) *Occurrence*—World-wide
(2) *Organisms*—Brucella abortus, B. melitensis, B. suis
(3) *Reservoir of infection*—Animals, e.g. cattle, goats, sheep and swine
(4) *Modes of transmission*—Ingestion, contact
(5) *Control*— (i) Pasteurisation of milk
       (ii) Elimination of brucellosis from herds

Bacterial Food Poisoning
Food poisoning in the tropics is commonly due to three species of bacteria: *Salmonella* spp. which are the most important, *Staphylococcus aureus* and *Clostridium welchii*.

(1) Salmonella Food Poisoning
Salmonella food poisoning typically presents with diarrhoea, vomiting and fever. The *incubation period* is usually 12 to 24 hours.

Medical geography
This is world-wide, but infection is commoner in tropical communities with low hygiene standards.

Bacteriology
Salmonellae have been subdivided into many types, the majority being named after the place where they were first isolated. The

commonest type causing food poisoning is *S. typhimurium* which is widely distributed in the animal, bird and reptilian kingdoms.

Epidemiology
The source of infection is usually *Salmonella*-infected animals, e.g. cattle, poultry, pigs, dogs, cats, rats and mice.

Meat is the common mode of transmission either as a result of illness in cattle or by contamination from intestinal contents in unhygienically maintained abattoirs. Other vehicles of infection are eggs and egg products, as a result of faecal contamination of the shell, and milk and milk products. Foodstuffs can be infected at any stage from the abattoir to the home by rats and mice, by human carriers of *Salmonellae* or subclinically infected persons during the processing or preparation of food. Typically explosive small epidemics occur among groups of people who have eaten of the same food.

Laboratory diagnosis
Serological agglutination methods are needed to identify the type of *Salmonella*, but the genus is readily recognised by standard bacteriological techniques.

Control
This is essentially a matter of food hygiene to be applied from the abattoir to the home.

(a) *The individual*
No individual should handle foodstuffs except after thorough washing of hands. Any person suffering from diarrhoea should be debarred from handling or preparing food. High standards of personal hygiene must be maintained by any person connected with food whether cooked or uncooked.

(b) *The community*
Veterinary inspection of abattoirs must be thoroughly and scrupulously carried out and inspection of animals done both before and after slaughter. Carcasses of animals suffering from salmonellosis must be condemned from human consumption. The abattoirs should be hygienically maintained in order to avoid infection or contamination from intestinal contents. Meat and meat products should be thoroughly cooked and if possible refrigerated if they are to be served cold. If no refrigeration facilities are available, foods should be carefully stored away from rats, mice, flies and kept as cool as is feasible in the circumstances. Health education is needed to raise the general standards of personal and food hygiene.

Salmonella Food Poisoning—Summary

(1) *Occurrence*—World-wide
(2) *Organism*—*Salmonella* spp.
(3) *Reservoir of infection*—Animals
(4) *Mode of transmission*—Meat and meat products
(5) *Control*— (i) Personal and food hygiene
            (ii) Inspection of abattoirs
            (iii) Health education of caterers and food handlers
            (iv) Refrigeration

(2) *Staphylococcus Food Poisoning*

Staphylococcus food poisoning is characterised by an abrupt onset with nausea and vomiting sometimes accompanied by diarrhoea and shock. The *incubation period* is from 1 to 6 hours, i.e. very short, which is a differential point from *Salmonella* food poisoning.

Medical geography
The disease is world-wide.

Bacteriology
Certain strains of coagulase-positive staphylococci which produce a heat resistant enterotoxin are responsible for this type of food poisoning. They must be differentiated from the non-enterotoxin producing *Staphylococcus aureus* and *albus*.

Epidemiology
The source of infection is man, i.e. food handlers carrying the organism in the nose, throat, hand and skin lesions such as boils, carbuncles and whitlows. Food is contaminated either by droplet infection or by direct contact with infected cutaneous lesions. The mode of transmission is through manufactured semi-preserved foods eaten cold such as hams, tinned meats, sauces, custards, cream fillings of cakes and unpasteurised milk due to staphylococcal infection of cattle. A sudden outbreak of vomiting and diarrhoea in a group of persons who have partaken of the same meal within a few hours suggests staphylococcus food poisoning. Any occasion for mass feeding as occurs in funerals, weddings, schools and other institutions, is liable to result in staphylococcus food poisoning. In these instances food is often pre-cooked, stored and then served cold or after rewarming.

Laboratory diagnosis
If an unconsumed portion of the suspected food is still available this should be sent to the laboratory for examination of enterotoxin-producing staphylococci.

Control
This consists in the proper education of food handlers and high standards of food hygiene.

(a) *The individual*
All food handlers should be educated in personal hygiene and excluded from contact with foodstuffs if they suffer from purulent nasal discharges or pyogenic skin lesions until they are cured.

(b) *The community*
High standards of catering should be maintained and hygienic techniques for handling, preparation and storage of foods used. Whenever possible, cooked foods should be refrigerated and the adequate heat-treatment of all milk and milk products is essential.

Staphylococcus Food Poisoning—Summary
(1) *Occurrence*—World-wide
(2) *Organisms*—Enterotoxin-producing staphylococci
(3) *Reservoir of infection*—Man
(4) *Mode of transmission*—Semi-preserved foods
(5) *Control*— (i) Personal hygiene of food handlers
       (ii) Food hygiene and refrigeration

(3) *Clostridium welchii* Food Poisoning
Clostridium welchii food poisoning presents with diarrhoea and pain, vomiting is not very common. The *incubation period* is 12 to 24 hours.

Medical geography
The condition is world-wide. A diffuse sloughing enteritis of the jejunum, ileum and colon known as '*enteritis necroticans*' or '*pigbel*' is very common in New Guinea.

Bacteriology
There are many serotypes of *Cl. welchii*. The rod-like organisms require anaerobic conditions in which to grow. They are Gram-positive and produce endospores. In New Guinea *Cl. perfringens* (*Cl. welchii*, type C) is thought to be associated aetiologically with 'pigbel'.

Epidemiology
The source of infection can be human, animal, or fly faeces, and the spores of *Cl. welchii* survive for long periods in soil, dust, clothes and in the environment generally. The carrier rate in human populations varies from 2 per cent to 30 per cent. The mode of transmission is by ingestion of meat which has been pre-cooked and eaten cold, or reheated the next day prior to consumption.

In New Guinea the disease is both epidemic and sporadic forms, is related to pig feasting, which is an integral and complex part of the indigenous cultures of all highland tribes. Males are affected more often than females. The fatality rates vary from nil to 85 per cent.

Laboratory diagnosis
   Cl. welchii can be isolated from the stools of individuals suffering from the disease and from food remnants.

Control
A proper standard of food hygiene is the most effective method of controlling *Cl. welchii* food poisoning.

All meat dishes should be either cooked and eaten immediately or refrigerated until required. Reheating of foodstuffs should be avoided and in New Guinea special precautions should be taken when pig-feasting occurs.

Clostridium Food Poisoning—Summary
   (1) *Occurrence*—World-wide, New Guinea (special type)
   (2) *Organism*—*Cl. welchii*
   (3) *Reservoir of infection*—Man, animals
   (4) *Mode of transmission*—Ingestion of meat
   (5) *Control*—Cooking and storage of meat

III. Protozoal Infections
The most important protozoal infections transmitted by the faeces/oral route are (i) amoebiasis, (ii) the flagellate infestations and (iii) toxoplasmosis.

Amoebiasis
Amoebiasis is caused by the protozoan *Entamoeba histolytica*. The parasite lives in the large intestine causing ulceration of the mucosa with consequent diarrhoea.

Medical geography
Amoebiasis has a world-wide distribution, but clinical disease occurs most frequently in tropical and subtropical countries. In temperate climates the infection is often non-pathogenic and symptomless.

Applied biology
   The amoeba multiplies by binary fission. It lives in the lumen of the large intestine where under suitable conditions it invades the mucous membrane and submucosa. If red blood cells are available, the amoeba will ingest them. When diarrhoea occurs, amoebae are expelled to the exterior as such, and then are found in the freshly passed fluid stools. Amoebae are very sensitive to environmental changes, and so are short lived outside the body. When there is no diarrhoea and other conditions are favourable for encystation, the amoebae cease

feeding, become spherical, secrete a cyst wall and the nucleus divides twice to form the characteristic mature four-nucleate cyst.

There are two other characteristic structures, a glycogen vacuole which acts as a carbohydrate reserve, and chromatoid bodies which are a ribosome store. Cysts kept cool and moist remain viable for several weeks.

The cyst is the infective form, and when ingested hatches in the lower part of the small intestine or upper part of the large intestine and a four-nucleate amoeba emerges from the cyst. After a series of nuclear and cytoplasmic divisions, each multinucleate amoeba gives rise to eight uninucleate amoebae, which establish themselves and multiply in the large intestine.

The sizes of the cysts produced by individual strains are uniform; they vary from 7 μm to 15 μm in diameter; they can be divided into two groups, those strains producing cysts over 10 μm and those below 10 μm in diameter. The strains producing small cysts are now held to belong to a separate species, *E. hartmanni*. Infections with *E. hartmanni* are symptomless.

Epidemiology

Infection with *E. histolytica* occurs throughout both temperate and tropical climates, although the incidence of overt disease is high only in the tropics and subtropics. The disease is spread by cyst passers, who may be divided into two main groups:

(*a*) convalescents who have recovered from an acute attack

(*b*) individuals who can recall no clinical evidence of infection.

The latter possibly are the more common source of infection, even in countries with high standards of hygiene. Bad sanitation is more important than climate in the predominance of overt infection in the tropics. Carrier rates of *E. histolytica* among symptomless subjects have varied from 5 per cent in temperate areas with good hygiene to 80 per cent in some tropical communities. The parasite can be transmitted by direct contact through the contaminated hands of cyst carriers, e.g. in institutions; it is also transmitted indirectly by means of contaminated food, such as raw vegetables fertilised with fresh human faeces; and through the intermediaries of food handlers and flies. Infected water has occasionally been held responsible for the transmission of large outbreaks of the disease.

Although several animals harbour *E. histolytica*—monkeys, dogs, pigs rats, cats—they are thought to be of no epidemiological importance in human infections. Amoebic dysentery is not infrequently a house or family infection. Among other factors influencing the epidemiology of the disease we have to consider the following: (i) age and sex, (ii) race, (iii) immunity and (iv) diet.

Any differences that have been reported in the incidence of the disease between males and females are probably related to exposure rather than a true sex susceptibility to the infection. The disease seems to appear in fulminating form in pregnant and puerperal women. This may be a corticosteroid effect. Amoebiasis in childhood is not uncommon. It usually occurs in the age-group nil to 6 years, as those between the ages of 7 and 16 years seem to enjoy a greater immunity to ill effects from *E. histolytica* infection than others.

All races are susceptible to the disease. Although the infection is often milder in Europeans, this is probably related to sanitary standards, diet, and freedom from debilitating disorders, rather than to a genuine racial factor. Reports from Madras indicate that amoebiasis was twenty times more frequent in Hindus than in Muslims, while in Durban the incidence and severity of amoebic dysentery is greater in Africans than in Indians or Europeans.

There is no evidence that amoebiasis confers any protective immunity and the infection can persist for many years after its establishment. The general condition of patients plays an important role; thus, severe cases of amoebiasis are often seen among soldiers on active service.

Laboratory diagnosis

The clinical diagnosis of amoebiasis has to be confirmed by identification of *E. histolytica*. During an attack of amoebic dysentery the motions are loose, offensive, and contain mucus and blood, faecal elements are always present. On microscopical examination motile amoebae, some with engorged red cells, will be found in the freshly passed stool or in specimens removed at sigmoidoscopy or proctoscopy.

In asymptomatic infections, and during remission, the stool is semiformed and contains *E. histolytica* cysts. They can be seen to contain one or more bar-shaped chromatoid bodies and staining with iodine reveals one to four nuclei and a glycogen mass. Repeated stool examinations (six specimens collected at weekly intervals) should be made before absence of infection can confidently be assumed. Concentration techniques for cysts are available, and cultural methods may assist diagnosis in scanty infections.

Until recently, immunological methods for the diagnosis of intestinal and extra-intestinal amoebiasis have been equivocal. Complement-fixation, precipitin, and intradermal tests have all been used with varying success. New techniques, e.g. latex agglutination and amoebic gel-diffusion tests, with improved antigens promise better results, although they are not yet generally available. The fluorescent antibody test has proved very reliable.

Control

The main control measure is the provision and use of sanitary disposal of faeces coupled with personal cleanliness.

(a) *The individual*
Raising the standards of personal hygiene through health education is
the only method that can be applied to the individual, e.g. advice on
washing of hands, especially after defaecation. Food handlers, e.g.
cooks, are a specially important group to train. Adequate treatment of
individual infections with metronidazole or other amoebicides reduces
the reservoir of infection.

The community
The provision of a safe water supply and facilities for sanitary disposal
of faeces are the main control measures applicable to the community.
The use of human faeces as fertilisers should be discouraged. In areas
where a pure water supply is not available, water should be boiled and
raw vegetables and fruit thoroughly washed and dipped in boiling
water. Food should be protected from flies.

Amoebiasis—Summary
(1) *Occurrence*—World-wide
(2) *Organism*—E. histolytica
(3) *Reservoir of infection*—Man
(4) *Modes of transmission*—Contaminated hands, food
(5) *Control*— (i) Sanitary disposal of faeces
     (ii) Personal hygiene

Other Amoebae
Infection of the human gut may occur with other amoebae, namely
E. coli; *Dientamoeba fragilis*; *Endolimax nana*; and *Iodamoeba butschlii*.
There is controversy, however, concerning the actual pathogenicity of
these organisms. *Naegleria fowleri* has been reported as causing a fatal
necrotising meningo-encephalitis.

Flagellate and Other Intestinal Protozoa
A number of flagellate protozoa commonly parasitise the human
intestine and genito-urinary tract, e.g. *Trichomonas hominis*; *Chilomastix
mesnili*; *T. vaginalis*; and *Giardia lamblia*. The ones with real claims to
pathogenicity are *G. lamblia* and *T. vaginalis* whch are found both in
the tropics and in temperate countries. *T. vaginalis* urethritis is common
in males (see p. 130).

(1) *Giardiasis*
Heavy infection with *G. lamblia* is often accompanied by diarrhoea or
steatorrhoea.

Applied biology
The trophozoite lives in the upper part of the small intestine particularly the duodenum and jejunum. In appearance it resembles a

half-pear split longitudinally measuring 12-18 μm in length. It reproduces itself by a complicated process of binary fission. The cysts —which are the infective forms—occur in the faeces, often in enormous numbers. They are oval in shape, contain at first two nuclei which divide, giving rise to four in the mature cyst.

Epidemiology
Man is the source of infection. *G. lamblia* is harboured by many animals, but these play little part in the epidemiology of human infections. The infection is transmitted by the ingestion of cysts, as a result of insanitary habits or contaminated food. It is common in children and in adults, sometimes causing symptoms of malabsorption in both, due to mechanical irritation rather than invasion of the mucous membrane. Giardia infections may persist for years and the parasite may invade the biliary tract.

Laboratory diagnosis
Diagnosis of infection is made by finding cysts of the parasite in formed stools and vegetative forms in fluid stools.

Control
The main control measures are the provision and use of a safe method of excreta disposal and the raising of personal standards of hygiene.

(2) *Trichomonas hominis and T. vaginalis*
T. hominis inhabits the caecum and large intestine. The body is pear-shaped, 10-15 μm in length. The single ovoid nucleus is situated in the rounded-anterior end and there are three flagellae. There is no cystic phase. The presence of these flagellates in diarrhoeic stools has no pathogenic significance. *T. vaginalis* is found in the vagina and male urethra. It is larger than *T. hominis*, reaching 27 μm in length, and usually has five anterior flagella. No cysts are known. The flagellate is commonly found during the reproductive period in women, and men play an important part in the transmission of the infection. The incidence of infection in the vagina may be high and the presence of the parasite is associated with lowered vaginal acidity.
In the female vaginitis is usual and an anterior urethritis may occur. Posterior urethritis is rare and the bladder is never affected.

Diagnosis is made by finding the flagellate in vaginal and prostatic secretions or in the urine.

Control
This involves the treatment of both marriage partners simultaneously with metronidizale, 200 mg tds for 5 days.

(3) *Isosporiasis*

The coccidia *Isosopora belli* and *I. hominis* are widely distributed in the tropical world. No pathological accounts are available and the pathogenicity of these organisms is mild and controversial.

(4) *Balantidiasis*

Balantidiasis in man has been recorded from most parts of the world, and is caused by infection with the ciliate protozoon, *Balantidium coli* which is a common parasite of the pig.

Applied Biology

The large ovoid cysts are passed in the faeces and contain the parasite which may be seen moving actively. The enclosed balantidium then loses its cilia, and sometimes two individuals are found in the same cyst. *B. coli* reproduces asexually by transverse fission. Transmission of infection takes place by ingestion of cyts, but the subsequent life cycle is not known.

Epidemiology

B. coli has been found in the intestinal contents of man and a large number of animals—wild boars, sheep, horses, rats, frogs, monkeys, etc., but domestic pigs are much the most important reservoir hosts. Infection in man is comparatively rare despite man's close contact with pigs in many countries, and in more than 50 per cent of human cases there may be no history of contact with pigs.

It is possible that man is most often infected by fingers, food, drinking water, or soil contaminated by pigs' faeces containing balantidia, usually in the encysted form. Handling of the intestines of infected animals or flies are other possible modes of transmission. Furthermore, the possibility of infection from green vegetables grown in soil fertilised by pig excrement must be borne in mind, especially as cysts may remain viable for weeks in moist faeces.

The reported incidence in man is very variable (0·5-5·1 per cent) and depends on whether freshly collected specimens of faeces are examined or not. Epidemics have been reported from mental institutions, and in New Guinea a high incidence of infection has been recorded.

Laboratory diagnosis

The stools are bloody and mucoid. Examination of faeces will reveal the typical large ovoid cysts 45-60 μm in length containing the parasite. The trophozoites may also be seen in freshly collected stools. The protozoon is oval in shape and of variable size—20-30 μm in length by 40-60 μm in breadth. The body is clothed with a thick covering of cilia arranged in longitudinal rows. Both the direct and indirect fluorescent antibody techniques have recently been applied in the diagnosis of *B. coli*.

Control

High standards of personal hygiene must be maintained, especially among persons in close contact with pigs—gloves should be worn when handling the intestines of potentially infected animals. Green vegetables should be washed and dipped in boiling water. Environmental sanitation of piggeries should be encouraged. Sanitary disposal of faeces and purification of water are the main control measures for the community.

Toxoplasmosis

Toxoplasmosis is caused by the intracellular sporozoon *Toxoplasma gondi*. The infection may be congenital or acquired. Clinically there are four types of acquired toxoplasmosis: (i) asymptomatic, (ii) acute, (iii) glandular and (iv) chronic.

Medical geography

Toxoplasmosis has a world-wide distribution. In the tropics it is probably commoner than is generally realised.

Applied biology

The life cycle of *T. gondii* is similar to that of coccidian parasites and its taxonomic status is now considered to be a coccidian parasite related to the genus *Isospora*. When extracellular, the organism is crescent shaped, about 6 μm long. The cytoplasm stains blue with Giemsa and the eccentric nucleus red. In the intracellular stages *T. gondi* appears singly or in clusters within the reticulo-endothelial cells. Aggregations of the organisms may form pseudocysts. The cystic form of the parasite reaches 100 μm in diameter. Reproduction of the organism is by binary fission. Toxoplasma trophozoites and cysts characterise acute and chronic infections respectively, but cysts may form early in the acute stage and trophozoites may remain active for years in some chronic infections.

Epidemiology

Man is the main reservoir of human infection. The method of transmission of *T. gondii* from person to person is unknown except in congenital infections. Surveys of various populations have shown that a high incidence of asymptomatic infection occurs in the warm or hot humid areas, and a low incidence in the cold areas and hot dry areas. In general, there does not appear to be any differences in infection rate between urban and rural populations, between sexes or between races in the same environment. *T. gondii* is widely distributed in the animal kingdom, being particularly common in cats, dogs and rabbits. However, in spite of the circumstantial evidence indicating a possible transmission between animals and man, it is probable that both may become infected from a common source or sources. Ingestion of raw beef and pork meat are a recognised mode of infection and it has been demonstrated that infection was particularly high in a tuberculosis hospital in France, where the children were fed raw or underdone meat. Antibodies, however, are found just as frequently in vegetarians as in meat eaters in India. High infection rates have also been found in sewage workers, rabbit trappers, laboratory workers and nurses. The role of droplet infection and mechanical subcutaneous inoculation by biting, or blood-sucking arthropods, in the transmission of toxoplasmosis, has yet to be proved. *Toxoplasma* can be transmitted inside the egg of the cat roundworm *Toxocara cati*, but this is not likely to be the main mode of infection in man.

Laboratory diagnosis

In the blood there may be a leucocytosis or leucopenia. An eosinophilia has been described. There may be a mild degree of anaemia and a leukamoid reaction and atypical lymphocytes may be seen.

Toxoplasma may be isolated from blood, cerebrospinal fluid, saliva, sputum, lymph nodes, skin, liver and muscle by intraperitoneal injection of the biopsy or other material into mice, guinea-pigs or hamsters. Mice are most suitable as they do not suffer from toxoplasmosis as a laboratory infection.

A number of serological tests have been described for the detection of antibodies to *T. gondii*, the cytoplasm-modifying test of Sabin-Feldman (dye-test) is the one most widely used. It is a sensitive test which shows the presence of antibody in many of the normal adult population, and the most convincing method of diagnosing active toxoplasmosis is by the demonstration of at least a fourfold rise in titre, coupled with the isolation of toxoplasma in tissues or body fluids by inoculation of mice.

Other serological tests in common use are:
(i) complement-fixation tests
(ii) direct agglutination test
(iii) haemagglutination test
(iv) fluorescent antibody test.

Recently a toxoplasma neutralisation test and a micro-agglutination test have been described.

Control

The most effective treatment for both man and animals is a combination of pyrimethamine and sulphonamides. Intimate contact with sick animals should be avoided, and ingestion of raw meat discouraged.

Toxoplasmosis—Summary
(1) *Occurrence*—World-wide
(2) *Organism*—*T. gondii*
(3) *Reservoirs of infection*—Man, other mammals
(4) *Modes of transmission*—Raw beef and pork
(5) *Control*— (i) Personal hygiene
            (ii) Thorough cooking of meat of animal origin

IV. Helminthic Infections

Many important helminths are transmitted through the gastro-intestinal tract and the infections they give rise to can be classified as follows:

Nematodes	*Cestodes*	*Trematodes*	
Ascariasis	Taeniasis	Paragonimiasis—Lung fluke	
Toxocariasis	Diphyllobothriasis	Clonorchiasis	
Trichuriasis	Hymenolepsiasis	Opisthorchiasis	Liver flukes
Enterobiasis	Hydatid disease	Fascioliasis	
Dracontiasis		Fasciolopsiasis	
Trichinosis		Heterophyiasis	Intestinal flukes
Angiostrongyliasis		Metagonimiasis	
Gnathostomiasis			

Ascariasis

This disease, due to *Ascaris lumbricoides*, is often symptomless and infection is discovered incidentally; occasionally it causes intestinal obstruction in children.

Medical geography
A. lumbricoides, the large intestinal roundworm, has a world-wide distribution the incidence of which is largely determined by local habits in the disposal of faeces. Its highest prevalence is in the hot humid climates of Asia, Africa and tropical America.

Applied biology
The adult worms live in the small intestine. Their colour is yellowish-white and they may reach a length of 40 cm. The female is prolific, laying up to 200 000 eggs a day. The typical egg has a yellowish-brown mamillated appearance.

The eggs are passed in the faeces, and providing the environment is suitable a larva develops within the egg and becomes infective in about 10 days. After eggs containing larvae are swallowed by man, the young worms hatch, are set free in the small intestine and begin the migration. This takes them through the wall of the small intestine, and by way of the hepatic portal system to the liver. They are then carried by the bloodstream to the right heart and to the lungs, where they remain for several days, after which they migrate passively up the bronchi and trachea to the pharynx. They are now swallowed and re-enter the small intestine where they become sexually mature in about 2 months.

The migratory phase of larval development in the liver and lungs requires 8-15 days and is associated with fever, allergic dermatitis, eosinophilia and pneumonitis or pneumonia.

Epidemiology
Man is the reservoir of infection which is spread by faecal pollution of the soil. The eggs are swallowed as a result of ingestion of soil or contact between the mouth and various inanimate objects carrying the adherent eggs. Contamination of food or drink by dust or handling is also a source of infection. Eggs of *Ascaris* pass unaltered through the intestine of coprophagous animals and can thus be transported to locations other than human defaecation sites. The well-protected eggs withstand drying and can survive for very lengthy periods.

Although all age-groups show infection in endemic areas, the incidence and intensity are highest in the younger age-groups. Infants may be parasitised soon after birth by ova on the mother's fingers. In human subjects the observed differences in incidence and intensity at different ages are probably due to differences in behaviour and occupational activities between children and adults, as well as to the development of acquired resistance.

Ascaris eggs are resistant to cold and to disinfectants in the strengths in normal use. They are killed by direct sunlight and by temperatures above 45 °C. Under optimum conditions eggs may remain viable for as long as 1 year. *A. suis*, which infects pigs, is morphologically identical and can mature in man, but cross-infection has not been proved. In epidemiological studies, serological tests (e.g. larval microprecipitation test) are useful to detect early infections as well as the lung manifestations of the larval stages of *Ascaris* infection.

Laboratory diagnosis
The microscopical diagnosis of ascariasis can be confirmed by examination of faeces samples. Because of their characteristic morphology and colour the ova can be found relatively easily in 'direct smears'. Concentration and quantitative techniques are available.

Control
The main method of control is the sanitary disposal of human excreta.

(a) *The individual*
Health education should be directed towards raising standards of

personal hygiene especially among mothers, who should be encouraged to train young children not to defaecate indiscriminately.

(b) *The community*
A method of sanitary disposal of faeces, i.e. some type of latrine acceptable to the people and best suited to the terrain, should be introduced and the people encouraged to use it. Human faeces should not be used as fertiliser unless previously composted so that the resulting high temperature can kill the eggs. Sanitary facilities should be provided for persons who spend long hours at work out of doors and such persons, e.g. farmers, should be encouraged to use the facilities provided. Mass treatment of pre-school and school children may be undertaken using a single dose of one of the piperazine compounds (2 g-5 g) or levamisole (40 mg-80 mg).

Ascariasis—Summary
(1) *Occurrence*—Hot humid climates of the world
(2) *Organism*—*A. lumbricoides*
(3) *Reservoir of infection*—Man
(4) *Modes of transmission*—Contaminated hands, food, drink
(5) *Control*— (i) Sanitary disposal of faeces
         (ii) Personal hygiene

Toxocariasis (visceral larva migrans)
Evidence has now accumulated that human disease due to larval migration of *Toxocara canis* and *T. cati* constitutes an important public health problem, and although the majority of reports to date have emanated from the more developed countries we believe that it is merely a question of time before these infections are widely reported from the tropics as a major cause of some of the otherwise unexplained clinical syndromes seen in these areas.

Medical geography
The majority of human cases have been reported from the eastern half of the United States, but the disease has been recognised in the Philippines, Mexico, Hawaii, Turkey, Puerto Rico and other countries. Toxocaral infection of dogs has been reported from Malta, Nigeria, Uganda, Kenya, Tanzania, Mexico and India.

Applied biology
    T. canis and *T. cati* are parasites of dogs and cats and their presence in the human host is an abnormal migration of their larval phase.
    Under favourable conditions, the eggs passed in the dog's faeces become infective in 2-3 weeks. From the swallowed eggs emerge the contained second-stage larvae which penetrate the intestinal walls and reach the liver. The majority of larvae remain in the liver but others may pass on to the lungs or other organs of the body, includ-

ing the central nervous system and the eye. Occasionally the larvae complete their cycle of development in the human host, resulting in infection with adult *T. canis* or *T. cati*.

Epidemiology
The reservoir of infection is the dog, or less frequently the cat. Infection is acquired by ingesting soil which has been contaminated, usually by dogs' faeces. Young children are particular susceptible to toxocariasis because of their habit of eating dirt, and of handling soiled fur of puppies and then putting the fingers in the mouth. The severity of the disease depends upon the numbers of worms that have invaded the body and the duration of infection. It has been shown that puppies are more infected than adult dogs and that the incidence among bitches is lower at all ages. It is possible that nematode larvae other than *Toxocara* may be involved in visceral larva migrans. Viral encephalitis due to larval migration has been reported and the transmission of poliomyelitis virus by larvae of *Toxocara* has been suspected.

Laboratory diagnosis
A high, stable persistent eosinophilia reaching levels of 60 per cent is a prominent feature. *Toxocara* larvae can be identified in biopsy material and provide the most certain means of making a definite diagnosis. The fluorescent antibody test has also been used.

Control
Elimination of infection in puppies and dogs is the most effective way of controlling the disease. Puppies used as household pets should be regularly examined and treated. Children should be instructed in habits of personal hygiene. Treatment of pets can be effectively carried out with one of the piperazine compounds.

Toxocariasis—Summary
(1) *Occurrence*—World-wide
(2) *Organisms*—T. canis and *T. catis*
(3) *Reservoir of infection*—Dogs and cats
(4) *Mode of transmission*—Handling infected household pets
(5) *Control*— (i) Treatment of household pets
        (ii) Personal hygiene

Trichuriasis
This infection is due to the whipworm *Trichuris trichiura* and it is often symptomless. Heavy infections of over 1000 worms, however, may cause bloody diarrhoea with anaemia and prolapse of the rectum.

Medical geography
Trichuriasis occurs throughout the world but is more prevalent in the warm humid tropics.

Applied biology

The sexually mature worms, which are about 5 cm long, have a whiplike shape and live in the caecum and upper colon of man. After fertilisation the eggs are passed in the faeces within 4 weeks of infection and embryonic development takes place in the soil. Under favourable conditions of moisture and temperature the larvae develop inside the eggs within 2-5 weeks. The embryonated eggs are infective.

When the eggs are ingested by man the larvae escapes into the upper small intestine and migrate directly to the caecum, where they become adults within 1-3 months.

Epidemiology

Man is the reservoir of infection. Soil pollution is the determining factor in the prevalence and intensity of infection in a community, and clay soils are more favourable than sandy soils. Transmission occurs through the insanitary habit of promiscuous defaecation; and infection usually results from the ingestion of infective ova from contaminated hands, food or drink. Although *Trichuris* infection of domestic and other animals occurs, it is unlikely that animal reservoirs play a part in the epidemiology of human infection. Coprophagous animals can transport *Trichuris* eggs to locations other than human defaecation sites, since the eggs are passed unaltered through their intestine. The higher prevalence in children is probably due to greater exposure to infection.

Laboratory diagnosis

Direct smear examination of faeces will reveal the characteristic lemon-shaped ova. An egg count on an ordinary wet faecal smear (containing about 2 mg of faeces) of more than 100 ova is indicative of a heavy infection. Concentration and quantitative techniques can be applied.

Eosinophilia (10-20 per cent) is usually present, especially in massive infections. An associated microcytic hypochromic anaemia may be seen and the mucoid sticky stools may contain a preponderance of eosinophil cells and Charcot-Leyden crystals.

Control

(1) Sanitary disposal of faeces
(2) Personal hygiene.

Enterobiasis

This infection is due to the pinworm *Enterobius vermicularis* and is prevalent throughout the world and is probably less common in the tropics than in countries of the temperate zone. The infection may be symptomless or there may be mild gastro-intestinal discomfort and pruritus ani.

Applied biology

The female worm is about 8-13 mm long while the male worm—which is rarely seen—is only 2-5 mm. They both live in the caecum, where copulation takes place. The gravid females then migrate to the colon and rectum and at night pass through the anus to deposit their eggs on the perianal skin and genitocrural folds. Within a few hours larvae develop within the eggs, which are now infective. Upon ingestion by man, the larvae hatch in the duodenum and mature in the caecum. The life cycle from egg to adult lasts 3-7 weeks. The survival of the ova depends upon temperature and humidity; viability being greatest in cool, moist surroundings.

Epidemiology

Man is the reservoir of infection. The highest incidence of enterobiasis is in school-children from 5 to 15 years. It is very prevalent in crowded districts with faulty hygiene, in institutional groups, and among members of the same family.

The ova from the perianal region are transferred to night clothes, towels and bedding, and infection may follow when these are handled. Infective ova may be present in the dust and infection can therefore take place by inhalation. The intense pruritus around the perianal regions results in scratching and the hands, especially beneath the finger nails, become contaminated and ova are transferred directly to the mouth or indirectly through food and other objects which have been handled. Occasionally the larvae, after hatching in the perianal regions, re-enter the anus and migrate to the caecum, where they mature (retroinfection). There may be a racial susceptibility to infection, thus Puerto Rican children living in crowded conditions in New York had a lower incidence of infection than white, non-Puerto Rican children.

Laboratory diagnosis

Adult female worms may be found in the faeces or perianal skin. The method of choice making for a diagnosis is the Scotch adhesive tape swab applied to the perianal region in the morning before bathing or defaecation. Ova are identified by their asymmetrical shape and well-developed embryo when the tape is mounted on a slide for examination. The Scotch tape can be also applied to that part of the person's clothing which has been in contact with the perianal region. At least three examinations should be carried out before a negative diagnosis is made. Enterobiasis is very infectious and if one person is infected in a household all other members of the family should be suspect.

Control

Because enterobiasis is a family or institution infection, all members should be examined and those positive treated simultaneously. Scrupulous cleanliness, frequent washing of the anal region, the hands and the nails, especially after defaecating, controls the infection. Cotton drawers and gloves should be worn at night and boiled daily. The drug treatment of choice is Viprynium (Vanquin) in a single dose of 5 ml-30 ml.

Dracontiasis

The guinea-worm *Dracunculus medinensis* has been known since ancient times. It results in the formation of ulcers with extrusion of embryos on contact with water.

Medical geography

It occurs in local distributions in Africa, the Middle East, India, Pakistan, the Caribbean islands, Guyana and Brazil.

Applied biology

The sexually mature female is up to 1 m long and 2 mm in diameter; the uterus, which occupies most of the body, contains millions of embryos. The male is small and its fate after copulation is not known.

When the gravid female is ready to discharge the larvae, the cephalic end of the worm approaches the skin and secretes a substance which causes a blister to form. When the surface of the blister comes in contact with water, the anterior end of the vagina protrudes and the uterus expels the embryos into the water until the supply is exhausted. The female worm then shrivels and dies.

The larvae liberated in water must be taken up by suitable species of *Cyclops*, in which they develop into infective forms in about 3 weeks. Man becomes infected by drinking water containing infected *Cyclops*. These are digested by the gastric juices and the freed larvae penetrate the wall of the digestive tract and eventually migrate to the subcutaneous tissues. The female worm requires about 1 year before it is ready to discharge her embryos.

Epidemiology

Contamination of water with larvae from infected persons takes place when such persons draw drinking water from shallow ponds or wells. The water in these ponds, being stagnant with a high organic content, favours the presence of the vector species of *Cyclops*. In the dry season in some areas these ponds are much frequented since they often provide the only readily accessible source of water, thus creating a high *Cyclops/* man contact ratio. In other places, transmission may occur during the rains when surface pools exist which disappear in the dry season. Infection can also be contracted when drinking water while bathing in contaminated pools or during ritual washing of the mouth in the performance of religious ablutions.

It has been suggested that gastric acidity may be responsible for resistance to infection in some exposed persons, but this hypothesis has been repudiated.

Laboratory diagnosis
A microscopical diagnosis can be made by placing a few drops of water on the guinea-worm blister. This stimulates the discharge of embryos which can be seen on examination of the water under a $\frac{2}{3}$-inch objective.

Control
Transmission can be interrupted by the provision of a piped water supply, providing wells with a sanitary well-head, straining or boiling all water for human consumption. DDT at 1 part per million, chloride of lime or 'Abate' (Cyanamid) will achieve immediate though temporary control of infected waters by killing the cyclops intermediate host. Treatment of individual infections with niridazole or thiabendazole has given excellent results.

Trichinosis
Trichinosis is a disease caused by encysted larvae of *Trichinella spiralis*. This parasite is more prevalent in temperate than in tropical countries and is mainly confined to those countries where pork is eaten.

Applied biology
The adult worms are found in the small intestine of a number of carniverous animals including the pig, bush-pig, rats, hyenas and other hosts. Their life span in the intestine is approximately 8 weeks.

After fertilisation, the female worms bury themselves in intestinal mucosa and each produces about 1500 larvae. The larvae migrate via the intestinal lymphatics to the thoracic duct and into the bloodstream, whence they are distributed to the muscles. Here they develop and become encysted between the muscle fibres in 5-7 weeks. Calcification occurs in about 18 months but the encysted larvae remain alive for many years. When food containing encysted larvae is ingested by a suitable host the larvae are released by the action of digestive juices on the capsule and the cycle is repeated in the new host. In susceptible animals the larvae grow into sexually differentiated adults which on mating produce larvae which then invade striated muscle. In man, infection terminates at the cystic stage.

Epidemiology
Pigs are the chief reservoir of infection. Trichinosis in man results from eating raw or inadequately cooked pork or pork products, e.g. sausage meat. In Kenya, the bush-pig is a common source of infection.

Pigs become infected chiefly from eating uncooked slaughter-house refuse containing infected meat scraps; occasionally rats, which have a high natural infection rate of trichinosis, can be a source of infection when they are eaten by pigs.

Serological tests have shown that in many communities the incidence of infection is apparently higher than the number of clinically diagnosed cases, and it is obvious that many light infections pass unnoticed. In recent years small and large epidemics have occurred. Congenital trichinosis has been reported.

Laboratory diagnosis

One of the most constant, single, diagnostic aid in trichinosis is a rising eosinophilia 10-40 per cent; while parasitological diagnosis is based on the finding of the encysted larval worms in a thin piece of muscle biopsy compressed between two glass slides and examined under a low magnification of the microscope. In light infections, when direct examination is negative, the biopsy specimen should be incubated overnight in an acid-pepsin mixture and the centrifuged deposit examined for larvae.

Recently, intradermal and serological tests have been widely used. They include:

  (i) complement fixation
 (ii) bentonite agglutination
(iii) latex agglutination
 (iv) cholesterol agglutination
  (v) fluorescent antibody.

The CFT can provide a diagnosis in the first week of the disease—the specificity of the test is high. The bentonite, latex, cholesterol agglutination tests are excellent tests for diagnosing recent infections, but are unreliable in chronic infections.

Control

Adequate cooking of pork meat will essentially protect the individual. Legislation compelling all pig food containing meat to be cooked virtually stops transmission of trichinosis to the pig.

Angiostrongyliasis

Eosinophilic meningitis due to the nematode worm *Angiostrongylus cantonensis* occurs sporadically and occasionally in small epidemics in certain Pacific Islands, including Tahiti and Hawaii, and in South-East Asia including Vietnam and Thailand.

Applied biology

A. cantonensis is essentially a parasite of rats and only occasionally infects man. The eggs hatch in the faeces of the rat in which they are expelled, and the infective larvae invade certain snails or slugs. These are later eaten by rats, which thereby become infected. The life cycle in man is unknown, but young adult worms have been found in the cerebrospinal fluid and the brain where they measured 8-12 mm in length.

Epidemiology
Human infection results from the accidental ingestion of infected snails, slugs and land planarians (worm-like creatures) found on un-washed vegetables, such as lettuce. Freshwater prawns may become infected from snails and slugs washed into rivers and estuaries during rainy weather. This was thought to be the main source of local, human infection in Tahiti. Eating raw or pickled snails of the genus *Pila* is considered the mode of infection in Thailand; the percentage of posi-tive snails for *A. cantonensis* infections varying from 1·8 to 72 per cent. The peak incidence of eosinophilic meningitis occurs in the cooler, rainy months between July and November, during this period lettuces and strawberries are most consumed, and when unwashed lead to infection. In Thailand males are affected twice as frequently as females, the highest attack rate occurring in the second and third decade. It has been suggested that *A. cantonensis* originated in the islands of the Indian Ocean—Madagascar, Mauritius, Ceylon—and then spread eastwards to South-East Asia and so to the Pacific area, and the giant African snail *Achatina fulica* might have been instrumental in the spread of the para-site. In Malaysia, the shelled slug *M. malayanus* has been shown to shed infective third-stage larvae, but no human cases have yet been reported.

Laboratory diagnosis
Examination of the cerebrospinal fluid reveals increase in protein and a strikingly high eosinophilia (60-80 per cent)—larval worms are sometimes found in the CSF and can be identified as *A. cantonensis*.

Control
The infection is prevented by not eating unwashed vegetables and strawberries and uncooked snails, slugs and prawns infected with larvae. Efficient rat control will reduce the reservoir of infection.

Gnathostomiasis
Gnathostoma infection may present as 'creeping eruption', transitory swellings or eosinophilic meningitis.

Medical geography
The normal hosts for *Gnathostoma spinigerum* are domestic and wild felines, dogs and foxes. Human infections have, however, been reported from Israel, the Sudan, India and the Far East. The majority of human

cases to date have occurred in Thailand. One per cent of dogs in Bangkok are infected with gnathostomiasis.

Applied biology

The life cycle in the definitive animal hosts is well known, and involves two intermediate hosts—a *Cyclops* and a fish or an amphibian. Man is an unnatural host and the immature worms may locate either in the internal organs or near the surface of the body, but as the larvae rarely develop into adults the life cycle in man is not known. Adults have, however, been reported in the intestine and ova passed in human faeces.

Epidemiology

Gnathostoma infection in human beings is not uncommon in Thailand and a substantial animal reservoir of *G. spinigerum* has been reported. The parasite has been isolated from cats, dogs, domestic pigs, freshwater fish, eels, snakes, frogs, leopards, chickens and fish-eating birds. Human infection usually results from eating fermented fish, which is a Thai delicacy much liked by women. The dish known as *Somfak* is made up of raw freshwater fish, cooked rice, curry, salt and pepper and then wrapped in banana leaves. Recently it has been shown experimentally that penetration of the skin by the 3rd stage infective larva can occur. There is a possibility therefore that in addition to *ingestion*, human infection is possible during the preparation of raw fish dishes or raw chicken dishes by the 3rd stage larva penetrating the bare skin of the hands of individuals preparing these meals. Other ways for man to acquire the infection is by eating other forms of raw fish, frogs, and possibly snakes infected with encysted larvae.

Human infection has occasionally been attributed to *G. hispidum*, the definitive host in this instance is the pig.

Laboratory diagnosis

Diagnosis in human infections depends on finding the immature worms and identifying them. Cutaneous tests with antigens from larval or adult worms as well as the precipitin test have been used for diagnosis. Eosinophilia is present.

Control

The infection is prevented by not eating uncooked fish and meats of other animals infected with encysted larvae. Ancylol (disophenol) kills both the larval and adult forms of *Gnathostoma* in dogs and cats. Unfortunately the compound is too toxic for man.

Taeniasis

Taeniasis occurs in all countries where beef or pork are eaten. The larval stage of *T. solium* produces cysticercosis.

Medical geography
The beef tapeworm *Taenia saginata* has a cosmopolitan distribution and is particularly common in the Middle East, Kenya and Ethiopia. The pork tapeworm *T. solium* is also widely distributed and its larval stage, *Cysticercus cellulosae*, produces cysticercosis in man.

Applied biology
The life cycle and pathogenesis of *T. saginata* and *T. solium* are similar, with the exception of the classical intermediate hosts which are cattle and pigs respectively.

The adult worms live in the small intestine of man only. The respective intermediate hosts become infected by swallowing eggs or mature segments passed in the faeces. The embryos hatch, penetrate the intestinal wall and are carried by the bloodstream to the skeletal muscles, as well as to the tongue, diaphragm and liver. The sites of predilection appear to vary in different areas, and in these sites the larvae invaginate, grow and encyst to become the infective *C. bovis* and *C. cellulosae* in about 10 weeks.

The encysted bladder-like larval forms are pearly-white in colour and contain the invaginated heads of the future adult worms. The cysts of *C. bovis* live for about 9 months, while those of *C. cellulosae* remain viable for 3-6 years.

When infected beef or pork is ingested by man, the cysts are dissolved by the gastric juices; the worms pass to the small intestine, and the heads evaginate and attach themselves to the intestinal wall, where they develop into adult worms and within 2-3 months gravid segments are discharged.

The adult *T. saginata* is from 4 to 10 m long, the head contains four suckers but no hooks, and the uterus has 20 to 25 compound lateral branches on each side; while *T. solium* is only 2-8 m long, the head contains four suckers as well as a double crown of large and small hooks, and the uterus has only 7 to 12 lateral branches on each side. Each mature segment of either worm contains a set of male and female reproductive organs. The ova of *T. saginata* and *T. solium* are indistinguishable from each other morphologically.

Epidemiology
Man is the only reservoir of infection.

The world incidence of *T. saginata* is much higher than that of *T. solium* and it is estimated that in some parts of Kenya infection rates of taeniasis in man may approach 100 per cent and that 30 per cent of cattle may harbour cysticerci.

T. saginata is uncommon in young children and the incidence increases with age. The sexes are equally susceptible—man acquires infection by eating raw or partially cooked beef, while cattle are infected while grazing on pastures, fertilised by human faeces, which are flooded with sewage-laden water. The role of birds in the transmission of the disease is not clear.

T. solium is spread by the insanitary disposal of faeces, thus providing the pigs with a ready opportunity for infection when they ingest human excreta. Man is infected when eating uncooked or insufficiently cooked pork.

Laboratory diagnosis

'Direct smear' examination of the faeces occasionally reveals the typical *Taenia* ova. The intact segments which usually are passed can be compressed between two glass slides and the branches of the uterus at their origin from the main uterine stem can be counted and a differentiation easily made between *T. saginata* (20 to 35) and *T. solium* (7 to 12). The haemagglutination test is positive in about 50 per cent of patients.

Cysticercosis

The adult *T. solium* is a parasite of man alone and the worm lives in the small intestine while the larval worm encysts in pork flesh as *Cysticercus cellulosae*. The pig acts as the classical intermediate host. Man can, however, become infected with the larval worm, and this condition is known as cysticercosis.

Epidemiology

Direct infection of man by larval worms of *T. solium* can occur by ingestion of water and food contaminated by faeces or flies or by unclean hands transferring eggs from the adult worm carrier. Moreover, auto-infection can occur by a person carrying eggs from the anus to the mouth on the fingers, or by massive regurgitation of ova from the small intestine into the stomach.

The liberated larvae penetrate the intestinal mucosa and are then carried by the bloodstream to various parts of the body where they encyst, the commonest sites being the subcutaneous tissues, skeletal muscles and the brain. The cysticercus takes about 4 months to develop and becomes enveloped in a fibrous capsule, which eventually calcifies and may be seen radiologically. *C. cellulosae* are small, oval or spherical, whitish bodies with an opalescent transparency and denser spot on one side where the scolex (tapeworm head) is invaginated. The life span of the cysticercus varies from a few months to 35 years. The geographical distribution of cysticercosis is necessary similar to that of *T. solium*.

Control

Transmission of taeniasis and cysticercosis can be controlled by the sanitary disposal of human faeces, the thorough cooking of meat and raising the standards of personal hygiene.

(a) *The individual*
All persons suffering from taeniasis should be dewormed with niclosamide given in a single dose of 2 g or dichlorophen (6 g) on each of two successive days. The thorough cooking of all beef and pork meat affords personal protection and health education should be carried on to raise the standards of personal hygiene, especially among persons harbouring *T. solium*.

(b) *The community*
Sanitary disposal of human excreta is essential. Untreated human faeces should not be used as fertilisers and if possible human faeces should be avoided altogether as a means of manuring crops.

Strict abattoir supervision resulting in adequate inspection of carcasses and condemnation of infected meat should be carried out. If meat containing cysticerci has to be consumed it should be thoroughly cooked under the close supervision of a health officer.

Taeniasis—Summary
(1) *Occurrence*—World-wide
(2) *Organisms*—Taenia solium, T. saginata, Cysticercus bovis
(3) *Reservoir of infection*—Man
(4) *Modes of transmission*—Uncooked meat, auto-human infection
(5) *Control*— (i) Sanitary disposal of faeces
           (ii) Thorough cooking of meat
           (iii) Personal hygiene
           (iv) Individual specific treatment

Diphyllobothriasis
Infection by the fish tapeworm *Diphyllobothrium latum* is characterised by a megaloblastic anaemia due to vitamin B_{12} deficiency.

Medical geography
Diphyllobothriasis is more common in the temperate zones than in the tropics, where it has only been reported from the Philippines, Madagascar, Botswana, Uganda and southern Chile.

Applied biology
The adult, which may be 10 m long, lives in the ileum of man or of other mammals, and may have as many as 4000 segments. The gravid segments disintegrate and the ova are passed in the faeces. On reaching water the ciliated embryo escapes and is swallowed by the first intermediate host—a freshwater crustacean (*Cyclops* or *Diaptomus* species)—in which it develops as a *procercoid*. When the infected

crustaceans are swallowed by various freshwater fishes (salmon, pike, etc.) further development takes place in the musculature of these second intermediate hosts to form *plerocercoids*. When man and other animals eat raw fish the plerocercoid is liberated and attaches itself to the small intestine, where it grows into an adult in about 6 weeks.

Epidemiology

Man and a number of fish-eating mammals, e.g. dog, cat, fox, pig, bear, seal, etc., are the reservoir of infection. Man is infected by eating raw or insufficiently cooked fish; the latter having acquired their infections in waters contaminated by faeces containing ova of *D. latum*. As with the other tapeworms, the adult fish tapeworm is long lived. The export of raw fish may cause infection outside the endemic areas.

Laboratory diagnosis

If segments are passed in the faeces or vomitus, diagnosis can be made by seeing the typical rosette-shaped uterus when the segment is crushed between two glass slides. More commonly, however, 'direct smear' examination of the faeces will reveal the characteristic operculate ova.

Control

Thorough cooking of fish affords personal protection and all infected persons should be treated with niclosamide (Yomesan) or dichlorophen (Antiphen) in the same dosage as for taeniasis. Control of export of smoked fish should be exercised. Sanitary disposal of the human faeces will reduce infection of fish, and fishing should be forbidden in infected waters.

Hymenolepiasis

Three dwarf tapeworm infections can occur in man due to *Hymenolepis nana*, *H. diminuta* and *Drepanidotaemia lanceolata* respectively. They all occur in the tropics and subtropics.

Applied biology

The adult *H. nana* measures about 20 mm in length and contains 100-200 segments; it lives in the upper ileum attached to the intestinal mucosa by its globular head. The gravid segments rupture in the intestine and the eggs containing an infective embryo are passed in the faeces. When ingested by man, the embryo penetrates a villus and develops into a cysticercoid larva. On maturity it ruptures the villus, returns to the intestine and attaches itself to the mucosa, giving rise to segments. About a month is required from the time of infection to the first appearance of ova in the faeces.

The adult of *H. diminuta* also inhabits the small intestine and is larger than *H. nana*. The ova containing the embryo are passed in the faeces and it undergoes a cycle of development in rat fleas and other insects. When man ingests food contaminated with these insects, the liberated larva attaches itself to the intestine.

D. lanceolata is an infection of birds and man has only very rarely been accidentally infected.

Epidemiology
H. nana is a common tapeworm of man in the south-eastern United States, parts of South America, and India. Man becomes infected by ingesting the ova in food or water that has been contaminated by human or rat faeces. The infection can also be transmitted directly from hand to mouth. Owing to the unhygienic habits of children, *H. nana* is more prevalent in them, with the highest incidence occurring between 4 and 9 years. Although rats and mice are commonly infected, man is the chief source of human infections, infection being spread directly from patient to patient without utilising an intermediate host.

H. diminuta is an infection of rats and mice, man being an incidental host. The principal source of infection is food contaminated by rat and mice droppings on which the intermediate insect hosts also thrive. When man eats food containing these insect vectors he gets accidentally infected. Human infection is chiefly in children who ingest rat fleas.

Laboratory diagnosis
A moderate eosinophilia (4-16 per cent) occurs in both *H. nana* and *H. diminuta* infections. Diagnosis is made by finding the characteristic ova in the faeces.

Control
Personal hygiene, sanitary disposal of faeces and food hygiene will control these infections with dwarf tapeworms. The treatment of the individual is as for taeniasis, but it is advisable to repeat the dose after an interval of 3 weeks to kill any further tapeworms which may have emerged from their larval state in the intestinal villi.

Hydatid Disease
This disease can be caused by any one of three species of the genus *Echinococcus*—*Echinococcus granulosus*, *E. multilocularis* and *E. oligaettas*. Since the epidemiological and pathological features of these three tapeworms are very similar, a detailed description of only *E. granulosus* is given here.

Medical geography
Hydatid disease—caused by the larval form of *E. granulosus*—has a

cosmopolitan distribution, being particulary prevalent in the sheep- and cattle-raising areas of the world.

Applied biology

The adult *Echinococcus* is a small tapeworm about 5 mm in length which inhabits chiefly the upper part of the small intestine of canines, especially dogs and wolves.

When the ova, which are passed in the faeces, are swallowed by man or other intermediate hosts (e.g. sheep, cattle, horses, etc.) the enclosed embryo is liberated in the duodenum. It penetrates the intestinal mucosa, reaches the portal circulation, and is usually held up in the liver within 12 hours to develop into a hydatid cyst. If the embryo passes the liver filter, it enters the general circulation, and thus reaches the lungs and other parts of the body. It then develops into a hydatid cyst wherever it eventually comes to rest. Two main varieties of cysts occur—the unilocular and the multilocular. The unilocular hydatid cyst develops a wall with two layers, the outer layer is thick, laminated and elastic, while the inner layer is made up of a protoplasmic matrix containing many nuclei. Around the cyst there is a connective-tissue capsule formed by the tissues of the host. From the inner or germinal layer bulb-like processes arise which are termed brood capsules. By a process of localised proliferation and invagination of the wall of the brood capsules numerous scolices (tapeworm heads) are produced. Each scolex is borne on a pedicle and has suckers and two rows of hooklets. Some of the brood capsules separate from the walls and settle to the bottom of the cyst as a fine granular sediment, 'hydatid sand'. As the hydatid cyst enlarges invaginations of the wall may give rise to daughter cysts and from them granddaughter cysts may arise in a similar manner.

In some cases in which no effective encapsulation occurs the daughter cysts develop as a result of evagination of the cyst wall producing the *multilocular* or *alveolar* hydatid cyst. This variety of hydatid cyst is due to *E. multilocularis.* When the hydatid is eaten by definitive hosts—dogs, foxes, wolves and certain other carniverous animals— the numerous larvae develop into sexually mature worms in a few weeks. Dogs are usually infected when they eat the infected viscera of sheep or cattle.

Epidemiology

Dogs are the main reservoir of human infection. Infected ova may live for weeks in shady environments but they are quickly destroyed by sunlight and high temperatures. Man acquires hydatid disease when he swallows infected ova as a result of his close association with dogs, and the insanitary habit of not washing his hands before ingesting food. Although infection is usually acquired in childhood, clinical symptoms do not appear until adult life. The dog faeces contaminating fleeces of sheep can also be an indirect source of human infection. It has been shown that in Kenya hydatid cysts are present in more than 30 per cent of cattle, sheep and goats, though the disease in man occurs infrequently, except in the areas of Turkana. Canines are heavily infected while light infections have been recorded in wild carnivores, e.g. jackals and hyenas. The main cycle of transmission in Kenya is between dogs and domestic livestock. Turkana tribesmen are the most heavily infected people in Kenya because of the intimate contact between children and the large number of infected canines in the area—here dogs are used to clean the face and anal regions of babies.

Laboratory diagnosis

If the hydatid cysts rupture, its contents—hooklets, scolices, etc.—may be found in the faeces, sputum or urine. Eosinophilia is present but is usually moderate in degree (300-2000 per mm^3) and there may be hypergammaglobulinaemia.

Intradermal and serological tests have greatly increased the chances of diagnosis. In patients known to have hydatid disease the sensitivity of the *intradermal Casoni* test has varied from 57 to 100 per cent. A positive test may persist for 5 years or more after excision of a cyst. It has recently been suggested that the crude sterile hydatid fluid used in Casoni antigen may contain too much nitrogen to give specific results. An intradermal test antigen made up from an extract of lyophilised cyst material of *E. multilocularis* from experimental secondary infections in gerbils seems preferable.

The *complement-fixation test* is positive in 70 per cent of patients and may persist for 2 years after elimination of the infection. The *indirect haemagglutination test* is positive in 90 per cent of cases and only 2 per cent of control sera give measurable titres. Other serological tests used are the bentonite flocculation test, 71 per cent sensitive; the latex flocculation test; precipitin tests; and conglutination tests. In general, serological diagnosis of hydatid lung cysts is not very satisfactory and only 33-50 per cent of those infected give positive tests. It has been suggested that separation of the hydatid cyst from host tissue in the lung is so complete that little to no antigen escapes from the cyst to stimulate antibody production in the host. Moreover, cysts in the lungs are frequently found to be infertile, which may be a contributory factor to the lack of antigenicity. The indirect immunofluorescent reaction has also been successfully used in the diagnosis of hydatid disease.

Control

This depends on raising the standards of personal hygiene, deworming of infected dogs (with arecoline hydrobromide) and adequate supervision of abattoirs. Infected offal and meat should be destroyed, dogs excluded from slaughterhouses, and infected carcasses deeply buried or incinerated.

(a) *The individual*
Persons must be warned of the danger of handling dogs or sheep and the importance of washing their hands immediately afterwards.

(b) *The community*
Deworming of all infected dogs, if possible, is the best means of getting rid of the main reservoir of infection. The most suitable drugs for this purpose are the arecoline compounds or niclosamide. All meat or offal containing hydatid cysts should be disposed of and thus be made inaccessible to dogs. Abattoir supervision and hygiene will exclude dogs from the premises and infected carcasses should be incinerated. In sheep-rearing areas burial or incineration of dead sheep should be carried out.

Hydatid Disease—Summary

(1) *Occurrence*—World-wide
(2) *Organism*—Genus *Echinococcus*
(3) *Reservoir of infection*—Dogs
(4) *Mode of transmission*—Ingestion of infected ova
(5) *Control*— (i) Personal hygiene
           (ii) Deworming of dogs
           (iii) Abattoir hygiene

Paragonimiasis
This infection is characterised by cough, expectoration of bloody sputum and, later, signs of bronchiectasis or lung abscess.

Medical geography
Paragonimiasis is due to the lung fluke *Paragonimus westermani*, which has a wide geographical distribution. It occurs focally throughout the Far East, South-East Asia, the Pacific Islands, West Africa and parts of South America. A new species, *P. africanus*, which is considered to be the local causative agent of paragonimiasis, has been described from the Cameroons. Other species responsible for human infections are *P. siamensis* and *P. heterotremus*.

Applied biology
The adult worm is a reddish-brown, oval fluke (about 10 mm long and 5 mm wide) which lives mainly in cavities in the lungs. From these pulmonary pockets the ova escape through the bronchioles and are discharged in the sputum or in the faeces if the sputum is

swallowed. In other anatomical sites the ova reach the outside world only when abscesses are formed and rupture.

The contained miracidia hatch in water and enter a suitable species of snail (e.g. *Melania* spp.) in which they develop into cercariae. The cercariae emerge from the snail and penetrate the flesh of certain freshwater crabs and crayfish, where they encyst. Man and susceptible animals are infected by eating these raw or partially cooked crustaceans.

After ingestion, the larvae encyst and penetrate the wall of the jejunum into the peritoneal cavity. They can pass through the diaphragm into the pleural cavity and finally burrow into the lungs where, enclosed in a cystic cavity, they grow to adult worms 5-6 weeks after ingestion.

Epidemiology

Man is the reservoir of infection. Although a considerable domestic and wild animal reservoir of *Paragonimus* infection exists, the part it plays in the epidemiology of human disease has yet to be fully determined.

Transmission is maintained by faecal and sputum pollution of water in which the appropriate snails and vector crustaceans live, and by the custom of eating uncooked crabs and crayfish soaked in alcohol, vinegar, brine or wine. Infection can also occur during the preparation of such food, when encysted cercariae can be left on the knife or other utensils.

Although in most areas infection is higher in males than in females, in the Cameroons women are infected three times as often as men. The peak age of incidence is between 11 and 35 years of age. It has been reported that during a measles epidemic in Korea 80 per cent of *Paragonimus* infections were produced by the administration of the fluid extract of crushed crabs given medicinally to the patients. The infection may persist for many years after leaving endemic areas.

Laboratory diagnosis

The infected sputum is characteristically sticky and bloody, usually of a dark, brownish-red colour. The characteristically shaped eggs are usually found in the sputum or in the faeces on 'direct smear' examination or by concentration techniques. In the first year of infection eggs are seldom found but there is usually an eosinophilia of about 20-30 per cent.

Precipitin reactions with crude and fractionated antigens, intra-dermal tests and complement-fixation tests have all been used for diagnostic and epidemiological purposes. Cross reactions with other trematodes limit the usefulness of these tests, although the weal is larger and more closely defined with the homologous antigen.

D

Control

Crabs and crayfish should be cooked before eating. Faecal pollution of water should be prevented. Elevation of standard of personal and public hygiene and the provision of latrines will reduce transmission.

Clonorchiasis

This infection is caused by the oriental liver fluke *Clonorchis sinensis* and may be symptomless or result in severe liver damage with the possibility of malignant change.

Medical geography

Clonorchiasis is mainly found in the Far East. Endemic foci occur in Japan, South Korea, South Eastern China, Taiwan and Vietnam.

Applied biology

The adult *C. sinensis* is a flat, transparent fluke which inhabits the bile ducts and sometimes the pancreatic ducts of man and other fish-eating mammals. It is from 10 to 25 mm long and 3 to 5 mm in breadth.

Self-fertilisation is the common means of fecundation and the ova are carried down the common bile duct to the duodenum and are passed in the faeces. On reaching water the ova are ingested by a suitable snail (e.g. genus *Bithynia*) and hatch in the snail's digestive tract. The enclosed miracidia develop in the snail host into sporocysts and rediae within which cercariae develop. These eventually break out of the mother redia and escape into the water.

The cercariae with unforked tails penetrate the scales of one of several freshwater fishes (e.g. Cyprinoid) and encyst in their flesh, skin, and gills. Here they develop into numerous encysted metacercariae which are the infective forms, and which remain viable for 2 months after the death of the fish.

When ingested by man the metacercariae are freed by the action of the gastric and duodenal juices, and the larvae migrate to the common bile duct and then into the smaller biliary radicles where they mature into adults.

Epidemiology

Man is the reservoir of infection. As with paragonimiasis many animals harbour *C. sinensis*, but their importance in the epidemiology of the human disease has yet to be fully assessed.

Man and other mammals are infected by eating raw or undercooked fish containing metacercariae. Fish ponds fertilised with fresh human faeces are a common source of infection. Infected fish exported to other countries can result in the spread of the disease to areas where the parasite is not normally found.

Clonorchiasis is rare in infants under 1 year of age, it begins, however, at about 2 years, rising to 65 per cent in those aged 21-30 years and to a peak of 80 per cent in those dying between the ages 51 and 60 years. Males are more frequently infected than females, but there are no social differences in the prevalence of the disease because of the universal custom of eating raw fish. The life span of the worm is 25-30 years.

Laboratory diagnosis
A definitive diagnosis is made by finding the typical operculated ova by 'direct smear' examination of the faeces or duodenal aspirate.
There is usually a leucocytosis (23 000-48 200) with eosinophilia. In severe cases with secondary infection of the bile ducts there may be severe hypoglycaemia with blood sugars of 22-45 mg per cent; bilirubin levels of 3-10 mg per cent and a raised alkaline phosphatase.

Control
Fish should not be eaten raw and the use of human faeces in fish ponds should be avoided. Sanitary disposal of faeces and raising the standards of personal and community hygiene will reduce transmission.

Opisthorchiasis
This infection is very similar to clonorchiasis, resulting in enlargement of the liver and eventually malignant change.

Medical geography
This disease is due to two parasitic trematodes—*Opisthorchis felineus* and *O. viverrini*. In the tropics the former is prevalent in the Philippines, India, Japan and Vietnam, while the latter has been reported from north and north-east Thailand and Laos.

Applied biology
The life cycle and pathogenesis of these two human hepatic trematodes are similar to that of *C. sinensis*. The adults inhabit the distal bile ducts and the ova are passed out in the faeces. After ingestion by the appropriate snails (e.g. *Bithynia*) the miracidia develop into cercariae, which in turn penetrate the flesh of suitable species of freshwater fishes (e.g. Cyprinoid family) in which they encyst and develop into metacercariae. When the metacercariae are ingested by a suitable host—man, domestic, wild and fur-bearing animals—they encyst in the duodenum and migrate to the distal bile ducts particularly those of the left lobe of the liver. The entire life cycle takes about 4 months.

Epidemiology
Man, domestic, wild and fur-bearing animals are the reservoir of infection. The chief reservoir of *O. felineus* is the cat. Man and the reservoir hosts are infected by the consumption of raw or insufficiently

cooked fish. Snails and fish are infected by faeces deposited on the sandy shores and washed into the streams.

In north-east Thailand 90 per cent of people over the age of 10 are infected with *O. viverrini* and it is estimated that over 3·5 million persons in Thailand harbour the parasite. The source of infection is a popular dish called 'Keompla', consisting of raw fish, roasted rice, and vegetables seasoned with garlic, lemon juice, fish sauce and pepper. Chinese residents of Thailand who do not eat raw fish are free from infection. The largest number of human infections occur during the latter portion of the rainy season and the first part of the dry season, i.e. from September to February.

Laboratory diagnosis
This is made by finding the ova on 'direct smear' examination of faeces or duodenal aspirate.

Control
(i) Raw fish should be avoided; fish should be eaten only if cooked.
(ii) Sanitary disposal of faeces and a raised standard of personal and public hygiene will reduce transmission.

Fascioliasis
This infection may be silent or may present with symptoms of chronic liver disease and portal hypertension.

Medical geography
Fascioliasis is caused by the trematode *Fasciola hepatica* (sheep-liver fluke), which has a world-wide distribution in ruminants, being especially prevalent in the sheep-rearing areas of the world. In some areas, e.g. Hawaii, the causative agent of fascioliasis is *F. gigantica*.

Applied biology
The adult worm, which is large (30 mm long and 13 mm broad), flat and leaf-shaped, lives in the bile ducts of liver parenchyma of sheep, cattle, goats and other animals, and man. The eggs are passed in the faeces and hatch in a moist environment. The released miracidia then enter the appropriate species of snails (*Limnaea*), and develop successively into sporocytes, rediae and cercariae. The cercariae then leave their snail host and encyst on various grasses and water plants. When this water vegetation is ingested by the appropriate hosts, the larvae excyst in the intestine, penetrate the mucosa, enter the liver through the portal circulation, and eventually reach the bile ducts, where they mature in about 3 months.

F. hepatica obtains its nourishment from the biliary secretions and can absorb simple carbohydrates.

Epidemiology
The reservoir of infection is ruminants especially sheep. Man usually contracts infection by eating lettuce or water cress contaminated by sheep or other animals' faeces. The highest incidence of infection occurs in low, damp pastures where the grasses and the water are infected with encysted cercariae.

Laboratory diagnosis
The finding of the typical operculated eggs in faeces (150×90 μm) is diagnostic, but unfortunately these do not appear till about 3 months after infection. Duodenal intubation may reveal the ova in biliary secretions at an earlier stage of the disease. There may be a leucocytosis (12 000-40 000 per mm^3) and an eosinophilia of 40-85%.

Intracutaneous and serological tests are useful but not specific or sensitive enough, the haemagglutination test is reputed to be the most sensitive.

Control
Lettuce or water cress should be sterilised by momentary immersion in boiling water, this will destroy the encysted cercariae.

Fasciolopsiasis
This infection is often symptomless, but with heavy infections abdominal pain with alternating diarrhoea and constipation may occur.

Medical geography
Fasciolopsiasis is caused by the large, fleshy fluke—*Fasciolopsis buski*—which is found mainly in China, but also in India, Indo-China, Thailand, Malaysia, Indonesia, Taiwan and Europe.

Parasitology
F. buski is normally an intestinal parasite of the pig and of man and inhabits the small intestine. The eggs are passed in the faeces and the miracidium is released and swims in water until it penetrates a suitable mollusc host of the genus *Segmentina*—where it develops into a sporocyst, redia and cercariae. When the cercariae leave the snail they encyst on aquatic plants. When the encysted cercariae are ingested by man, the cyst wall is dissolved in the duodenum and the liberated larvae attach themselves to the mucosa, where they develop into adult worms whose nourishment is derived from the duodenal secretions. The egg output per worm is very high, averaging 25 000 eggs per day.

Epidemiology
Man, who is a source of infection, is infected when he eats raw water-plants contaminated with encysted cercariae. Pigs are also an important animal reservoir, infecting the stagnant ponds in which edible water plants grow. The commonest source of infected edible water plants are

the water caltrops and water chestnuts which are often cultivated in ponds fertilised by human faeces. In China, these tubers are eaten raw and fresh from July to September and, as they are peeled with the teeth, an easy entry of the cercariae to the mouth is provided.

Laboratory diagnosis

The diagnosis can be made by finding the characteristic operculated ova in the faeces, there may be a leucocytosis and eosinophilia. Occasionally, adult flukes are vomited or found in the faeces.

Control

This consists in adequate cooking of the potentially infected foods and prevention of faecal pollution of the water in which they grow. Provision of latrines and the raising of standards of personal and public hygiene by health education helps to reduce transmission.

Heterophyiasis and Metagonimiasis

These conditions are due to infection by two very minute flukes— *Heterophyes heterophyes* and *Metagonimus yokogawai*. In the tropics the former is found in Egypt, Tunisia, South China, India and the Philippines, while the latter occurs in the Far East and Indonesia.

The **life cycle** and **epidemiology** of both flukes is similar. The adults live in the upper part of the small intestine embedded in mucus or in the mucosal folds. The eggs containing miracidia are passed in the faeces and, on ingestion by suitable snails, develop into sporocysts, rediae and cercariae. The cercariae then leave the snails and enter the appropriate fish, in which they encyst into infective metacercariae. When the fish are eaten raw or partially cooked the metacercariae are liberated and the larvae develop into adult worms in the small intestine.

The first snail intermediate hosts for *H. heterophyes* are brackish water snails (e.g. *Pirinella conica*), while the second intermediate hosts are mullets; for *M. yokogawai* the hosts are snails of the *Semisulcospira* species and salmonoid and cyprinoid fishes.

The pathogenicity of these parasitic infections is very low, unless aberrant ova enter the circulation when the spinal cord may be affected.

In addition to man, other mammals are also infected and, like clonorchis infection, heterophiasis is acquired by eating raw or partially cooked infected fish.

Diagnosis is made by finding the characteristic ova in the faeces. There may be eosinophilia.

Control

Control depends on avoiding eating raw and partially cooked infected fish and raising the standards of personal and community hygiene.

Food hygiene. See p. 282.   *Disinfection.* See p. 282.

Chapter Five

Infections through Skin and Mucous Membranes

In one group, transmission of infection occurs by contact with contaminated persons or objects. In the other groups, infection may be acquired by exposure to infected soil (hookworm), water (schistosomiasis, leptospirosis), by the bites of animals (rabies) or through wounds (tetanus).

Contact Infections

Table 5.1 gives examples of disease which are spread by contact.

TABLE 5.1
Examples of infections acquired through skin and mucous membranes

VIRUSES	BACTERIA	FUNGI	PROTOZOA	HELMINTHS	ARTHROPODS
Smallpox	Gonorrhoea*	Superficial fungal infection e.g. ringworm	Trichomonas vaginalis	Schistosomiasis	Scabies
				Hookworm	
Chicken-pox	Syphilis*				
Trachoma	Yaws				
Inclusion conjunctivitis	Endemic treponematoses				
Lymphogranuloma venereum*	Leprosy				
	Tetanus				

* Venereal diseases.

The Infective Agents

The infective agents include viruses, bacteria, fungi and arthropods.

Physical and biological characteristics
Some of the agents which are transmitted by direct person-to-person contact are notably delicate organisms which do not survive long outside the human host and cannot become established in any part of the environment, neither in an alternate host nor in an inanimate object such as soil or water. The venereally transmitted diseases such as gonorrhoea and syphilis are the best examples of this group; the usual mode of infection is therefore through intimate contact, mucous membrane to mucous membrane, or skin to skin. Some of the other infective agents which can survive in the environment for relatively longer periods, may be spread indirectly through the contamination of inanimate objects.

In most of these infections man is the sole reservoir of infection, although some of the superficial fungal infections may be acquired from lower animals.

Mode of transmission
This may be by *direct contact* from touching an infected person; also through kissing and sexual intercourse, especially in the case of venereally transmitted diseases.

It may be by *indirect contact* through the handling of contaminated objects such as toys, handkerchiefs, soiled clothing, bedding or dressings.

Environmental factors which aid the transmission of these infections include high population density as in urban areas, overcrowding and poor environmental and personal hygiene.

Epidemiological features of contact infections
A contact infection would tend to spread from an infected source to susceptible persons in the same household and to others who make contact with him at work and in other places. There is therefore a tendency for cases of contact infections to occur in clusters among household contacts, and within groups of persons who have close contacts, e.g. children's play groups, schools and factories.

In the case of venereal diseases, the clustering occurs in relation to those who are in sexual contact.

Host Factors

The behaviour of the human host is an important factor in the occurrence of certain contact infections. For example, a high level of personal cleanliness discourages the spread of some superficial infections. Age is another important factor, as for example in infections such as scabies and tinea capitis to which children are generally more susceptible than adults. The occurrence of venereal diseases is largely determined by the sexual behaviour of the host.

In some of the infections, e.g. smallpox, one attack confers lasting immunity but this is not a general rule for all the contact infections. Thus, repeated attacks of gonorrhoea may occur. The herd immunity that is derived from the high frequency of an endemic treponemal infection such as yaws may protect the community, though not the individual, from venereal syphilis.

Control of Contact Infections

1. *Infective agent*
   (*a*) Elimination of the reservoir by case finding, selective or mass treatment.

2. *The route of transmission*
   (*b*) Improvement of personal hygiene.
   (*c*) Elimination of overcrowding.
   (*d*) Avoidance of sexual promiscuity.

3. *The host*
   (*e*) Specific immunisation, e.g. smallpox.
   (*f*) Chemotherapy and chemoprophylaxis, e.g. yaws.

Variola (Smallpox)

This is an acute viral infection which typically presents with severe prodromal constitutional symptoms (fever, backache, headache, prostration), and a characteristic skin rash. It usually causes a severe illness with a high case fatality rate in non-immune subjects. In classical smallpox (variola major), the case fatality rate may be as high as 30 per cent, but in the milder form, Alastrim (variola minor) the case fatality rate is below 5 per cent. Since it is highly infectious, massive epidemics tend to occur in populations which have not been vaccinated. The *incubation period* is usually 10 to 12 days, but may be as short as 7 days or as long as 16 days.

Medical geography

The disease is still endemic in parts of Africa, Asia and South America but many parts of the world—North America, Western Europe—are free from infection except when it is introduced by infected travellers.

Virology

The infectious agents is the variola virus, a member of the pox group of viruses.

Laboratory diagnosis

The following methods are in use:

1. *Culture of the organism* on chick embryo chorio-allantoic membrane
   (*a*) From blood in the pre-eruptive phase.
   (*b*) From skin lesions at all stages from macule to scab.

2. *Microscopy of smears of skin lesions*
   This is a simple test which can provide a rapid diagnosis. Material from a papule or from the base of a vesicle is smeared to a clean dry slide and stained with 1 per cent gentian violet and 2 per cent sodium bicarbonate. The presence of large numbers of elementary bodies is presumptive evidence of smallpox infection.
3. *Demonstration of the antigen*
   The antigen may be demonstrated from skin lesions by using a complement fixation test or the fluorescent antibody test.
   Laboratory tests are most valuable in confirming the diagnosis in atypical cases.

Epidemiology
Man is the reservoir of infection. Transmission is by direct contact with infected persons, or indirect contact with soiled clothing or other contaminated objects. The organisms may survive in dried scabs for long periods—a few months to several years. The infection may also be by droplets or may be airborne over short distances in a confined space. The disease is highly infectious; transmission may occur after a very brief, slight exposure. Massive outbreaks with high attack rates tend to occur in non-immune populations. One attack of smallpox confers lifelong immunity. All age-groups are susceptible, but the illness tends to be very severe in pregnant women.

Control and Eradication
The control of smallpox involves the protection of susceptible persons in the endemic areas, and the prevention of the introduction of the disease into non-endemic areas. The control of this infection depends on active immunisation of the susceptible population with the live vaccine; it also depends on an efficient surveillance programme which is designed to detect any outbreak as early as possible, confining it to the smallest possible area and clearing the focus in the shortest possible time.

Control measures in dealing with an outbreak:
1. Isolate the sick patients until the lesions are healed.
2. Trace and vaccinate all contacts and keep them under surveillance for three weeks.
3. Identify the source of infection
4. Notify the appropriate health authority

Vaccination against Smallpox
The vaccine contains live vaccinia virus; it is usually manufactured by infecting healthy calves with cowpox, and the skin lesions are harvested and purified. Alternatively, the vaccinia virus may be cultured in the

chick embryo. The latter procedure has overcome the objections of those who, on religious grounds, cannot accept the vaccine that is manufactured from lesions on the cow. The glycerinated fluid vaccine must be stored at low temperatures if it is to retain its potency; this has usually proved very difficult under field conditions in the tropics. The fluid vaccine has been largely replaced by the freeze-dried vaccine, which retains its potency very well without refrigeration.

Effective smallpox vaccination consists of the introduction of the vaccine into the superficial layers of the skin. This can be achieved by the scratch method, multiple-pressure method or by using the jet injector gun. The first method consists of making a superficial scratch in the deltoid region after cleaning and drying the skin. The scratch should not be deep enough to draw blood. The vaccine is then rubbed into the scratch mark. The multiple pressure technique is now preferred; it consists of making multiple rapid pressures (20 to 30 times) with the side of a needle through a drop of vaccine which is placed on clean, dry skin. For mass immunisation, the multiple-jet injector gun with the special intradermal nozzle is very useful. Provided that there is good crowd control, one team with a foot-operated jet injector gun can vaccinate 500 persons an hour. Moreover, compared with other methods, the jet injector gun gives a consistently high (99 per cent) success rate.

Vaccination Reactions

(a) In a successful primary vaccination, the local skin lesion evolves from a macule, to papule, vesicle, and a pustule. It dries and the scab comes off leaving a scar. In this *vaccinia reaction*, the maximum area of redness occurs on the 7th day. Two other types of lesions have been described:

(b) *The accelerated or vaccinoid reaction*—the area of maximum redness occurs between the 3rd and the 7th day. This type of reaction with vesicle formation indicates some degree of host immunity.

(c) *The early (immediate or vaccinoid) reaction*—consists of the development of a lesion with the maximum areas of redness by the 3rd day. This type of reaction may indicate a high level of host immunity if one is satisfied that the vaccine is potent and that the vaccination technique was correct. This type of reaction also occurs when the vaccine has lost its potency. If in doubt, one should re-vaccinate using a vaccine of known potency.

Complications of Smallpox Vaccination

(a) *Local*
(i) Secondary infection including tetanus or staphylococcal infection.
(ii) Vaccinia gangrenosum (or necrosum)—a progressive necrotic lesion at vaccination site.

(b) *Distant and general*
(i) *Disseminated vaccinia* may result from mechanical accidental transfer of the infection from the vaccination site to other parts of the body. Accidental vaccination of the eye may be dangerous.
(ii) *Eczema vaccinatum* (Kaposi's varicelliform eruption) may occur in persons suffering from allergic eczema, if they are vaccinated or if they come into contact with someone who was recently vaccinated.
(iii) *Encephalitis*. This is a serious complication which is fortunately rare. The risk is highest in adults receiving primary vaccination.

Contra-indications to Smallpox Vaccination
The following persons should not be routinely vaccinated against smallpox:
(*a*) Pregnant women, but vaccination is strongly indicated if a pregnant woman is exposed to infection.
(*b*) Persons suffering from leukaemia, hypogammaglobulinaemia and those receiving treatment with corticosteroids and other immuno-suppressive drugs.
(*c*) Persons suffering from allergic eczema; they should also avoid close contact with anyone who has been recently vaccinated.
(*d*) Sick, febrile persons; postpone vaccination until after recovery from acute illness.

If any of these persons has been exposed to infection, or if for any other reason, vaccination is necessary it may be carried out whilst protecting them from the risk of disseminated lesions with immune anti-vaccinial globulin.

Vaccination Programme
In endemic areas, routine smallpox vaccination should be commenced in early infancy preferably before the 3rd month. Vaccination should be repeated periodically, at least every 3 years.

Surveillance of Smallpox
Until global eradication of smallpox, all communities have to maintain a state of watchfulness to prevent the introduction of the disease into non-endemic areas and also to detect and deal with any outbreak promptly. In the endemic areas, all health personnel should be taught how to recognise or suspect cases of smallpox; they must also know the various measures which must be taken urgently including notification to the appropriate authority, in order to combat the outbreak. Non-endemic areas can be safeguarded against the introduction of the infection by strict adherence to the international regulations and by maintaining vigilance at points, such as airports or seaports, through which the infection is likely to be introduced. Any traveller coming from, passing through or going into an endemic country, must have

a valid certificate indicating that he has been vaccinated or re-vaccinated within the 3 years.

The World Health Organisation co-ordinates the global surveillance of smallpox. All member nations are required to report cases regularly by cablegram to WHO headquarters in Geneva; the information is analysed and disseminated to member nations.

Smallpox—Summary

(1) *Occurrence*—Mainly Asia, Africa and South America
(2) *Organism*—Smallpox virus
(3) *Reservoir of infection*—Man
(4) *Mode of transmission*—Contact, droplets
(5) *Control*— (i) Routine vaccination with live vaccinia virus
       (ii) Isolation of patients
       (iii) Vaccination and surveillance or quarantine of contacts
       (iv) Epidemiological control—notification of cases—identification of the source of infection—mass immunisation of the public

Chickenpox

Chickenpox is an acute febrile illness with a characteristic skin rash. The *incubation period* is usually from 2 to 3 weeks.

The main importance of chickenpox lies in its differentiation from smallpox. The typical clinical features of chickenpox and smallpox are compared in Table 5.2. The clinical diagnosis should be confirmed by laboratory tests if these are available. In any case, public health measures should be carried out and precautions maintained until the diagnosis of smallpox can be firmly excluded.

Medical geography
Chickenpox is a common infection all over the world.

Virology
The aetiological agent is the varicella-zoster virus.

Epidemiology
Man is the reservoir of infection. Transmission is from person to person, either directly through contact with infectious secretions from the upper respiratory tract and through droplet infection or indirectly through contact with freshly soiled articles. The patient remains infectious for about 1 week from the onset of the illness.

Host factors play an important part in determining the clinical manifestations of this infection. In most cases, it is a mild, self-limiting disease. It tends to be more severe in adults than in children. The overall case fatailty rate is low, but it is high in cases complicated with

TABLE 5.2

Clinical features of smallpox and chickenpox compared

	SMALLPOX	CHICKENPOX
PRODROMAL SYMPTOMS	Fever, headache, severe prostration for 2 to 4 days before rash appears	Mild or no marked constitutional signs until just before rash appears
SKIN RASH Pattern of appearance	Only one crop, all lesions appearing within 1 to 2 days	Lesions appear in crops over several days to one week
	Lesions are at the same stage of development	Many stages of the lesions from vesicles to scabs are seen together on same part of the body
Distribution	*Centrifugal*—most numerous on the face and the distal parts of arms and legs	*Centripetal*—more numerous on the body than on the limbs
	Involves the palms and soles	Palms and soles not often involved
Individual lesions	Axilla usually spared	Axilla usually involved
	Evolution from macule to scab takes at least one week	Lesions evolve more rapidly—scabs appear within 3 to 4 days
	Circular	Oval
	Deep set	Superficial
	Vesicles are multilocular	Vesicles are unilocular
	Become umbilicated with rupture of central lobes	Vesicles collapse and become flat with rupture of vesicle
SCAR	Depressed	Superficial

primary viral pneumonia. Fulminating infection with haemorrhagic bullae may occur in patients on corticosteroid therapy.

One attack of chickenpox usually confer lifelong immunity; the patient may subsequently exhibit a recrudescence of infection in the form of herpes zoster from latent infection.

Laboratory diagnosis

The organism may be isolated from the early skin lesions or from throat washings. A rising titre of complement-fixing antibodies in acute and convalescent sera is also diagnostic.

Control

The disease is usually notifiable, the main interest being in investigating cases and outbreaks to exclude smallpox. No specific immunisation against chickenpox is available. Infected persons may be isolated from other susceptibles, rigid isolation being enforced until the differentiation from smallpox is established.

Chickenpox—Summary

(1) *Occurrence*—World-wide
(2) *Organism*—Varicella-zoster virus
(3) *Reservoir of infection*—Man
(4) *Modes of transmission*—Contact, droplets, fomites
(5) *Control*—Exclude smallpox

Trachoma

Trachoma is a major cause of blindness in the tropics and is characterised by a mucopurulent discharge initially progressing to a chronic kerato-conjunctivitis, with the formation of follicles, with hyperplasia, vascular invasion of the cornea and, in the late stage, gross scarring with deformity of the eyelids. Vision may be impaired, and in severe cases it may lead to blindness. The *incubation period* is from 4 to 12 days.

Medical geography

The occurrence of the infection is world-wide, including tropical, subtropical, temperate and cold climates, but the distribution of disease is uneven, being mostly in the Middle East, Mediterranean coast, parts of tropical Africa, Asia and South America. In the United States of America, it selectively affects certain groups such as American Indians and Mexican immigrants. It is estimated that throughout the world, 400 million persons are infected with trachoma and 20 million are blind.

Virology

The organism responsible for trachoma is termed TRIC agent (trachoma inclusion conjunctivitis agent). It belongs to the PLT (psittacosis, lymphogranuloma venereum, trachoma) group of atypical viruses which are midway between true viruses and bacteria. The causal agent was first isolated with certainty in Peking and confirmed in the Gambia.

Epidemiology

Man is the reservoir of infection. The infective agent is present in the purulent and mucoid discharges of the infected eyes, nasal discharges and tears. Transmission is by mechanical transfer or from the infective discharges either by direct contact or through contaminated clothing or cosmetics. Flies, particularly the Musca species (e.g. *Musca sorbers*), may also transmit the infection.

Children are more susceptible than adults. Infection is particularly common where there is poor personal hygiene; exposure to sun, wind and sand may aggravate the clinical manifestations.

Infection does not confer effective immunity. The disease traces a variable course with spontaneous healing in some cases or progressive damage in others. In countries with a high incidence of bacterial conjunctivitis, particularly of the seasonal epidemic variety, the severity of the trachoma is enhanced and disabling complications are more frequent. In other areas, e.g. the Gambia, the disease is mild, and serious sequelae uncommon.

Laboratory diagnosis

Intracytoplasmic inclusion bodies 0·25-0·4 μm in diameter, staining purple with Giemsa or reddish-brown by iodine, may be seen in conjunctival scrapings. These elementary particles have been termed Halberstaedter-Prowazek bodies and are the principal microscopic diagnostic feature in trachoma but are also seen in inclusion conjunctivitis of the newborn. The number of inclusions tends to be proportional to the intensity of the infection and are most numerous in scrapings from the upper lid.

In early lesions neutrophils may be abundant. In later lesions plasma cells, lymphoblasts and macrophages containing necrotic debris (Leber cells) may be seen.

The agent may be cultured in the yolk of the sac of the embryonated egg.

Control

Improvement of living standards and mass treatment campaigns are the most effective methods for the prevention of trachoma.

(a) The individual

Active disease in individuals is treated with sulphonamides or tetracyclines. Treatment can be given systematically, locally or preferably by both methods. Soluble or long-acting sulphonamides can be used for systemic treatment while 1 per cent tetracycline ointment is an effective ophthalmic preparation. Hygienic measures include improvement in personal cleanliness, and the avoiding of the sharing of handkerchiefs, towels and eye cosmetics. It involves health education and the provision of adequate water supply.

(b) The community

The prevalence of trachoma has been reduced in some areas by 'intermittent' mass treatment with 1 per cent tetracycline ointment. The ointment is applied twice daily for 3-6 consecutive days each month for 6 months. This regime is most effective in schools 'a captive population' where it has been successfully used both curatively and prophylactically. It is important to bear in mind, however, that in areas of high endemicity the main reservoir of infection is the pre-school child and suitable mass campaigns against this particular age-group are also vitally important. Active research on vaccination is making slow progress.

Trachoma—Summary

(1) *Occurrence*—World-wide, uneven distribution, mainly tropical and sub-tropical
(2) *Organism*—Trachoma virus
(3) *Reservoir of infection*—Man
(4) *Modes of transmission*—Contact, fomites, mechanically by flies
(5) *Control*— (i) Improvement in personal hygiene
            (ii) Mass treatment with antibiotic eye ointment

Inclusion Conjunctivitis

This infection manifests itself as an acute purulent conjunctivitis of neonates or as follicular conjunctivitis of adults. The *incubation period* is from 5 to 12 days.

Medical geography
The distribution of infection is probably world-wide but the frequency of the infection is not fully appreciated except in places where interested clinicians have adequate laboratory facilities.

Virology
The causative agent is a virus which is closely related to the trachoma virus, both being referred to jointly as the TRIC agents.

Epidemiology
Man is the reservoir of infection, the usual habitat of the organism being the genital tract in the female cervix or the epithelium of the male urethra. The genital infection is asymptomatic.

The newborn baby is infected from its mother's genital tract during delivery; the infection may also be transmitted mechanically from eye to eye, but adults often acquire the infection in the swimming pool.

Control

Topical treatment with tetracycline ointment is usually effective but sulphonamides may also be administered by the oral route. Routine eye toilet of newborn babies is of no apparent value. Chlorination of swimming pools is useful in preventing adult infections.

Inclusion Conjunctivitis—Summary

(1) *Occurrence*—World-wide
(2) *Organism*—A TRIC virus
(3) *Reservoir of infection*—Man, mainly carriers with genital infection
(4) *Modes of transmission*—Intrapartum, contact, swimming
(5) *Control*— (i) Early treatment
                (ii) Chlorination of swimming pools

Venereal Diseases

These are infections which are specifically transmitted during sexual intercourse. Although various other infections may be transmitted during sexual intercourse, the commonly recognised venereal diseases are:

Syphilis
Gonorrhoea
Lymphogranuloma venereum
Granuloma inguinale (Donovanosis)
Soft sore
Non-gonococcal urethritis
Herpes genitalis.

Epidemiology of venereal diseases

The infective agents include viruses, bacteria and protozoa, but most of them share the characteristic of being delicate, being easily killed by drying or cooling below body temperature, with the reservoir exclusively in man. Hence, transmission is mainly through direct close contact but rarely indirectly through fomites.

Route of transmission

Lesions are generally present on the genitalia, and the infective agents in the secretions and discharges from the urethra and the vagina, but extragenital lesions may occur through haematogenesis dissemination as in syphilis or through inoculation of the infective agent at extra-genital sites. Transmission occurs:

(a) mainly through genital contact
(b) through extragenital sexual contact such as kissing
(c) through non-sexual contact, e.g. congenital syphilis, gonococcal ophthalmia neonatorum, or accidental contact as when doctors, dentists or midwives handle tissues infected with syphilis
(d) through fomites, e.g. soiled moist clothing such as wet towels, may transmit vulvovaginitis to pre-pubescent girls.

It is not uncommon for patients to claim that they contracted the venereal infection through some indirect contact such as the lavatory seat; such mechanism is extremely unlikely and the patient will usually admit to sexual exposure once his confidence has been obtained.

Host

The most important host factor is sexual behaviour, the significant feature being sexual promiscuity. The transmission of a venereal disease almost always implies sexual activity involving at least three persons. For if A infects B, it implies that A has also had sexual contact with at least one other person X, who infected A. Thus, venereal diseases have the highest frequency in those who are most active sexually, particularly those who indulge in promiscuous sexual behaviour with frequent changes of partners. Thus, young adult males away from home (sailors, soldiers, migrant labourers, etc.) are often at high risk.

Cultural attitudes to sex also play an important role. In some communities sexual matters are treated on a system of double standards in that whilst young unmarried girls are expected to remain chaste, young men are permitted or even encouraged to indulge in promiscuous sexual activities often with a small group of notorious women including prostitutes. Even after marriage, similar standards may apply; married women may be veiled, confined to special quarters in the household, or chaperoned on outings but with little or no restrictions on the extramarital sexual activities of the male. A more permissive attitude to sexual relations has developed in some communities which now tend to take a liberal view of all forms of sexual relations regardless of the sex or the marital status of the partners.

Promiscuity before marriage and infidelity after marriage represent the major behavioural factors underlying the transmission of venereal disease, whilst sexual abstinence and marital fidelity are protective.

The factors which influence the pattern of sexual behaviour (see Fig. 5.1) include:

(1) *Fear*—of God, parents, public opinion, pregnancy, venereal diseases
(2) *Absorbing interests*—sublimation through work or leisure pursuits
(3) *Masturbation*—self release
(4) *Sex for gain*.

Control

The general guide-lines for the control of venereal diseases are as follows:

A. Infective Agent

(1) Eliminate the reservoir of infection
The reservoir is exclusively human; it includes untreated sick patients but inapparent infection especially in women represents the most important part of the reservoir. The identification and treatment of the promiscuous female pool is of great importance. Regular medical examination and treatment of known prostitutes, inhabitants of brothels, and other places where promiscuous sexual behaviour is

known to occur. Such medical supervision of prostitutes cannot entirely eliminate the risk of infection.

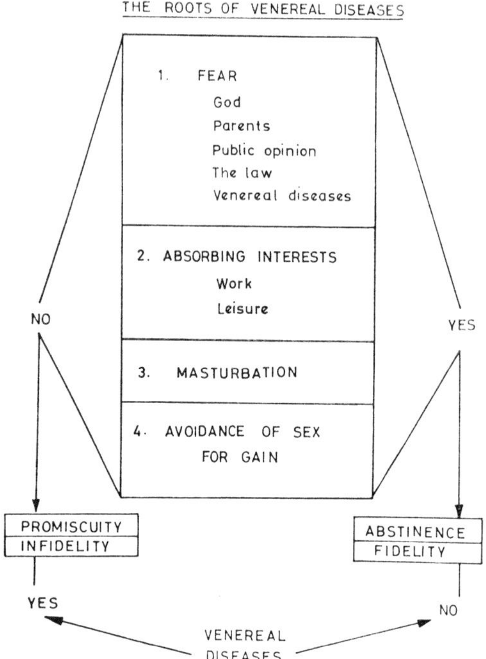

FIG. 5.1   The roots of Venereal Diseases (*after* R. R. *Wilcox*).

B. *Route of Transmission*

(2) *Discourage sexual promiscuity*
Through sex education, make the community aware of the dangers of sexual promiscuity. One objective would be to influence young persons before their sexual habits become established.

Encourage stable family life by providing married quarters in work camps, etc.

(3) *Local prophylaxis*
The use of rubber condoma diminishes but does not eliminate the risk of infection of the male.

Careful toilet of the genitals with soap and antiseptic creams immediately after exposure also gives partial protection.

C. *Host*

(4) *Specific prophylaxis*
Specific immunisation is not available against any of the venereal diseases. Although a measure of protection can be obtained by using

antibiotic chemoprophylaxis, this approach can be dangerous for the individual and the community. Chemoprophylaxis may suppress the acute clinical manifestations but the disease may remain latent and progress silently to late complications. The widespread use of a particular antibiotic in sub-curative doses may encourage the emergence and dissemination of drug-resistant strains.

(5) Early diagnosis and treatment
   Patients—This is one of the most important measures for the control of venereal diseases. Facilities for the diagnosis and treatment of those diseases must be freely accessible to all infected persons. Experience has shown that in order to reach the whole community everyone must have access to a free and confidential service.
   Contacts—In addition to treating the patient, his sexual contacts must be investigated and treated. In highly promiscuous groups where sexual activities occur in association with the use of alcohol or drugs, the details of the chain of transmission may be difficult to unravel. In such cases, one may use the technique of 'cluster tracing'. Apart from seeking a list of sexual exposures with dates, the patient is asked to name friends of both sexes whom he feels may profit from investigation for venereal diseases.

Lymphogranuloma Venereum

This is a chronic infection of the genitals which spreads to involve regional lymph nodes, and the rectum. Typically it produces ulcerative lesions on the genitalia with induration of the regional lymph nodes ('climatic bubo'). Anal and genital stricture may occur at a late stage; so also may elephantiasis of the vulva. Extragenital lesions and general dissemination occasionally occur.

Medical geography
The infection is endemic in many parts of the tropics and subtropics.

Virology
The causative agent is a large virus of the psittacosis group.

Laboratory diagnosis
   Stained smears of pus and other pathological material may show virus particles. The organism can be identified on culture in the yolk sacs of embryonated eggs. The complement fixation test becomes positive some 2 to 4 weeks after the onset of the illness. A skin test, the Frei test, is available, but cross-reactions with other viral infections of the psittacosis group may occur depending on the purity of the antigen. It tends to remain positive for long periods.

Epidemiology
Man is the reservoir of infection, the source being the open lesions in patients with active disease. Transmission is mainly by sexual contact but also by indirect contact through contaminated clothing and other fomites.

As with other venereal diseases, the sexual behaviour of the host is a major factor determining the distribution and spread of this infection. Recovery from a clinical attack does not confer immunity.

Control

The main principles are as for other venereal diseases. The early stages of infection respond to sulphadiazine, but tetracyclines are the drugs of choice especially for the severe or advanced cases.

Lymphogranuloma Venereum—Summary

(1) *Distribution*—Tropics and subtropics mainly
(2) *Organism*—Lymphogranuloma venereum virus
(3) *Reservoir*—Man
(4) *Transmission*—Genital sexual contact—indirect contact
(5) *Control*—As for other venereal diseases; the organism is sensitive to sulphonamides and broad-spectrum antibiotics

Chancroid

This is an acute venereal infection which typically presents as a ragged painful ulcer on the genitalia; the inguinal lymph nodes become enlarged and may suppurate. Extragenital lesions may be found on the abdomen, fingers or other sites.

The *incubation period* is usually from 3 to 5 days but it may be very short (24 hours) where the lesion affects mucous membrane.

Medical geography
The infection occurs in many parts of the world, especially in tropical seaports.

Bacteriology
The causative agent is *Haemophilus ducreyi*, a Gram-negative non-sporing bacillus.

Epidemiology
Man is the reservoir of infection. The open lesions are the most important source of infection although it has been suggested that the carrier state may exist in women.

Sexual contact is the usual mode of transmission but extragenital lesions may occur from non-sexual infection of children or accidental infection of doctors, nurses or other medical personnel who come into contact with infected lesions.

Laboratory diagnosis
Microscopy of the stained smear of the exudate from ulcers or pus from the regional lymph nodes may show a mixed flora including Gram-negative bacilli. The organism can be isolated on culture of pus from the ulcer or bubo. An intradermal skin test is available but it does not differentiate active infections from previous attacks.

Biopsy of the regional lymph nodes may also provide useful information.

Control
The general measures for the control of venereal diseases apply to the problem of chancroid. Active infections usually respond to treatment with sulphonamides but in resistant cases, antibiotics such as streptomycin, tetracycline, or chloromycetin may be used.

Chancroid—Summary
(1) *Occurrence*—Tropics, especially seaports
(2) *Organism*—Haemophilus ducreyi
(3) *Reservoir of infection*—Man
(4) *Modes of transmission*—Sexual contact, accidental infection through non-sexual contact
(5) *Control*—As for other venereal diseases

Granuloma Inguinale
This is a chronic infection which presents with granulomatous lesions of the genitalia; regional lymph nodes may be affected and metastatic lesions occur.

The *incubation period* is 1 week to 3 months.

Medical geography
The infection occurs in various parts of the tropics and subtropics, particularly in poorer communities.

Organism
The aetiological agent is *Donovania granulomatis.*

Epidemiology
Man is the reservoir of infection. Transmission may be by sexual contact, but non-sexual contact may also be important.

Laboratory diagnosis
Stained smears from active lesion show the typical Donovan bodies. A skin test is available and the complement fixation test can also be used in diagnosis.

Control

General hygienic measures are important. Known cases should be treated with antibiotics (streptomycin, tetracycline, chloramphenicol or erythromycin). Contacts should be examined and treated if indicated.

Granuloma Inguinale—Summary

(1) *Distribution*—Tropics and subtropics
(2) *Organism*—Donovania granulomatis
(3) *Reservoir of infection*—Man
(4) *Transmission*—Contact, including sexual contact
(5) *Control*—General hygienic measures—as for other venereal diseases

Gonorrhoea

This disease is caused by infection with *Neisseria gonorrhoeae*. In the male, it usually presents as an acute purulent urethritis with spread in some cases to involve the epididymis and testis. Late complications include urethral stricture, urethral sinuses and sub-fertility. A high proportion (80-90 per cent) of infected females are unaware of the infection; the others present with symptoms of urethritis and urethal or vaginal discharge. Complications in the female include Bartholinitis, salpingitis, pyosalpinx and pelvic inflammatory disease. Late complications include sub-fertility resulting from tubal obstruction. The *incubation period* is usually between 2 and 5 days, occasionally shorter (1 day), but may be as long as 2 weeks. It is usually notifiable nationally.

Geographical distribution

The distribution is world-wide with particular concentrations at seaports, and in areas having a high concentration of migrant labour or military personnel.

Bacteriology

N. *gonorrhoea* is a Gram-negative diplococcus, with a characteristic bean shape. It dies rapidly outside the human body, being susceptible to drying and heat.

Epidemiology

Man is the reservoir of infection; the most important part is the female pool with asymptomatic infection.

Transmission of the infection is mostly by:

(a) *Sexual genital contact*
(b) *Indirect contamination*. This may produce infection in prepubertal females. Vulvo-vaginitis may occur in a young girl who is infected by sharing towel or other clothing with an infected older relative. Post-pubertal girls do not become infected in this way; some cases of vulvo-vaginitis in young girls are the result of sexual contact with infected males.

(c) *Ophthalmia neonatorum.* This infection occurs in the course of delivering the baby of an infected mother.

All persons are susceptible. There is no lasting immunity after recovery; repeated infections are common. As with other venereal diseases, the most important host factor is sexual behaviour.

Laboratory diagnosis

Clinical diagnosis can be confirmed by bacteriological examination of stained smears of urethral discharge, cervical discharge or other infected material; the characteristic diplococci, some within pus cells, can be seen. The organisms can also be cultured on chocolate agar as a form of enrichment medium or on selective media such as the Thayer-Martin medium which contains antibiotics which suppress the growth of other organisms. Fluorescent antibody techniques are also available for diagnosis.

Control

The control of gonorrhoea is posing a difficult problem in most parts of the world. Various factors have contributed to this difficulty:

(*a*) Revolutionary change in sexual modes

(*b*) Replacement of the condom by effective contraceptive techniques which do not provide a mechanical barrier to infection

(*c*) Emergence of drug resistant strains

The control of gonorrhoea is based on the principles set out in the section on venereal diseases.

Gonococcal ophthalmitis can be prevented by treating all infected pregnant women and by toilet to the eyes of all newborn babies. The latter consists of instilling one drop of 1 per cent silver nitrate into the eyes of every newborn baby.

Gonorrhoea—Summary

(1) *Occurrence*—World-wide

(2) *Organism*—*Neisseria gonorrhoeae*

(3) *Reservoir of infection*—Man

(4) *Modes of Transmission*—Sexual contact. Rarely through fomites. Eye infection during delivery

(5) *Control*— (i) As for other venereal diseases
(ii) Toilet to the eyes of newborn babies

Treponematoses

The treponematoses are diseases caused by spirochaetes which belong to the genus *Treponemata*. The most important diseases in this group are:

(*a*) Venereal syphilis (*Treponema pallidum*)

(*b*) Yaws (*T. pertenue*)

(*c*) Pinta (*T. carateum*)
(*d*) Non-venereal syphilis (*T. pallidum*)

There has been much speculation about the origin and differentiation of these organisms. One view regards the organisms as being virtually identical but apparent differences in clinical manifestations result from epidemiological factors; the other view regards the organisms as separate but related entities. In practical terms, the pattern of treponemal diseases is still evolving with the eradication of the non-venereal treponematoses from endemic areas and with the rise in the frequency of venereal syphilis in some areas where the disease was previously not recognised as an important public health problem.

Venereal Syphilis

This is a chronic infection which is characterised clinically by a localised primary lesion, a generalised secondary eruption involving the skin and mucous membranes, and a later tertiary stage with involvement of skin, bone, abdominal viscera, cardiovascular and central nervous systems. The *incubation period* is usually 2 to 4 weeks but may be from 9 to 90 days. The primary lesion is usually a painless sore associated with firm enlarged regional lymph nodes. The initial lesion tends to heal spontaneously after a few weeks. Six weeks to 6 months or even a year later, secondary lesions appear usually as generalised non-itchy, painless and non-tender rash, shallow ulcers on the oral mucosa, widespread lymphodenopathy and mild systemic disturbance, including fever. These manifestations regress spontaneously, and the infection enters a latent phase which may last for 10 years or more before the tertiary lesions appear, although spontaneous healing may occur during the latent stage.

Although venereal syphilis was previously unknown or was not recognised in some parts of the world, the distribution of the venereal infection is now virtually world-wide.

Bacteriology
T. *pallidum* is a spirochaetal organism, a thin organism, 1-15 μm long with tapering ends; there are about 5-20 spirals. It is a motile organism, fresh preparations under dark-ground illumination show characteristic movements.

The organism is delicate, being rapidly killed by drying, at high temperature (50°C), disinfectants such as phenolic compounds, and by soap and water. It may survive in refrigerated blood for 3 days. The organism may remain viable for several years if frozen at −78°C.

Epidemiology
Man is the reservoir of infection, the sources of infection being moist

lesions on the skin and mucosae, and also tissue fluids and secretions such as saliva, semen, vaginal discharge and blood.

Transmission is mainly venereal through genital or extragenital contact, but it may be non-venereal.

(i) *Venereal transmission*

Genital contact may lead to infection with the organisms penetrating normal skin and mucous membranes. In the male, the infection may be quite obvious in the form of a primary chancre on the penis but the infective female may be unaware of a similar lesion on her cervix. Inapparent infection in the female, especially the promiscuous female, is an important source of infection.

Infection may also be transmitted during sexual play from extra-genital sites such as the mouth during kissing; the infected partner may develop primary lesions on the lips, tongue or breast.

(ii) *Non-venereal transmission*

This may be accidental, through touching infected tissues as in the case of dentists or midwives.

Congenital infection may occur in a child who is born to an infected mother, even though the mother is at a latent phase. Intra-uterine syphilitic infection may be associated with repeated abortions, still-births, or congenital infection in a live child, who may show lesions at birth, but more commonly clinical signs appear later.

The most important host factor in the epidemiology of syphilis is sexual behaviour, a high frequency of infection being associated with sexual promiscuity. A current infection with syphilis may provide some immunity, but if super-infection occurs, the clinical manifestations may be modified. There is some degree of cross-immunity to syphilis in persons infected with the other non-venereal treponematoses but such immunity is not absolute.

Laboratory diagnosis

(1) *Dark-field microscopy* of exudates of primary and secondary lesions usually reveal the spirochaete.

(2) *Serological tests* on blood and cerebrospinal fluid. A variety of serological tests for syphilis are in use, but they fall into two main groups:

(a) *Non-treponemal antigen*

These tests are based on the presence of the antibody complex—reagin, in syphilitic infections. This complex may be detected by using a flocculation test, e.g. VDRL slide test, Kahn test, Mazzine cardiolipin, or Kline cardiolipin. Alternatively, a complement-fixation test may be used, e.g. Kolmer test.

(b) *Treponemal antigen tests*
These include the Treponema Pallidum Immobilisation test (TPT),
Fluorescent Treponemal Antibody (FTA) and the Reiter Protein
Complement-Fixation test (RPCFT).

The serological tests usually become positive 1-2 weeks after the
appearance of the primary lesions, and are almost invariably positive
during the secondary stage of the illness but may later become negative spontaneously or after successful chemotherapy at any stage.

False positive reactions
Using non-treponemal antigens false positive serum reactions are
encountered in some persons who have not been infected with syphilis
or other treponemal organism. Such *biological false positive* reactions are
particularly associated with certain infections: protozoal (malaria,
trypanosomiasis), spirochaetal (leptospirosis, relapsing fever), bacterial
(leprosy, tuberculosis) and viral atypical pneumonia, glandular fever,
lymphogranuloma venereum. It has also been noted in cases of collagen
vascular disease and following vaccination against smallpox or yellow
fever.

Tests based on treponemal antigens, being more specific, are less
liable to give such biological false positive reactions. Neither type of
test can, however, differentiate syphilis from other treponemal infections.

A positive serological test therefore indicates the probable presence
of a specific treponemal infection, the nature of which can be determined
on clinical and circumstantial evidence.

Control
The general principles for the control of venereal diseases apply to
the control of syphilis:

(1) *General health promotion*
Through health and sex education make the population aware of the
danger of promiscuous sexual activity. Young persons especially should
be encouraged to take up diversional activities in the form of games,
interesting hobbies and other absorbing interests. Although the provision of good recreational facilities is highly desirable, it cannot however, by itself, make a significant change in sexual habits.

(2) *Control of prostitution and promiscuous sexual behaviour*
There are conflicting views about the best way to deal with the problem
of prostitution in relation to venereal disease. At the one end it is
suggested that prostitution being a social evil should be totally abol-
ished, if necessary, by imposing severe penalties. An alternative view
holds that whilst it may be desirable to abolish prostitution, it is not

feasible to do so, and that harsh laws merely drive the practice under-ground and discourage the prostitutes and their partners from seeking appropriate medical treatment. In place of clandestine prostitution, licensed brothels are allowed to operate under the close supervision of the health authorities. Neither method provides a satisfactory solution.

The role of prostitutes in the transmission of syphilis varies from community to community. In some societies, professional prostitutes make a major contribution but, in others, much of the transmission results from promiscuous behaviour not involving immediate financial gain.

(3) *Early diagnosis and treatment*

Serology plays an important role in the detection of cases of syphilis, especially in the latent phase. Whenever feasible, there should be routine serological screening of pregnant women, blood donors, those who are about to get married, immigrants, hospital patients, prisoners and other groups.

Where there is a high probability that a person has been infected, such as the contact of a patient with open lesions, 'epidemiological treatment', i.e. treatment on the basis of presumptive diagnosis, should be given. Penicillin is the drug of choice; given early and in appropriate doses, syphilitic infection can be eradicated. Other antibiotics, e.g. tetracyclines, may be used if the patient is allergic to penicillin. There is as yet no effective artificial immunisation against syphilis.

Syphilis—Summary

(1) *Occurrence*—World-wide
(2) *Organism*—*Treponema pallidum*
(3) *Reservoir of infection*—Man
(4) *Modes of transmission*—sexual contact, non-sexual contact, trans-placental
(5) *Control*— (i) Control of sexual promiscuity
     (ii) Early detection and treatment of infected persons, including serological screening

Non-venereal Treponematoses
Yaws

This non-venereal treponemal infection mainly affects skin and bones, rarely if ever affecting the cardiovascular or the nervous system. The skin lesions may be granulomatous, ulcerative or hypertrophic; destructive lesions of bone and hypertrophic changes are late lesions of bone. The *incubation period* is usually about 1 month, varying from 2 weeks to 3 months.

The disease was highly endemic in many parts of the tropics and subtropical zones of Africa, South-East Asia, the Pacific, the Caribbean and Central and South America. There has been a marked fall in the incidence of the disease.

Bacteriology
The infective agent, *Treponema pertenue*, cannot be distinguished from *T. pallidum* on microscopy (light, phase contrast or electron).

Epidemiology
Man is the reservoir of infection, the source of infection being the often moist skin lesions in the early phase of the disease. Transmission is mainly by direct contact, but flies, especially *Hippelates pallipes*, may carry the infection from a skin lesion to a susceptible host.

Most early cases are seen in children under 15 years. The disease occurs predominantly in rural communities where there is the combination of poverty, low level of personal hygiene, warm humid climate, and where children especially usually wear little clothing. Transplacental transmission does not occur.

Laboratory diagnosis
(1) *Dark field microscopy* of the exudates from moist lesions will reveal the spirochaete.
(2) *Serological tests* of blood become positive at an early stage of the infection, but tend to become negative when the disease has been latent for several years. None of the serological tests can differentiate syphilis from other treponemal infections.

Control
Yaws has been successfully controlled and virtually eradicated from some parts of the world where it had been highly endemic. The successful programme was backed by the World Health Organisation and it consisted of:

(a) *Epidemiological survey* by clinical examination of the entire population.
(b) *Mass chemotherapy with penicillin* of patients, including those with latent infection, and contacts. Specific treatment is with a single intramuscular injection of long acting penicillin in oil with 2 per cent aluminium monostearate (PAM).
(c) *Surveillance* through periodic clinical and serological surveys.

Apart from such specific campaigns, general improvement in personal hygiene and in level of living standards has contributed greatly to the disappearance of the disease.

Yaws—Summary
(1) *Occurrence*—Tropics and subtropics of Africa, South-East Asia, Philippines, Pacific Islands, Caribbean, Central and South America. Mainly rural. Now well controlled in or eradicated from most areas

(2) *Organism—Treponema pertenue*
(3) *Reservoir of infection*—Man
(4) *Mode of transmission*—Direct contact
(5) *Control*— (i) Mass survey and chemotherapy
           (ii) Improvement of personal hygiene

Pinta

This is a spirochaetal infection which initially presents as a superficial non-ulcerating papule. Later flat hyperpigmented skin lesions develop, and these may become depigmented and hyperkeratotic. The *incubation period* is from 7 to 20 days.

Medical geography
It occurs predominantly in the dark-skinned people of Mexico, Central and South America, North Africa, Middle East, India, the Philippines and some areas in the Pacific.

Bacteriology
The infective agent is *Treponema carateum* a spirochaete which is morphologically indistinguishable from *T. pallidum*.

Epidemiology
Man is the reservoir of infection; the patients with early active lesions are the sources of infection.

Transmission is mainly from direct non-venereal contact, or through indirect contact. It has been suggested that certain biting insects play a role but this is not proven.

Infection is commoner in children than in adults. The relatively high frequency of cases in negroid persons may be related to socio-economic factors and personal habit, rather than to genetic factors. There is some cross-immunity with syphilis and other treponemal infections but protection is partial and syphilis may co-exist with pinta.

Pinta—Summary

(1) *Occurrence*—Tropics and subtropics—America, Africa, Middle
         East, India, Philippines
(2) *Organism—Treponema carateum*
(3) *Reservoir of infection*—Man
(4) *Mode of transmission*—Direct and indirect contact
(5) *Control*—As for yaws

Endemic (Non-venereal) Syphilis

This refers to a manifestation of infection with *Treponema pallidum* in an epidemiological situation in which the infection is highly endemic with non-venereal transmission occurring predominantly in young persons. A primary chancre is not commonly encountered and it is mainly extragenital. In the secondary stage, mucosal lesions (mucous patches) occur in the mouth, tongue, larynx and nostrils. Condylomata lata are also found in the moist areas: ano-genital area, groins, axillae, below the breast and the angles of the mouth. A variety of other skin lesions may also be present at this stage. Late lesions include skin gummata, nasopharyngeal ulceration, and bone lesions (osteitis, gummata). Cardiovascular and neurological involvement may occur but are apparently rare. Congenital infection is also rare.

The *incubation period* is 2 weeks to 3 months.

Medical geography
The infection is found in remote rural areas in parts of tropical Africa, the Middle and Near East, and southern Europe. It has virtually been eliminated from most of these areas where it was formerly endemic.

Bacteriology
The causative organism, *T. pallidum*, is indistinguishable from the aetiological agent of venereal syphilis.

Epidemiology
The distribution of the disease is associated with poverty, overcrowding and poor personal hygiene. Early infections occur predominantly in childhood.

Man is the reservoir of infection. Transmission is by close person-to-person contact; indirect transmission may occur through indirect contact from sharing pipes, cups and other utensils.

With improvement in social conditions, the endemic syphilis recedes, few children become infected but adults acquire venereally transmitted syphilis.

Laboratory diagnosis
The organism can be seen under dark-field microscopy from wet lesions such as mucous patches and condylomata. Serology becomes positive by the time that secondary lesions occur.

Endemic Syphilis—Summary

(1) *Distribution*—Tropical Africa, Middle and Near East, Southern Europe
(2) *Organism*—Treponema pallidum
(3) *Reservoir of infection*—Man
(4) *Mode of transmission*—Direct and indirect contact
(5) *Control*— (i) Mass survey and chemotherapy with penicillin
      (ii) Improvement in personal hygiene

Leprosy*
This is an infection due to the specific micro-organism, *Mycobacterium leprae*, which is of low invasive power and pathogenicity. The four main clinical forms described are: indeterminate leprosy; tuberculoid leprosy; borderline leprosy (probably the commonest form) and lepromatous leprosy.

Medical geography
The disease is common in the Indian subcontinent, tropical Africa, South-East Asia and South America. Small foci of infection exist in southern Europe and in the countries bordering the Mediterranean. Leprosy has been introduced by immigrants into countries that have been free of indigenous cases for many years, e.g. the United Kingdom.

Bacteriology
M. leprae is a slender rod-like organism which is both acid and alcohol fast and Gram-positive. It is found singly or in masses (globi). The bacilli are scanty in some clinical forms of leprosy (indeterminate and tuberculoid), while they are very numerous in the lesions of lepromatous leprosy. The organism has never been consistently cultured on artificial media. *M. leprae* has been successfully inoculated into the footpads of mice. The viable organism stains deeply and uniformly; irregular staining or beading indicates non-viability.

Epidemiology
The incubation period of leprosy is long and indefinite. Man is the only source of infection. The infectiousness of leprosy is not high, and repeated skin to skin contact seems to be necessary. The mechanism of contagion probably consists of the transfer of living *M. leprae* from skin to skin, and the introduction of the bacilli into the corium by some slight and unremembered trauma. There is no positive evidence for the existence of an extrahuman reservoir of leprosy bacilli; nor for different strains. The role of fomites contaminated by skin squames or by nasal secretions is not clear. Conjugal infections are usually 5 per cent or less.

While prolonged and intimate contact is classically considered to be necessary for infection to develop, there are well-authenticated cases of patients acquiring the infection after a brief passing contact with a person suffering from leprosy. It is quite rare, however, for workers in leprosaria to contract leprosy. Although leprosy is commonest in moist and humid lands, climatic factors *per se* are probably not important. Children and adolescents are commonly held to be more susceptible than adults, as are males more than females, but these

* We are grateful to Dr S. Browne for the liberal use of his writings in the preparation of this section.

E

generalisations are not as definite as they are sometimes made out to be. Hormonal influences may play a part, since there seems to be an increased incidence at puberty in both sexes, and clinical exacerbation of the disease may occur during pregnancy and particularly after parturition. Racial and genetic susceptibility affect the pattern of the disease from Central Africa since, as one moves eastwards or westwards from this central point, the ratio of lepromatous to tuberculoid patients increases.

The natural history of leprosy can conveniently be represented as follows:

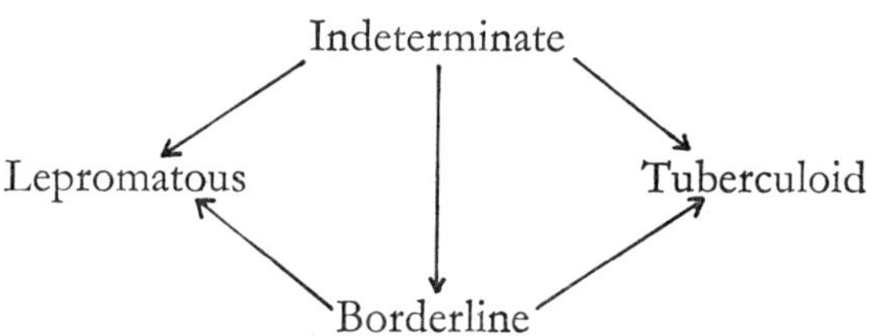

All persons exposed to repeated contact with open cases of leprosy do not contract the disease, and, moreover, a variable proportion of those who do develop leprosy, suffer from a self-healing form. Many persons infected with leprosy manifest a vigorous response to the organism, while a variable proportion develop the severe progressive form of the disease characterised by minimal response (lepromatous).

Recent work has emphasised the complex nature of the immune response in leprosy. Both immunoglobulins and lymphocyte-mediated immune mechanisms are involved. Patients whose resistance is impaired lack cell-mediated immunity.

The lepromin test

The antigens used for the lepromin test are prepared by the maceration of tissue containing great numbers of bacilli, such as a nodule obtained from a patient suffering from active lepromatous leprosy. The organisms are killed by heat or by other means. A refined lepromin is obtained by treating the tissue with chloroform and ether, and then centrifuging at high speed. The deposit is suspended in carbol-saline. The test is performed by injecting 0·1 ml of antigen intradermally; the site of injection is inspected after 24 hours, and daily thereafter. There are other methods of preparing a suitable antigen from bacillus-containing material and sundry modifications of the test.

There are two types of cutaneous response to the lepromin test. The early reaction of *Fernandez* consists of an erythematous infiltrated area which appears 24-72 hours after injection, while the *Mitsuda* reaction is nodular in form and most intense 21-30 days after injection.

The early reaction is now interpreted as a response to soluble substances of the bacillus, and the late reaction as resistance to the bacillus excited by insoluble substances. Variation of the intensity of the lepromin test occurs among leprosy patients as well as among contacts. The best site for the inoculation is the anterior aspect of the forearm.

The Mitsuda reaction is negative in pure lepromatous leprosy, strongly positive in major tuberculoid leprosy, and variably positive in intermediate forms. BCG vaccination may result in conversion of a negative lepromin reaction to positive, this conversion occurring in a variable proportion of subjects to a variable degree.

Neither an early nor a late lepromin reaction proves immunity. The lepromin test is essentially an allergic reaction, though many leprologists believe that the reaction tests both allergy and immunity to leprosy bacilli. The proportion of persons in endemic areas giving positive Mitsuda reactions increases with age from nil at birth up to 80 per cent in adults. It has been speculated that an intrinsic natural factor exists—which is called factor N (N for natural)—that gives an individual the capacity to react specifically to *M. leprae*. Thus about 20 per cent of the population, for no apparent reason, will not become lepromin-positive however strong the natural or artificial extrinsic stimuli may be, this minor group probably lacks intrinsic factor N.

Laboratory diagnosis

The cardinal point in diagnosis is the demonstration of *M. leprae* in a smear of clinical lesion stained by the Ziehl-Neelson method. The best sites for taking smears are the following:

(1) the active edge of the most active lesion
(2) the ear lobes
(3) the mucosa of the nasal septum.

Biopsy of typical macules, nodules, infiltrations or enlarged nerves is often used. Bacterial assessment of patients with leprosy is made by counts on skin smears or biopsy specimens, from which two indices can be derived—(*a*) the *Morphological Index* (M.I.), and (*b*) the *Bacteriological Index* (B.I.).

The *morphological index* is the average percentage of morphologically normal and viable (i.e. solid-staining or deeply staining) bacilli in smears from the various sites.

The *bacteriological index*, expressed by various notations (0 to 4 or 5 or 6), is a measure of the average concentration of recognisable bacillary forms in smears from various sites on the skin (and possibly nasal mucosa).

Control

Where determined and sustained efforts can be made, leprosy can be cured in the individual and controlled in the community.

(a) *The individual*

Dapsone (diaminodiphenylsulphone, DDS) is the sheet anchor of leprosy treatment in both the individual and the community. It is relatively non-toxic and cheap, is active in all kinds of leprosy, can be administered for long periods by trained medical auxiliaries and only rarely induces drug resistance. It is usually given orally at a dosage of 25 mg weekly rising continuously to a maximum of 100-200 mg weekly. DDS is given for at least 2 years in indeterminate or tuberculoid leprosy, and usually for at least 4 years in borderline or lepromatous patients. In the latter instance the drug should ideally be continued for life at half the therapeutic dose—i.e. the dose that causes cessation of all clinical and bacteriological activity. Clofazimine (Lamprene) is active in dapsone-resistant leprosy and in the treatment of acute exacerbation (lepra reactions).

(b) *The community*

The threshold below which leprosy ceases to be a public health problem depends on a number of factors and probably varies from country to country.

Although the factors that determine the persistence or disappearance of leprosy in a community are still unknown, the general principles of control of a slightly contagious bacillary disease can be applied to leprosy, namely:

   (i) reduction of contagious sources by chemotherapy to a level at which there is little danger of spread

  (ii) control of the frequency and duration of potentially infective contacts

 (iii) tracing and supervision of all persons exposed to infection.

Methods of control depend on the incidence of leprosy in the community, the state of the existing medical services and the willingness of the authorities to accord leprosy control the place its importance deserves.

In lands where leprosy is more highly endemic (namely most of the tropics and subtropics) its control is a most difficult problem. All the adverse factors are present in some degree, namely:

   (i) overcrowding and low standards of hygiene

  (ii) lack of medical services

 (iii) limited financial resources

 (iv) ignorance and prejudice

  (v) the existence of diseases that kill (malaria) or are more prevalent (schistosomiasis, onchocerciasis), more contagious (tuberculosis, cholera) or more amenable to control measures (poliomyelitis, water-borne diseases, trachoma).

The essence of leprosy control is survey, education and treatment. *Survey* may mean a whole-population survey, a pilot or sampling operation, or be limited to certain readily available groups such as school-children, schoolteachers, workmen and their families, or army and police recruits. When the prevalence is high, regular whole-population surveys conducted annually by teams of auxiliaries working under a doctor are essential. Clinical examination of stripped subjects, conducted with due regard to privacy and social habits, is the rule. Doubtful lesions are examined by the doctor in charge, smears are taken and either stained on the spot or fixed for subsequent staining at the central laboratory. If possible, contacts of known leprosy patients are seen even more frequently. Treatment is instituted at once for all patients in whom active leprosy has been diagnosed. Advantage is taken of the presence of relatives and fellow-villagers to establish good public relations and to embark on a suitable scheme of education. From the beginning, leprosy should be integrated into the comprehensive medical service for the control of transmissible diseases and treatment provided for leprosy patients suffering from other diseases as well. This also fosters good public relations, for duplication of services is avoided and the health of the whole community is improved.

The mainstay of the anti-leprosy campaign in an urban or rural area in the developing countries is the all-purpose dispensary in charge of a competent paramedical worker. After being instructed in the rudiments of leprosy diagnosis and treatment, the latter is able to recognise early leprosy, ensure regularity of treatment of all patients and participate in health education, simple physiotherapy, etc.

Leprosy patients are treated either at *static dispensaries* or in *mobile clinics*. The choice will be determined largely by local conditions, such as the status of the public health service, distribution of the population, the prevalence of leprosy, local communications, etc. The drugs used should be restricted to a few (the fewer the better) and they should be given according to a simple codified regime. The great majority of patients, whatever the form or stage of leprosy and whatever their age and sex, may be safely and satisfactorily treated in this fashion, and the risk of untoward side-effects is minimal.

The mobile clinic—whether for leprosy only or an all-purpose type—has proved its worth in Francophone Africa. The itinerary is planned so that regular visits are paid every so often along a certain route. Patients foregather at set points from surrounding villages and hamlets to receive a supply of drugs sufficient to last until the next visit. Paramedical workers travel on bicycles where the truck cannot go, rejoining it further along the route. The essential features of the service are diagnosis, examination of contacts and the taking of slit-smears. While the drawbacks and shortcomings of this system are obvious, it is the only way of tackling the leprosy problem in a scattered population with primitive and precarious communications. One real disadvantage of rural control schemes is that patients no longer suffering from active disease may have to walk long distances to receive a supply of anti-leprosy tablets that have no effect on their burnt-out disease, but with possible worsening of the ulcers on their anaesthetic feet. The campaign will inevitably suffer as a result.

In some circumstances, the *segregation village* has been advocated. When arable land is available and the patients can support themselves by farming, the temporary expedient of the segregation village has much in its favour, provided the goodwill of tribal chiefs and populace has been assured. Sometimes the local authorities themselves take the initiative. The village should fall within the purview of a resident medical auxiliary who may also have either a small ward for in-patients or access to beds in a local hospital. If such villages can be properly supervised and patients can return home when this is deemed advisable they may play a useful part in the leprosy campaign. However, they may also perpetuate false notions about leprosy; the inmates stay on and acquire a landed and vested interest in the village, perhaps holding the local population to ransom by begging. In some countries (for instance Korea) these communities, which include cured patients, raise enormous problems. Their upkeep makes heavy financial demands on the government, and special schools have to be set up for the children, thus strengthening the fears of the healthy population that leprosy sufferers transmit a taint.

The *central hospital* forms an essential element in a leprosy control scheme. At any one time about 1 per cent of the patients will be in-patients. Facilities for reconstructive surgery should be available, as also for pre- and post-operative physiotherapy, for training in the use of anaesthetic limbs, for occupational therapy or vocational training, and for the provision of prostheses.

In no other disease do social and psychological factors loom so large as in leprosy. Since no specific psychological changes can be attributed to leprosy *per se*, the factors determining the psychological changes that occur are rather the outcome of the patient's attitude to his disease and the attitude of society. In the patient, traditional beliefs as well as guilt feelings may result in either apathy and resignation or a resentful aggressiveness towards society. Leprosy in the present 'incarnation' may be regarded as retribution for misdeeds in a previous one, so that nothing can or should be done to ameliorate it. When seen as punishment for a sexual misdemeanour, leprosy may lead to such intense feelings of remorse and recrimination that suicide is contemplated or even committed. On the other hand, the person with leprosy may be led to believe that his only hope of cure is to deflower a virgin and thus pass on his disease to someone else.

Tolerance by society is the exception rather than the rule. As a result the patient tries to conceal his trouble for as long as possible, for the consequences may be compulsory segregation or shunning of the whole family by the community. Apparently healthy relatives are regarded as 'tainted' and may find it impossible to secure marriage partners, or those already married may be forced into divorce. Concealment of early (and treatable) leprosy lesions not only allows the disease to progress to irreversible deformity but also perpetuates an endemic situation.

BCG or *prophylactic dapsone* to contacts especially children offer good prospects for the successful control of leprosy, though further trials are needed to ascertain the exact role of both these methods of prophylaxis among susceptible communities. Thus, chemoprophylaxis with dapsone to children under 15 years of age who were contacts of lepromatous and other bacteriologically positive index cases, has recently given encouraging results in India and the Philippines.

Leprosy—Summary

(1) *Occurrence*—Indian subcontinent, tropical Africa, South-East Asia, South America
(2) *Organisms*—*Mycobacterium leprae*
(3) *Reservoir of infection*—Man
(4) *Mode of transmission*—Intimate contact
(5) *Control*— (i) Individual treatment with DDS
      (ii) Survey
      (iii) Static dispensaries or mobile clinics
      (iv) Education of society
      (v) BCG and/or prophylactic dapsone

Superficial Fungal Infections

A wide variety of fungi infect skin, hair and nails, without deeper penetration of the host tissues. The various clinical manifestations include favus, ringworm of the scalp, body, feet ('athlete's foot') and nails; some produce dyspigmentation, e.g. Tinea versicolor. The lesions are mostly disfiguring but apart from the aesthetic aspect some are disabling, e.g. athlete's foot could lead to splitting of the skin and secondary bacterial infection.

Medical geography
These infections have a world-wide distribution but some of the clinical manifestations such as ringworm of the feet tend to be more severe in the moist tropics. There are geographical variations in the incidence of various species, e.g. the predominant cause of tinea capitis in North America is *M. audouini* but it is *T. tonsurans* in South America.

The infective agents include species of *Epidermophyton*, *Trichophyton*, *Microsporon and Mallassezia furfur* (causative agent of Tinea versicolor).

Epidemiology
Man and animals represent the main reservoir of many of these infecttions but some of the fungi are also found in the soil. Domestic pets

play an important role for some infections, e.g. *M. canis* which is transmitted from dogs and cats.

Transmission may be from direct contact but also indirectly through contact with contaminated floors, barber's instruments, clothing, combs and other personal articles.

All age and racial groups are susceptible to these infections but some of the infections show variation with age and sex, e.g. ringworm of the scalp due to *Microsporon audouini* is most prevalent in pre-pubertal children. Subclinical infections occur; some of these organisms can be cultured from persons who do not show clinical signs.

Laboratory diagnosis

Specimens for examination include scrapings from the skin and nails, and also infected hairs. The organisms may be demonstrated on microscopy of skin scrapings which can be cleared with a solution of 10 per cent potassium hydroxide. Some of the organisms can be cultured on selective media such as Sabouraud's glucose agar at 20°C. Some of the fungal lesions in hairy areas display fluorescence when examined under ultraviolet light ('Wood's light') and this serves as a useful screening test.

Control

Prompt identification and treatment of infected persons will help to reduce the reservoir of infection, but the existence of subclinical infections may limit the value of this measure.

General hygienic measures in homes, schools and public places such as baths and swimming pools can help reduce the hazard of infection. The sharing of towels and other personal toilet articles should be discouraged. The handling of animals including domestic pets is also an avoidable risk.

Fungal Infections—Summary

(1) *Occurrence*—World-wide, but certain manifestations, e.g. clefts, are more severe in the tropics
(2) *Organisms*—Various species of *Epidermophyton*, *Trichophyton*, and *Microsporon*; also *Malassezia furfur*
(3) *Reservoir of infection*—Man, animals and soil
(4) *Transmission*—Direct contact, indirect contact with contaminated articles
(5) *Control*— (i) Personal hygiene
          (ii) Sanitation in baths and pools

Candidiasis

This is a mycotic infection which usually affects the superficial layers of the oral cavity (thrush), female genitalia, and other mucous membranes; lesions of the skin especially in the moist folds, may occur;

involvement of nails may present as chronic paronychia; and rarely the organism becomes disseminated systemically in debilitated persons, e.g. leukaemia and other neoplasms especially under treatment with corticosteroids, and broad-spectrum antibiotics.

The *incubation period* varies widely, but in children, it may be of order of 2 to 6 days.

Medical geography
It has a world-wide distribution.

Mycology
Candida albicans is the main pathogenic organism producing these lesions, rarely other organisms such as *Saccharomyces* may produce a similar oral lesion.

Epidemiology
Man is the reservoir of infection. Transmission is by contact with infected persons, both patients and carriers.

The carrier state is very common, the organism being found as part of the oral and intestinal flora. The occurrence of disease is therefore largely determined by host susceptibility. Newborn babies and infants, debilitated persons such as diabetics, cachectic patients with advanced cancer, and patients with advanced tuberculosis.

Ill-fitting dentures, tuberculous cavities and similar local factors may predispose to lesions of candidiasis. Treatment with broad-spectrum antibiotics may so alter the normal flora as to promote the overgrowth of these yeasts with consequent pathological manifestations. Housewives, cleaners and bartenders who soak their hands in water for long periods are liable to chronic paronychia due to candidiasis.

Transmission is by contact. The newborn infant may be infected by her mother during childbirth.

Control

This includes prompt treatment of infections using mycostatin, in severe cases. Genital infections should be treated in late pregnancy. Prolonged use of broad-spectrum antibiotics should be avoided.

Candidiasis—Summary

(1) *Occurrence*—World-wide
(2) *Organism*—Candida albicans
(3) *Reservoir of infection*—Man
(4) *Transmission*—Contact, during parturition
(5) *Control*— (i) Careful use of broad-spectrum antibiotics
        (ii) Elimination of local predisposing factors
        (iii) Treatment of pregnant women

Trichomoniasis
This is a chronic infection of the genital tract of both sexes. In the female, it presents with vaginitis accompanied by copious discharge; and with urethritis in the male.

The *incubation period* is from 1 to 3 weeks.

Medical geography
It has a world-wide distribution

Parasitology
The causative agent is *Trichomonas vaginalis*, a protozoan flagellate.

Laboratory diagnosis
Microscopy of wet film preparation of vaginal or urethral discharge may show the motile organism. The organism can also be identified in stained smears.

Epidemiology
Man is the reservoir of infection, the infected genital discharges being the source of infection. Transmission is by sexual intercourse or by indirect contact through contaminated clothing and other articles. Clinical manifestations occur more frequently in males than in females.

Control
Although the general principles for the control of venereal diseases apply, the main approach is the treatment of infected persons and their sexual partners. Improvement in personal hygiene is also important.

Trichomoniasis—Summary
(1) *Occurrence*—World-wide
(2) *Organism*—*Trichomonas vaginalis*
(3) *Reservoir of infection*—Man
(4) *Transmission*—Sexual contact—indirect contact through fomites
(5) *Control*— (i) As for other venereal diseases
          (ii) Improvement in general hygiene

Scabies
This is an infection of the skin by the mite, *Sarcoptes scabiei*. The skin rash typically consists of small papules, vesicles and pustules, characterised by intense pruritus. Another typical feature is the presence of burrows which are superficial tunnels made by the adult mite. Secondary bacterial infection is common. Lesions occur most frequently in the moist areas of skin, e.g. web of the fingers.

The *incubation period* ranges from a few days to several weeks.

Medical geography
The distribution of the disease is widespread in the tropics with particular concentration in poor overcrowded areas; it is also found in the temperate zones, especially in slums and where disasters such as wars have led to crowding and insanitary conditions.

Causative agent
The infective agent is the mite *Sarcoptes scabiei*. The female mite which is larger than the male, measures 0·3 to 0·4 mm. The gravid female lays its eggs in superficial tunnels. Within 3-5 days, the eggs hatch to larvae and nymphs which pass through four stages and finally moult after 3 weeks to become sexually mature adults. The adults pair and mate on the skin surface.

Epidemiology
Man is the reservoir of infection. There is a related species of mite in animals—*Sarcoptes mange*; man may acquire this infection on contact with infected dogs, but this mite cannot reproduce on human skin.

Transmission of scabies is by direct contact with an infected person or indirectly through contaminated clothing. Infection may be acquired during sexual intercourse.

All persons are apparently susceptible but infection is particularly common in children; several cases are commonly found within the same household.

Laboratory diagnosis
The adult mite can be seen using a hand lens, and identified under the microscope; the female mite can be brought to the surface by teasing the burrows with a sharp pointed needle.

Control
A high standard of personal hygiene must be maintained, with particular emphasis on regular baths with soap and water, frequent laundering of clothes, and the avoidance of overcrowding also help to prevent the spread of infection.

Infected persons should be treated by the application of benzyl benzoate emulsion or tetraethylthiuram monosulphide following a thorough bath. Other affected members of the family should be treated at the same time to prevent re-infection. Mass treatment may be useful in large institutions such as work camps.

Scabies—Summary
(1) *Occurrence*—World-wide, overcrowded poor areas
(2) *Organism*—*Sarcoptes scabiei*
(3) *Reservoir of infection*—Man

    (4) *Mode of transmission*—Direct contact; or indirectly through con-
taminated clothing

    (5) *Control*— (i) Improvement in personal hygiene
                (ii) Treatment of affected persons

Other Infections acquired through Skin and Mucous Membranes

Apart from infections transmitted by contact with infected persons, some infections are acquired through skin by exposure to infected soil (tetanus, hookworm), to water (schistosomiasis, leptospirosis) or animal bites (rabies).

Hookworm

This is an important intestinal parasite which occurs commonly in warm climates especially in communities with poor environmental sanitation. Anaemia secondary to blood loss is the most important clinical feature of hookworm infection. Although light to moderate loads of infection may be well tolerated in well-nourished persons who have an adequate intake of iron, heavy infection usually leads to iron-deficiency anaemia and occasionally to severe protein depletion. Thus, the occurrence of diseases in hookworm infection depends on the interaction of the load of infection, the state of the iron stores and the diet of the host.

Medical geography
The infection is endemic in the tropics and subtropics; it is receding from the more developed areas being most highly prevalent in the rural areas of the moist tropics. It occurs in various parts of tropical Africa, south-eastern USA, Mediterranean countries, Asia and the Caribbean. In parts of West Africa, N. *Americanus* is the predominant species, whereas *A. duodenale* is found in the Mediterranean area; in most other areas, in Asia, Central and South America, mixed infections occur.

Parasitology
The two main species which infect man are *Ancylostoma duodenale* and *Necator americanus*. The adult worms living in the intestine, are attached to the intestinal wall from which they suck blood; they migrate from site to site. The eggs are passed in faeces, and after hatching the larvae mature in the soil. The infective larvae may survive in the soil for many weeks. Man is infected on contact with soil, the infective larvae penetrating the unbroken skin and this may give rise to a pruritic rash (ground 'itch'). The larvae migrate to the lungs and ascend the trachea to be swallowed and carried to the intestine where the adult worms become established.

    The hookworms of cats and dogs, *Ancylostoma braziliense* and *A. caninum*, fail to achieve full maturity in man but may cause a serpiginous skin rash—cutaneous larva migrans.

Laboratory diagnosis
Hookworm infection is diagnosed by the identification of the eggs in stool; concentration methods are used for detecting light infections. Quantitative assessment of the load can be made by using a dilution method, e.g. the Stoll technique. The larvae can be cultured from stool on moist filter paper at room temperature, 25°C; the species of the worm can be identified from the larval stage or from expelled adults.

Epidemiology
Man is the reservoir of infection, the source of infection being the faeces of infected persons. Transmission is by contact with infected soil, usually in persons who walk barefoot. Light loads of infection are well tolerated, but anaemia will occur with larger loads, especially if dietary iron intake is low. In rural communities, adult male farmers have a high risk of severe infection.

Control
The most important measure is the sanitary disposal of faeces, thereby avoiding the contamination of soil.

The wearing of shoes is also protective but may not be practicable for poor peasant farmers.

Hookworm—Summary
(1) *Distribution*—Tropics and subtropical area of Africa, South America and Asia
(2) *Organisms*—*Necator americanus*; *Ancylostoma duodenale*
(3) *Reservoir of infection*—Man
(4) *Transmission*—Contact with contaminated soil.
(5) *Control*— (i) Sanitary disposal of faeces
         (ii) Wearing of shoes

Tetanus
This is an acute disease caused by the action produced by *Clostridium tetani*. The disease is characterised by an increase in muscle tone, and spasms, fever and a high mortality in untreated cases. Usually the hypertonia and the spasms are generalised, but in some mild cases, the muscle rigidity may be confined to a local area, e.g. a limb, and spasms may also be localised to the laryngeal muscles. Trismus is usually an early symptom. A peculiar grimace 'risus sardonicus' is often noted in these patients. In tetanus neonatorum, the first symptom is failure to suck in a baby who had sucked normally for the first few days after delivery.

The incubation is usually between 3 days and 3 weeks. The interval between the first symptom of stiffness and the appearance of spasms is known as the period of onset.

Medical geography
This is world-wide with a high concentration in some parts of the tropics. Farmers and others living in areas are usually more frequently affected than urban dwellers. With routine immunisation of children and prophylactic care of wounds, the disease is now rare in the developed countries.

Bacteriology
Clostridium tetani is a Gram-positive rod, an obligate anaerobe, which forms terminal spores giving it a characteristic drumstick shape. The spores are highly resistant to drying and to high temperatures; they may withstand boiling for short periods.

Epidemiology
The reservoir of infection is the soil and the faeces of various animals including man. The organism gains entry into the host through wounds; any wound may serve as the portal of entry for tetanus:

(a) *Post-traumatic*
Deep penetrating wounds especially when associated with tissue necrosis, and particularly when contaminated with earth, dung or foreign organic material. Superficial wounds including burns may also cause tetanus. The umbilical wound is the usual portal of neonatal tetanus.

(b) *Post-puerperal and post-abortal*
These arise from the use of contaminated instruments and dressings.

(c) *Post-surgical*
These may also be from instruments and dressings, but the infection may be endogenous, from the presence of the organism in the host's bowel or in his wounds.

(d) *Chronic ulcers and discharging sinuses*
Chronic ulcers, guinea-worm infections, chronic otitis media, infected tuberculous sinuses may serve as portals of entry.

(e) *Cryptogenic*
In a high proportion of cases, no focus is found, presumably some of of these are due to minor injuries which have healed.

All non-immune persons in all age-groups are susceptible. Infection does not confer immunity; repeated attacks occur.

Laboratory diagnosis
The diagnosis can be firmly made without laboratory tests. The isolation of the organism from the wound is of little value since it may be recovered from the wounds of persons who show no sign of tetanus.

Control

There are three main lines of prevention:

(1) *Antibacterial measures*
These include the protection of wounds from contamination, adequate cleansing of wounds and careful débridement. Antibiotics especially long-acting penicillin can also be given to suppress the multiplication of *Clostridium tetani*. If the wound is old, i.e. more than twelve hours, tetanus may occur despite an adequate dose of penicillin.

(2) *Passive immunisation*
Tetanus antitoxin (ATS) in the form of horse serum is used. 1500 units are given in the average case although a larger dose may be required for patients who present with heavily contaminated wounds. Repeated doses of ATS will lead to sensitisation of the patient creating the hazard of allergic reactions. These later doses are also rapidly eliminated from the body and therefore are less effective for prevention and treatment.

(3) *Active immunisation*
Active immunisation with tetanus toxoid is the most satisfactory method of preventing tetanus. Ideally everyone should be given a course of active immunisation. Booster doses can then be given periodically, e.g. every 5 years or whenever the person is injured. Special preparations are available for combined active-passive immunisation. Active immunisation of the pregnant woman will protect the infant from neonatal tetanus.

Tetanus—Summary

(1) *Occurrence*—World-wide, but very low incidence in developed countries as a result of immunisation programme
(2) *Organism*—*Clostridium tetani*
(3) *Reservoir of infection*—Man
(4) *Mode of transmission*—Through wounds
(5) *Control*— (i) Active immunisation with tetanus toxoid
     (ii) Toilet of wounds
     (iii) Penicillin prophylaxis
     (iv) Passive immunisation with antitetanus serum

Mycobacterium Ulcerans Infection (Buruli ulcer)

Mycobacterium ulcerans which results in the formation of chronic necrotising ulcers of the skin and subcutaneous tissues is being recognised as a common problem in many parts of the world. The predominance of lesions occur in the extremities.

Medical geography
The infection has been recognised in Australia, Uganda, Zaire, West Africa, Malaysia, Mexico and New Guinea. The condition is probably

more widespread in the tropics than is generally reported, being confused with tropical ulcer.

Bacteriology
M. ulcerans grows preferentially at a temperature of 32-33°C. It belongs to the group of slow-growing mycobacteria requiring 4-18 weeks to grow from initial isolation.

Epidemiology
The prevalence of Buruli disease varies considerably in the various reported areas. A careful recent study of the epidemiology of Buruli disease was carried out in Uganda, where the outstanding geographic feature was the distribution of Buruli lesions near the Nile. Thus, the section of the Kinyara refugee settlement closest to the Nile had the highest incidence of the disease. In these parts, more than 25 per cent of refugee children under 15 years of age developed Buruli lesions. The disease apparently is more common in sparsely settled areas, and may be related to the cultivation of previously undisturbed areas.

Buruli disease occurs from infancy to old age, but the highest incidence is in children from 5 to 14 years. Among adults it is more common among women than men. Two factors are mainly responsible for the age and sex distribution: immunity to the disease and exposure to the agent. People with a naturally positive tuberculin reaction are partially protected from Buruli disease. The most important reasons for the age, sex distribution and differences in anatomic sites are probably attributable to differential exposure. The method of transmission is unknown and the disease has only been tentatively included in this section until conclusive evidence of its mode of spread has been obtained. Atypical mycobacteria have been isolated from grasses in areas of high endemicity in Uganda. The usual *incubation period* is about 4 to 10 weeks. There is a peak seasonal incidence between September to November each year.

Laboratory diagnosis
Classically, histological examination of the lesions, reveals complete necrosis of subcutaneous tissue with numerous organisms in subcutaneous fibrous septa. There is a notable absence of inflammatory cells.

Control
(a) *The individual*
The first principle of surgical treatment is excision of all involved tissue; the second is early covering of the denuded area with skin.

(b) *The community*
BCG vaccination has given promising results. Health education emphasising to the communities the significance of the early lesion—a small nodule—has resulted in Uganda in an overall reduction in total hospitalisation and operative time, as well as the elimination of crippling deformities.

Schistosomiasis

This remains one of the most important parasitic infections in the tropics. Human infection, due mainly to *Schistosoma haematobium, S. mansoni* and *S. japonicum*, causes chronic inflammatory changes with progressive damage to various organs. The localisation of the worms varies from species to species. At first the lesions are granulomatous with damage to parenchymatous host cells; later fibrotic changes take place. Even after the worms have been eliminated, residual sequelae

TABLE 5.3

A classification of the course of Bilharziasis—based on parasitological, clinical and pathological aspects

STAGE	PARASITOLOGICAL	CLINICAL	PATHOLOGICAL
Stage of invasion	Migration and beginning of maturation	Incubation period, including cercarial dermatitis, if present	Slight inflammatory reactions in skin, lungs and liver
Stage of maturation	Completion of maturation and early oviposition	Toxaemic stage of the disease (or acute febrile stage) not always recognised or present	Allergic reactions, generalised and local to products of eggs and/or young schistosomes
Stage of established infection	Intensive oviposition accompanied by a corresponding egg discharge	Stage of early chronic disease, characterised for instance by haematuria, or intestinal and other digestive manifestations possibly with cardio-pulmonary or other complications	Local inflammatory reactions due to ova, resulting mainly in granuloma formation. Fibrosis is not a predominant feature
Stage of late effects	Prolonged infection (usually with reduced or discontinued egg extrusion)	Stage of late chronic disease, due to irreversible effects, and/or sequelae or complications	Progressing formation of fibrous tissue, with its consequences according to the organs involved intensity of infection and possibly other factors

may persist. Four clinical stages are identified (Table 5.3). Local dermatitis occurs at the site of penetration ('cercarial dermatitis'), fever and malaise may occur after the appearance of the skin lesions. Later during the migratory phase, more systemic manifestations may occur, fever, transient skin rashes, cough with radiological evidence of pulmonary infiltration and eosinophilia. These early manifestations of schistosomiasis are usually missed, and diagnosis is made only at the stage of established infection. *S. haematobium* mainly affects the urogenital system and classically presents with haematuria; later frequency and dysuria may occur.

The late effects of *S. haematobium* include contraction of the bladder, obstructive uropathy from involvement of the ureter and secondary bacterial infection; cancer of the bladder is associated with chronic vesical schistosomiasis.

Established infection due to *S. mansoni* and *S. japonicum* mainly affect the bowel with secondary changes in the liver. Initially, the patient may present with weakness, tiredness, loss of weight, anorexia, dysenteric symptoms, abdominal tenderness and hepatosplenomegaly. Late effects include progressive fibrosis of the liver and secondary portal hypertension. Infection with *S. japonicum* has been associated with cancer of the bowel. Ectopic lesions occasionally occur in the skin, brain, spinal cord and other sites. Pulmonary arteritis may lead to cor pulmonale in severe long-standing schistosomiasis.

Medical geography
It has been estimated that a total of about 200 million persons are affected in various parts of the world.

S. haematobium occurs in many parts of Africa, North, West, Central and East Africa, parts of the Middle East and a few foci in Southern Europe (Portugal).

S. mansoni is found in the Nile delta, West, East and Central Africa, South America and the Caribbean.

S. japonicum occurs in China, Japan, the Philippines and other foci in the Far East.

Parasitology
These worms are trematodes with the peculiar morphological feature in that the body of the male is folded to form a gynaecophoric canal in which the female is carried. The adult worms are found in the veins; *S. haematobium* are predominantly in the vesical plexus, *S. mansoni* in the inferior mesenteric veins and *S. japonicum* predominantly in the superior mesenteric veins.

Other schistosomes which infect man include *S. bovis*, *S. mattheei*, and *S. intercalatum*.

Life Cycle of the Schistosomes

The female lays eggs which pass through the bladder or bowel into urine and faeces respectively. A proportion of eggs are retained in the tissues and some are carried to the liver, lungs and other organs. If an excreted egg lands in water, it hatches and produces a free living form, the miracidium, which swims about with the aid of its cilia. It next invades an intermediate host, a snail of the appropriate species. Within the snail it undergoes a process of asexual multiplication, passing through intermediate stages of redia and sporocysts to become the mature cercaria. The cercaria, which is the infective larval stage for man, emerges from the snail and swims being propelled by its forked tail. On contact with man, the cercaria penetrates the skin, sheds its tail and becomes a schistosomule. The latter migrates to the usual site for mature adults of the species.

Intermediate hosts

All the intermediate hosts of schistosomes are snails belonging to the Gastropoda class in the orders Pulmonata and Prosobronchiata. Various species of *Bulinus* snails are the vectors of *S. haematobium*, whilst *Planorbid* snails, species of *Biomphallaria*, are the intermediate hosts of *S. mansoni*. Both *Bulinus* and *Biomphallaria* are aquatic snails which breed in ponds, lakes, streams, marshes, swamps, drains, dams, and irrigation canals. *Oncomelania* species, the intermediate host of *S. japonicum*, are amphibious snails, living in moist vegetation. These snail hosts are affected by physical factors such as temperature; and by chemical factors, pH and oxygen tension. The snails are hermaphrodite but not self fertilising; they lay eggs usually on vegetation; these hatch and grow to mature adult forms.

During the dry season, the aquatic snails aestivate in the drying mud, with the openings on the shells covered with dried mucus. Although snails with immature infections may survive the dry season, those with mature infections usually die. *Oncomelania*, being an operculated snail, survives drying much better than the non-operculated snails.

Laboratory diagnosis

Parasitological and immunological methods are used in the diagnosis of schistosomiasis. Eggs of *S. haematobium* are usually found in urine and occasionally in faeces. The optimal time for urine collection is around midday. For a quantitative assessment of the load of infection, a 24-hour collection of urine can be examined, or timed collection around midday (e.g. 11 a.m. to 1 p.m.) when egg count is highest, may be used. For *S. mansoni* and *S. japonicum* infection, examination of faeces may reveal the eggs; concentration techniques may be required for light infections; quantitative assessment should be based on the examination of 24-hour stool collections on two or more occasions. Eggs of *S. mansoni* are occasionally found in urine. Rectal biopsy ('rectal snip') is useful in diagnosing infections, particularly those due to *S. mansoni* and *S. japonicum* but it is also positive in some cases of *S. haematobium*; the specimen is easily obtained by curetting the superficial layers of the rectal mucosa and examining the material fresh between two glass slides; it can later be fixed and stained.

Other diagnostic techniques include cystoscopy, pyelography, liver biopsy, biochemical tests of hepatic and renal function. These are mainly used for the detailed assessment of individual patients but some have been adapted for field survey.

Immunological tests include a skin test in which antigen is injected intradermally and the size of the test wheal from the antigen is compared with a control.

A variety of serological tests, e.g. circumoval precipitin (COP), Cercariahüllen, fluorescent antibody tests, are used for the diagnosis of schistosomiasis; the tests are group specific and so cannot identify the particular infecting species. Some of the tests (e.g. COP) become negative after treatment or spontaneous cure, but others, e.g. the skin test, remain positive for indefinitely long periods. False positive results may occur in persons who have been exposed to avian and other non-human schistosomes.

Epidemiology
Man is the main reservoir of *S. haematobium* but naturally acquired infection with *S. mansoni* has been found in various animals including primates. *S. japonicum* is widely distributed in various mammals—cats, dogs, cattle, pigs and rats—and they constitute a significant part of the reservoir. Other schistosomes, e.g. *S. bovis* and *S. intercalatum*, are basically infections of animals with occasional infection in man.

Man acquires the infection by wading, swimming, bathing or washing clothes and utensils in the polluted streams. Certain occupational groups, e.g. farmers and fishermen, may be exposed to a high risk.

The age and sex distribution of schistosomiasis varies from area to area. One fairly common pattern is of high prevalence rates of active infection in children, who excrete relatively large quantities of eggs, and a lower prevalence rate of active infection among adults; the latter show late manifestations and sequelae. Epidemiological studies indicate that the load of infection is an important factor in determining the severity of pathological lesions and clinical manifestations.

Control
There are four basic approaches to the control of schistosomiasis:
  (*a*) Elimination of the reservoir
  (*b*) Avoidance of pollution of surface water

(*c*) Elimination of the vector
(*d*) Prevention of human contact with infected water.

(a) *Elimination of the reservoir*
Where the main reservoir of infection is human, mass chemotherapy would be a useful control measure provided a suitable drug is available. The ideal drug would be simple to apply, effective, safe and cheap. No schistosomicidal agent fulfils all these conditions. Limited success has been claimed for antimony drugs, for niridazole ('Ambilhar') in *S. haematobium* infection, and for *hycanthone* ('Etrenol') in *S. mansoni* infection. These drugs are rather expensive, often costing more than US $3 per patient per course, and all of them have significant toxic effects.

(b) *Avoidance of pollution of surface water*
This can be achieved by providing suitable sanitary facilities for the disposal of excreta and teaching people how to use them appropriately. It is important for the programme to include children since they usually have relatively high outputs of viable eggs. Unless the programme is highly successful, little benefit will be derived from these measures because infected communities usually produce many more eggs than are required to maintain infection in the snails.

(c) *Elimination of the vector*
Physical alteration of the habitat, e.g. drainage of swamps, may solve the problem by eliminating the breeding sites of the snails. Where such radical cure is not feasible, the situation can be improved by rendering the environment hostile to the snails, e.g. removal of aquatic vegetation, altering the flow rate of the streams, or building concrete linings to the walls of the drains.

Chemical measures are very useful now that more effective and safer molluscicides have been devised. The older chemicals, copper sulphate and sodium pentachlorophenate are being replaced by niclosamide ('Bayluscide') and N-trityl morpholine ('Frescon'); the latter two are safer and more effective. Molluscicides must be applied under the direction of those who have expert knowledge and experience to assure effective action against the snails and minimal risk to man and other living things. For the amphibian snail vectors of *S. japonicum*, calcium cyanamide or yuramin are very effective molluscicides.

Biological control has been attempted by the use of predatory fishes, e.g. *Astatoreochronics albiacide*. The most successful biological method has been through the use of the *Marisa cornuarietis* snail which feeds voraciously, thereby competing with *Biomphallaria glabrata*, and also it consumes their egg masses and their young. Great care needs to be applied in the use of this method lest the predator becomes a more serious menace.

(d) *Prevention of human contact with infected water*
This requires the provision of alternative supplies of safe water, thereby
eliminating the risk of exposure to infected streams. Where contact
with such waters is unavoidable, protective clothing such as rubber
boots should be worn; this may prove impractical for peasant farmers
or subsistence fishermen.

Schistosomiasis—Summary

(1) *Distribution*—*S. haematobium*—tropical Africa, Middle East
  S. mansoni—tropical Africa and South America
  S. japonicum—China, Japan and other areas in Far
  East
(2) *Organisms*—*S. haematobium*, *S. mansoni* and *S. japonicum*; also
  animal schistosomes including *S. mattheei*, *S. bovis*,
  and *S. intercalatum*
(3) *Reservoir of infection*—*S. haematobium*—man. *S. mansoni*—man,
  some primates and rodents. *S. japonicum*—
  man, various domestic and wild animals

Leptospirosis

This is an acute febrile illness usually accompanied by malaise, vomiting, conjunctival injection and meningeal irritation; in severe cases,
jaundice, renal involvement and haemorrhage may occur. The *incubation
period* is from 3 days to 3 weeks.

Medical geography
Various pathogenic species of leptospira are present in most parts of
the world. The occurrence of human disease is determined by the
distribution of the organisms in animal reservoirs.

Bacteriology
Leptospira are thin spirochaetal organisms, which can remain viable in
water for several weeks. Many different serotypes have been identified,
some of the common ones being *Leptospira icterohaemorrhagica* (the
agent of Weil's disease), *L. canicola* (canicola fever), *L. pomona*, and
L. bovis

Laboratory diagnosis
The organisms may be seen on microscopy of blood or centrifuged
specimen of urine using dark ground illumination, or of a thick blood
film stained with Giesma's technique. The organism can be isolated
on culture or by inoculation of blood intraperitoneally into hamsters
or guinea-pigs. The serotype is identified by serological tests.
Agglutinating and complement fixing antibodies can be detected in
infected patients.

Epidemiology
The reservoir of infection is in various vertebrates; both wild and domestic animals are involved—cattle, dogs, pigs, rats and other rodents, and reptiles. Urine is the source of infection.

The infection may be acquired by contact with infected water, the organism penetrating the skin, or by ingestion of contaminated water or food. Certain occupations carry the risk of exposure to leptospirosis, e.g. fish workers, persons working in sewers, rice paddies, or other collections of surface water, and soldiers who may have to wade across streams.

Control

Domestic animals should be segregated as far as possible from water sources for human use. The reservoir in wild animals should also be eliminated, e.g. by the control of rodents.

Human contact with potentially contaminated water should be avoided, and where such contact is unavoidable protective clothing be worn.

Immunisation for persons at high risk has been suggested using the local strain of leptospira as antigen; similarly pet dogs can be vaccinated.

Leptospirosis—Summary
(1) *Distribution*—World-wide
(2) *Organisms*—Leptospira species—various serotypes
(3) *Reservoir of infection*—Domestic and wild animals
(4) *Transmission*—Contact with polluted water—ingestion
(5) *Control*— (i) Limit animal contact with human sources of water
       (ii) Avoid contact with contaminated water
       (iii) Immunisation

Rabies

Rabies is a viral infection which produces fatal encephalitis in man. The clinical features include convulsions, dysphagia, nervousness and anxiety, muscular paralysis and a progressive coma. The painful spasms of the throat muscles make the patient apprehensive of swallowing fluids, even his own saliva ('hydrophobia'). Once clinical signs are established the infection is invariably fatal.

The *incubation period* is usually 4 to 6 weeks but it may be much longer, 6 months or more.

Medical geography
The infection is endemic in most parts of the world with the exception of Great Britain, Australia, New Zealand, Scandinavia, areas of the West Indies and the Pacific Islands. The disease is most commonly encountered in parts of South-East Asia, Africa and Europe.

Virology

The causative agent is a myxovirus which can be isolated and propagated in chick embryo or tissue culture from mouse and chick-embryos. The freshly isolated virus ('street virus') in experimental infections has a long incubation period (1 to 12 weeks) and it invades both the central nervous system and the salivary glands. After serial passage in rabbit brain, the virus ('fixed virus') multiplies rapidly solely in brain with a short incubation period of four to six days after experimental inoculation.

Epidemiology

Rabies is basically a zoonotic infection of mammals, especially the wild carnivores in the forest (foxes, wolves, jackals). The urban reservoir includes stray and pet dogs, cats and other domestic mammals, and in a part of South America, vampire bats play an important role in spreading infection to fruit bats, cattle, and other animals including man.

The transmission of the infection is by the bite of the infected animal, the virus being present in the saliva. It can also presumably be transmitted by the infected animal licking open sores and wounds. Airborne infection has been demonstrated in some special circumstances, notably in caves heavily populated by bats.

Rabies in Animals

With the exception of the vampire bat which tolerates chronic rabies infection with little disturbance, other mammals rapidly succumb to this infection once clinical signs develop. At first, there may be a change in the behaviour of the animal: restlessness, excitability, unusual aggressiveness or friendliness. Later, there are signs of difficulty in swallowing fluids and food. Paralysis of the lower jaw gives the 'dropped jaw' appearance in dogs. Finally the animal may become comatose and paralysed ('dumb rabies') but even at the terminal stage running around, attacking indiscriminately ('furious rabies').

Laboratory diagnosis

Various laboratory tests are used to establish the diagnosis in suspected animals or in human cases. The rabies virus may be demonstrated in the brain tissue, saliva, spinal fluid and urine, but brain tissue is most commonly examined. Microscopic examination of the brain may show characteristic cytoplasmic inclusion bodies (Negri bodies) in the nerve cells especially those of the hippocampal gyrus. These may be demonstrated on microscopic sections of the brain or by staining smear impressions from fresh brain tissue. The organism can be demonstrated by inoculation of suspected material into mice (intracerebral) or into hamsters (intramuscular), infection being identified by the presence of Negri bodies in the brains of the animals which die, by the fluorescent antibody technique or by neutralisation tests using specific antibody.

Control

In urban areas, the problem is best tackled by the control of dogs and also the appropriate management of cases of dog bite; stray dogs should be impounded and destroyed if unclaimed. Pet dogs, and preferably also cats, should be vaccinated every 3 years. In rabies-free areas, the importing of dogs, cats and other mammalian pets should be strictly controlled, such animals being kept in quarantine for at least 6 months. Whenever a dog is found to be rabid, other animals that have been exposed to it should be traced so that they can be vaccinated, kept under observation or destroyed. The control of rabies in wildlife is much more difficult. The risk can be minimised by trapping and killing wild animals which serve as reservoir of rabies.

Post-exposure Treatment

(1) *Local treatment.* The wound should be cleaned thoroughly with soap or detergent; an antiseptic such as chlorine bleach should be applied.

(2) *Artificial immunisation.* Rabies can be prevented in persons who have been exposed to risk by the use of active immunisation alone or in combination with passive immunisation. The decision to use artificial immunisation should be based on a careful consideration of the risk in each case.

Broad guidelines are provided in Table 5.4, but three points need to be carefully considered:

(a) *Prevalence of rabies in the area*
Vaccine may not be indicated in areas which are consistently free of animal rabies.

(b) *Biting animal: its species and state of health*
Carnivores are particularly important in the spread of rabies.

In the case of a dog bite, the animal should be captured alive if possible, and kept under observation for 10 days. If the animal has been killed or if it dies during the period of observation, steps should be taken to find out if it was rabid; the animal should be decapitated and the head sent to the laboratory. In the case of a wild animal, it should be killed and the brain examined for rabies.

It must be assumed that there has been exposure to rabies in cases of unprovoked bites by wild animals, or if the biting animal has escaped or been destroyed without examination. A dog which has been adequately vaccinated is unlikely to be rabid.

(c) *The site and extent of the bite*
Severe exposure. This includes cases of multiple or deep puncture

TABLE 5.4

Post-exposure treatment for the prevention of rabies

BITING ANIMAL		TREATMENT		
		TYPE OF EXPOSURE		
SPECIES	STATUS AT TIME OF EXPOSURE	NONE	MILD	SEVERE
DOMESTIC: Dog Cat	Healthy	None	None Begin vaccine at first sign of rabies in biting animal	Anti-rabies serum Begin vaccine at first sign of rabies in biting animal
	Signs suggestive of rabies	None	Rabies vaccine Stop treatment if animal is normal on fifth day after exposure	Anti-rabies serum plus rabies vaccine Stop treatment if animal is normal 5 days after exposure
	Rabid	None	Rabies vaccine	Anti-rabies serum plus rabies vaccine
	Escaped, killed Unknown	None	Rabies vaccine	Anti-rabies serum plus rabies vaccine
WILD ANIMAL	Regard as rabid if un-provoked attack	None	Anti-rabies serum plus rabies vaccine	Anti-rabies serum plus rabies vaccine

wounds; bites on the head, neck, face, hands or fingers. After such a severe exposure, the incubation period tends to be very short. Therefore, passive immunisation with anti-rabies serum is indicated.

Mild exposure. Single bites, scratches and lacerations away from the dangerous areas listed under severe exposure; also the licking of open wounds.

Two types of vaccine are available for active immunisation: the Semple type nerve-tissue vaccine and the duck embryo vaccine. The Semple type vaccine consists of rabbit brain material inactivated with phenol, it provides effective protection but carries the risk of allergic encephalitis. The duck-embryo vaccine is a suspension of duck embryo tissue infected with fixed virus neutralised with beta-propiolactone.

The primary course of immunisation consists of at least 14 injections, given subcutaneously starting with two doses per day for the first 7 days. This may be followed by 7 daily doses. Allergic reactions may occur. If encephalitis complicates the use of the nerve tissue vaccine, treatment with corticosteroids is indicated.

Passive Immunisation

Hyperimmune serum (at least 40 International Units/kg) should be given in cases of severe exposure as soon as possible after the bite. The usual precautions should be taken to prevent and deal with allergic reactions to horse serum. Where combined active-passive immunisation has been used, booster doses of the vaccine of non-nervous origin should be given 10 to 20 days respectively after the last dose of the 14-day course.

Pre-exposure Treatment

Certain persons such as veterinarians, dog catchers and hunters who run a high risk of rabies can be protected by using the duck embryo vaccine, e.g. two doses of 1·0 ml given 1 month apart, followed by a third dose 6 to 7 months later.

Rabies—Summary

(1) *Occurrence*—Endemic in most parts of the world except Great Britain, Australia, New Zealand, Scandinavia and parts of the West Indies and the Pacific Islands

(2) *Organism*—Rabies virus

(3) *Reservoir of infection*—Wild animals, strays and pets

(4) *Modes of transmission*—Bite of infected animals. Airborne in restricted circumstances

(5) *Control*— (i) Immunisation of pet dogs and control of stray dogs
(ii) Passive and active immunisation after exposure
(iii) Prophylactic immunisation of high-risk groups

Anthrax
This is an acute infection which may present as a localised necrotic lesion of the skin (malignant pustule) with regional lymphadenopathy; further dissemination will cause septicaemia. Pulmonary and gastro-intestinal forms of infection occur from inhalation or ingestion respectively of the infected material.

The *incubation period* is usually less than 1 week.

Medical geography
The infection is endemic in most agricultural areas both tropical and temperate.

Bacteriology
The causative agent, *Bacillus anthracis*, is an aerobic spore-bearing organism. The resistant spore survives drying, routine disinfection and other adverse environmental conditions; it remains viable for long periods on hides, skins and hairs.

Epidemiology
Anthrax is a zoonosis, the reservoir of infection being farm animals, cattle, sheep, goats horses and pigs. The animal products such as hides, skins and hair (e.g. brushes) are potential sources of infection.

Transmission may be by contact with these infected materials or animals. The organism may also be inhaled (wool sorter's disease) or swallowed, for example in contaminated milk.

Laboratory diagnosis
A smear of the skin lesion may show typical organisms as chains of large, Gram-positive rods. The organism can be isolated from skin, sputum or blood, by culture on blood agar. Virulence is tested by intraperitoneal injection into mice.

Control
Sick animals should be isolated. The carcasses of animals which die should be burnt or buried in lime, avoiding any contamination of soil. Animals and human beings at high risk can be immunised using a live attenuated vaccine. Animal products such as hides, bone meal, and brushes, should be disinfected usually by autoclaving where feasible. Protective clothing especially gloves should be worn when handling potentially infected material.

Anthrax—Summary

(1) *Distribution*—Widespread in agricultural areas
(2) *Organism*—Bacillus anthracis
(3) *Reservoir of infection*—Farm animals

(4) *Modes of transmission*—Contact with infected animals or their products. Inhalation. Ingestion

(5) *Control*—
  (i) Isolation of sick animals
  (ii) Careful disposal of infected carcasses
  (iii) Disinfection of hides, skins and hairs
  (iv) Protective clothing, e.g. gloves

Chapter Six

Arthropod-borne Infections

Arthropods play an important, and in some cases a determinant role, in the transmission of some infections. The epidemiology of these infections is closely related to the ecology of the arthropod vector, and hence the most effective measures for the control of these infections often relate to the control of the vector. The arthropod vector introduces a further dimension to the complex host-parasite interrelationship, and for some of these infections, a fourth factor is added when there is a non-vertebrate animal reservoir.

The Infective Agents
These include a wide variety of organisms ranging from viruses to helminths. The viral infections are known under the collective term 'arbo viruses', a contraction of 'arthropod-borne viruses'. These arboviruses cause a variety of clinical syndromes:

   (i) Fever
   (ii) Aseptic meningitis
   (iii) Encephalitis
   (iv) Haemorrhagic fever.

Vector-parasite Relationship
The vector may be specifically involved in the biological transmission of the infective agent, in which case, this is an essential phase in the life cycle of the agent. The phase within the vector which is often referred to as the *extrinsic incubation period* may involve (a) *morphological development* of the agent without multiplication, e.g. filiarial worms, (b) *Asexual multiplication*, e.g. arboviruses, plague, (c) *Sexual multiplication*, e.g. malaria. The extrinsic incubation period is important epidemiologically for only after its completion is the infection transmissible. Usually, the arthropod acquires the infection from an infected host but in a few specific instances the vector may acquire the infection congenitally by transovarian passage, e.g. mites in scrub typhus.

The vector may bring about a simple mechanical transfer of the agent from the source to the susceptible host. The housefly and other filth flies are important mechanical vectors of various infections especially gastro-intestinal infections, e.g. shigellosis, which rely on the faeco-oral route of transmission, and are dealt with in Chapter 4.

Mode of Transmission

In the case of mechanical tranfer of infections, the vector may carry the infective agent on its body or limbs, or the infective agents may be ingested by the vector passing through its body unmodified and excreted in faeces.

In most cases, biological transmission takes place when the vector bites the host. In this process, the vector may acquire the infective agents from the blood or skin tissues of the infected host or, alternatively, the infected vector may inoculate the infective agents from its salivary secretions into a new host, e.g. malaria.

In other cases, the host becomes infected through contamination of his mucous membranes or skin by the infective faeces of the vector, e.g. Chagas' disease; or by the infective tissue fluids which are released when the vector is crushed, e.g. louse-borne relapsing fever. The host may acquire infection by ingesting the vector; the transmission of guinea-worm occurs by this unusual route, when man ingests the infected cyclops, the crustacean intermediate host of this worm (see p. 75).

Host Factors

Many of the arthropod vectors which bite mammals show marked host preferences. Some of them bite man preferentially, and these are said to be *anthropophilic*; whereas others which bite animals preferentially are *zoophilic*. There is some evidence that mosquitoes are attracted to and bite some persons more often than others, but the basis for this preference is not as yet clearly understood.

Acquired immunity plays an important role in the epidemiology of some of the arthropod-borne infections. For example, previous exposure to the yellow fever virus may confer lifelong immunity; some protection from yellow fever may also be derived from exposure to related viruses of the B group. In other cases, immunity is of short duration and is not absolute, e.g. plague.

Control of Arthropod Infections

(1) Infective Agent.

(*a*) Destruction of animal reservoir, e.g. rats in the control of plague.
(*b*) Isolation and treatment of infected persons, e.g. yellow fever patient is nursed in a mosquito-proof room or bed.

(2) Route of Transmission

(a) *Control of vectors*
Preventing the vector from coming into contact with the human host.

    (i) *Biological barriers*, e.g. clearing an area to free it of breeding and resting places for the vectors; siting houses away from known breeding places of mosquitoes.

    (ii) *Mechanical barriers*, e.g. protective clothing, screening of houses, mosquito nets.

(b) *Destruction of the vectors*

    (i) *Trapping, collection and destruction of the vectors*. Various mechanical devices are in use, e.g. sticky strips to which flies adhere.

    (ii) *Chemical insecticides*. Some of these are active against the larval aquatic forms, others are directed against the adult vectors.

    (iii) *Biological methods*. These include the alteration of the physical constitution of the environment, and alteration of the flora and fauna.

Alteration of physical environment includes such things as the drainage of ponds, drying up of lakes and alteration in speed and course of a river. Alteration of the fauna may affect the food supply and shelter of the vector, e.g. by driving away the 'big game' from an area, there is a reduction in the food supply of *Glossina morsitans*, the vector of *Trypanosoma rhodesiense*. Alteration in the predator or parasite fauna may also affect the vector.

TABLE 6.1

Some examples of arthropod-borne infections

VIRUSES	RICKETTSIAE	BACTERIA	PROTOZOA	HELMINTHS
Arthropod-borne (ARBO-) viruses causing various diseases:	*R. prowazekii* var. *prowazekii* (louse-borne typhus)	*Pasteurella pestis* (Bubonic plague)	Malaria *Trypanosoma gambiense* *T. rhodesiense*	*Wuchereria bancrofti* *Brugia malayi*
(i) Fever	*R. mooseri* (murine typhus)	*Borrelia recurrentis*	*T. cruzi* *Leishmania donovani*	*Onchocerca volvulus*
(ii) Aseptic meningitis		*Bartonella bacilliformis*	*L. tropica*	*Ancanthocheilonoma perstans*
(iii) Encephalitis	*R. tsutsugamushi* (scrub typhus)		*L. mexicana* *L. braziliensis*	*A. streptocerca*
(iv) Haemorrhagic fever	*R. rickettsiae* (tick-borne typhus) *Coxiella burnetii*			*Mansonella ozzardi* *Loa loa*

Alterations in the flora may also affect food supply and shelter for the vector, as for example the clearance of low-level foliage to control *Glossina tachinoides* or the clearance of the water lily, *Pistia*, in the control of mansonia larvae and pupae.

(3) *Host*

Immunisation with an attenuated live virus gives protection against yellow fever, but specific immunisation is not generally available against other arboviruses. The use of specific chemoprophylaxis in the control of malaria and other arthropod borne infections is described in the section dealing with each infection.

The Arboviruses

The arthropod-borne viruses (arboviruses) may cause various syndromes in man or, alternatively, may present as atypical or subclinical infections only recognisable by antibody studies. The majority are zoonoses, and about 70 out of the 200 different arboviruses identified are known to cause disease in man. The definitive diagnosis depends upon isolation of the virus from patients early in the infection, with demonstration of a rise in titre of antibodies to the particular agent in at least two sera taken during the acute and convalescent stages of the disease.

Three main groups of arboviruses have been serologically defined as groups A, B and C, and the important viruses within these groups are listed in Table 6.2. The majority produce non-fatal infections. Control of the vector population where practicable will reduce the risk of infection. Steps can also be taken to avoid being bitten by vectors.

TABLE 6.2

Some clinically recognised arboviruses in the tropics. (After Horsfall and Tamm)

GROUP A	GROUP B	GROUP C	OTHER (grouped and ungrouped)
Chikungunya	Yellow fever	Apeu	Bunyamwera group
Mayaro	Dengue	Caraparu	Bwamba group
O'Nyong-Nyong	St Louis encephalitis	Itaqui	Phlebotomus fever
Venezuelian equine encephalitis	Japanese B encephalitis		Simbum group— Oporonche
Western equine encephalitis	Murray Valley encephalitis	Marituba	Tacaribe group— Junin
Eastern equine encephalitis	West Nile		Vesicular stomatitis group
	Ilheus	Nepuyo	Colorado tick fever
	Spondweni	Oriboca	
	Uganda S-H336	Ossa	
	Wesselsbron		
	Tick-borne encephalitis		Rift Valley fever
	Kyasanur Forest disease		California encephalitis complex
			Nairobi sheep disease
			?? Lassa fever

F

A number of arthropod-borne viruses infecting man, including sandfly fever and Colorado tick fever, do not fit into any of the groups so far described, which is indicative that other groups exist. Colorado tick fever is found in the United States, where small rodents are believed to be the normal hosts. Man, in whom it causes acute illness, becomes infected as the result of being bitten by the vector tick *Dermacentor andersoni*.

Because infection usually produces prolonged immunity, attack rates in all age-groups indicate the introduction of a new arbovirus, while disease confined to children implies reintroduction of virus or overflow from a continuous animal cycle to susceptible humans. Mosquitoes are the most common vectors of arboviruses, ticks the next most common, and *Phlebotomus* and *Culicoides* the least frequently involved.

Arboviruses: Group A

All the viruses in this group (about seventeen) have a number of general properties common to each other and to the rest of the arboviruses. The natural vectors or suspected vectors for all the known Group A viruses are mosquitoes. Clinically recognisable diseases of man have been described for:

   (i) *Chikungunya virus* which occurs in Africa, Thailand, Cambodia and India
  (ii) *Mayaro virus* which is found in Trinidad, Brazil and Bolivia
 (iii) *O'Nyong-Nyong virus* which produced an explosive epidemic disease in East Africa
  (iv) *Venezuelan equine encephalitis virus*. This is an apizootic of horses which affects man, and human outbreaks with fatalities have occurred in Venezuela, Colombia and Panama.

Arboviruses: Group B

The diseases most important to man result from infections with arboviruses of this group, most of which have mosquitoes as their vectors, with the exception of a subgroup which are tick-borne. Antigenic cross-reactivity is marked in the group B viruses, so that in areas where there is a high endemicity, e.g. tropical Africa, serological diagnosis may be difficult, and most rapid and definitive diagnostic method of active infection is by virus isolation. Many infections are symptomless. Clinically recognisable disease has been described for the following viruses in this group:

   (i) *Murray Vallay encephalitis virus* which occurs in Australia and New Guinea producing a high attack rate in children
  (ii) *West Nile virus* has been isolated in Africa, the Near East and India; it produces a dengue-like syndrome
 (iii) *Ilheus virus* is found in South and Central America and Trinidad

(iv) *Spodnweni, Uganda S-H336* and *Wesselsbron* viruses respectively occur in South Africa and Nigeria, Uganda and South Africa and in South Africa and Portuguese East Africa.

The most important diseases are (i) Yellow fever, (2) Dengnue fever, (3) Japanese B encephalitis, (4) Kyasanur Forest disease.

Diseases caused by Group B Arboviruses

(1) Yellow Fever

Yellow fever is an acute infectious disease of sudden onset and variable severity caused by a virus transmitted by mosquitoes. It is characterised by fever, jaundice, haemorrhagic manifestations and albuminuria. The *incubation period* in man is 3-6 days.

Medical geography
Yellow fever is endemic in large areas of South America and tropical Africa. The endemic zone in Africa approximately covers that part of the continent which lies between latitudes 15°N and 10°S. In South America the endemic zone stretches from south of Honduras to the southern border of Bolivia and includes the western two-thirds of Brazil, Venezuela, Colombia, and those parts of Peru and Ecuador which lie east of the Andes. Certain towns are considered as not forming part of these zones provided they maintain continuously an *Aëdes* index not exceeding 1 per cent. This index represents the proportions of houses in a limited, well-defined area in which breeding places of *Aëdes aegypti* are found. Epidemics occur from time to time and have comparatively recently been described from the Sudan, Ethiopia, the Senegal and Nigeria.

Yellow fever does *not* occur in Asia or the Pacific region, though the urban vector is widespread (*vide* South-East Asian haemorrhagic fever). It is not clear whether this is because the disease has not been introduced or because of a peculiar racial immunity, in any case the risk of introduction must be avoided at all costs. (Yellow fever *receptive areas*.)

Applied biology
Unmodified yellow fever virus attacks the cells of all three embryonic layers (pantropic). All strains show some degree of neurotropism, but the severity of the illness is largely due to the degree of viscerotropism shown; i.e. the degree of affinity shown for the abdominal viscera, particularly the liver. The degree of virulence shown by the virus can be modified by serial passage through mouse brain, or by culture in chick embryos or in tissue culture. The virus actually multiplies in the mosquito host: after biting an infected person or monkey, the mosquito itself becomes infective after an interval of about 12 days (extrinsic incubation period) and remains infective for the rest of its life. Mosquitoes are the only insects able to transmit infection.

Epidemiology

There are two main epidemiological forms of yellow fever:

(i) *Urban type.* The mosquito vector is *Aëdes aegypti*, which is primarily a domestic mosquito which breeds in or near houses, with the female preferring to lay her eggs in water collecting in artificial containers, such as old tins, etc.

The virus cycle in Man-Mosquito-Man; this method of spread requires large numbers of susceptible hosts, and hence tends to occur in

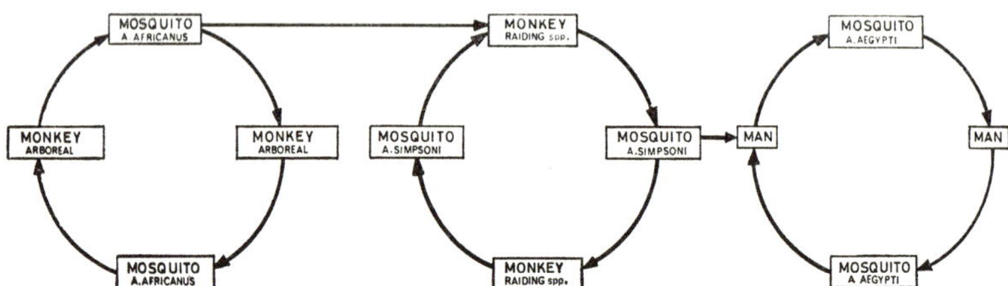

FIG. 6.1   Epidemiology of African yellow fever.

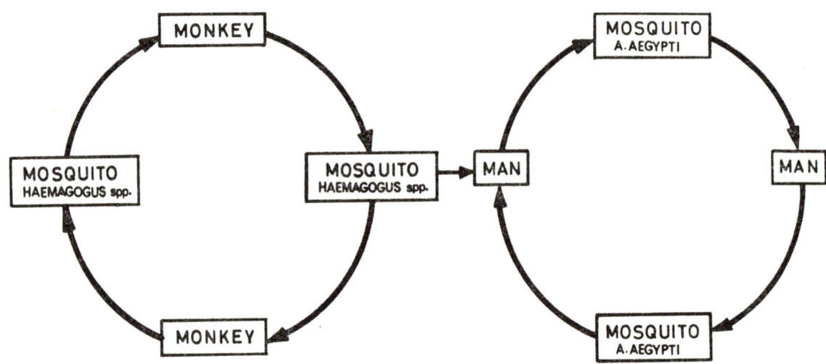

FIG. 6.2   Epidemiology of South American yellow fever.

large towns. Villages, with frequent passage of people from one village to another, will also be suitable for this type of spread. Urban-type yellow fever can effectively be controlled by anti-mosquito measures.

(ii) *Jungle type.* This may occur either in endemic or epizootic forms. In the endemic form, the disease, which is primarily one of monkeys, is almost constantly present, and sporadic cases of human infection occur from time to time. The primary spread of the virus is from monkey to monkey, via *A. africanus* in Africa and *Haemagogus* spp. in South America: both these mosquitoes live in the tops of trees. *Haemagogus* species will occasionally bite man, for example when a tree is felled, and South American jungle yellow fever is thus maintained.

In Africa, however, there is another way in which jungle yellow fever virus can be transmitted from the monkey to man. Certain monkeys have the habit of raiding crops, particularly bananas. Another mosquito, *A. simpsoni*, occurs on the edges of forests, and becomes infected by biting infected raiding monkeys, and then later bites the farmer when he collects his crop. *A. simpsoni* thus acts as a so-called 'Link-host'. It is important to remember that, in endemic areas, many cases of yellow fever are mild illnesses resulting in subclinical infections leading to immunity among the indigenous population.

Laboratory diagnosis

Virus isolation from the blood up to the 4th day of the disease is the diagnostic procedure of choice. Isolation of virus is by intracerebral inoculation of mice. After the 3rd day the mouse protection test can be used. This test involves demonstrating whether or not mice are protected from a challenge dose of the virus by antibodies in the patient's serum. A second protection test should be made some 5 days later. A significant rise of titre in the second sample would confirm the diagnosis, while an unaltered titre would only indicate an immunity due to a past infection or vaccination. It must be borne in mind that there may be cross-reaction with other viruses of the group B arbovirus group. Neutralisation, complement fixation, or haemagglutination inhibition tests are also employed, depending on the particular circumstances and the likelihood of previous exposure to other group B viruses. Histology of the liver in fatal cases establishes the diagnosis. Occasionally virus can be isolated from this organ.

Control

(a) *The individual*

Since the virus circulates in the blood during the first few days of the disease, a suspected case must be isolated for the first 6 days in a screened room or under a mosquito net. Steps should be taken at once to obtain laboratory confirmation of the diagnosis, but institution of control measures should not await results from the laboratory. Domestic contacts also should be isolated under screened conditions for 6 days, and the patient's house and all premises within a radius of 60 yards (55 m) should be sprayed with a residual insecticide. The first cases of yellow fever in an epidemic are likely to be mistaken for other illnesses, especially infective hepatitis. It is therefore very important always to remember the possibility of yellow fever in endemic areas and when in doubt to take blood for serological examinations or specimens of the liver (if necessary with a viscerotome) from corpses.

(b) *The vector*

In densely populated areas elimination of vector breeding must be undertaken at once. *A. aegypti* is a peri-domestic mosquito and will breed in practically anything that will hold water. This includes water containers such as jars and cisterns, as well as innumerable objects which may hold rain-water: defective gutters, old tins, jars and coconut shells (often hidden in the grass), and the bottoms of small boats and canoes. These breeding foci should be reduced as far as possible by suitable measures; water containers covered or screened, tins and other rubbish buried, and so forth. This is unlikely to prevent all breeding, but it will simplify treatment of the remainder by regular oiling or by addition of insecticidal briquettes.

Residual spraying of the interiors of all houses and out-buildings or of all surfaces close to breeding places (peri-focal spraying) will reduce the *Aëdes* population rapidly. Epidemic transmission will cease when the *Aëdes index* is reduced to below 5 per cent. To prevent introduction of an infected mosquito into countries where the disease is absent but conditions exist for transmission, aircraft coming from the endemic zone must be disinsecticised (by insecticidal aerosol) as specified by the World Health Organisation. This is particularly important in Asia, where vigorous antimosquito measures around airports should be carried out, international certificates of all persons coming from endemic zones scrupulously checked and adequate quarantine of animal reservoirs such as monkeys instituted. International notification provides health authorities with up-to-date information regarding the status of yellow fever throughout the world.

(c) *Immunisation*

Protection of scattered populations by vector control is, however, impracticable, and recourse must be had to vaccination of the whole community. This will afford protection for at least 10 years. Mass vaccination is advisable in epidemic conditions. Two vaccines are available: the 17D strain maintained by passage in chick embryo or in tissue culture and the Dakar strain maintained in mouse brain. This latter is prepared in a form which permits administration by scarification and is very suitable for use in scattered populations in rural areas. Infants under 1 year of age should preferably not be vaccinated, since encephalitis follows vaccination in this age-group more frequently than in adults. Some countries do not require vaccination certificates in the case of infants.

The spread of the disease is controlled by requiring all persons entering or leaving an endemic area to be in possession of a valid certificate of vaccination. Those not in possession of such a certificate may, on arrival in a non-endemic area, be subjected to quarantine for a period of 6 days from the date of last exposure to infection or until the certificate becomes valid. A vaccination certificate becomes valid 10 days after vaccination and remains so for 10 years. A certificate of re-vaccination done not more than 10 years after a previous vaccination becomes valid on the day of vaccination.

When vaccinations against both smallpox and yellow fever are needed, yellow fever vaccination should *precede* primary smallpox vaccination by a week. If primary smallpox vaccination is given first, then yellow fever vaccination should not be done before 3 weeks have elapsed. These intervals are advisable to lessen the risk of encephalitis, they are only applicable to persons being vaccinated for the first time or when many years have elapsed after a primary vaccination.

(2) *Dengue Viruses*

Dengue viruses produce, in general, a non-fatal, short, febrile illness, characterised by severe myalgia and joint pains. The occurrence of haemorrhagic phenomena with a significant mortality, especially in childhood, has been a feature of recent epidemics in South-East Asia. There are four main serotypes of Dengue viruses, numbers 1, 2, 3 and 4.

(a) *Dengue fever*

A. aegypti is the established mosquito vector of the dengue viruses responsible for dengue fever which is widely distributed throughout urban areas of the tropics and subtropics. The virus circulates in the blood at the onset of symptoms and for a few days. The extrinsic incubation period of the virus in *A. aegypti* is about 2 weeks. Infection confers immunity to the homologous strain for about a year. Diagnosis must be based on the clinical findings, intracerebral inoculation of blood in suckling mice, and other virological and serological tests. The only practical preventive measures are control of the vectors in their aquatic or adult stages as described for yellow fever. The prevention of mosquito bites by screening or repellents provides further protection.

(b) *South-East Asian haemorrhagic fever*

In recent years, epidemics of dengue with haemorrhagic phenomena have been reported from widely spaced regions—in Calcutta, the Philippines, Thailand, Malaysia and Singapore, and dengue viruses (3 and 4) have been isolated from *A. aegypti* during these epidemics. The epidemics have an urban distribution with cases clustered in the crowded, poorer, central districts of cities. The disease is usually seen in races of oriental origin; and haemorrhagic fatal manifestations are usually confined to persons under 15 years of age with a peak incidence in the 3-6 year group.

A fatal case of dengue haemorrhagic fever in an American child has recently been described from Thailand. Some outbreaks of haemorrhagic fever have been caused by the arbovirus *Chikungunya* (group A). On the whole the syndrome associated with chikungunya infection is milder than haemorrhagic dengue.

Control

Control of South-East Asian haemorrhagic fever is based on eradicating the urban vector mosquito *A. aegypti* as described for yellow fever.

(3) *Japanese B Encephalitis*

The majority of infections are inapparent or mild. The disease occurs in China, Taiwan, Korea, Japan, Malaysia, Singapore and India. The most efficient vector is *Culex tritaeniohynchus*, and the preferred vertebrate hosts are birds and domestic animals, e.g. pigs; man being only an incidental host. The virus is spread from rural to urban areas by viraemic birds. There are two peaks of incidence—under 9 years and over 60 years. Control of the vector mosquitoes is not practicable on a large scale. Isolation of pig sties from human habitats reduces the mosquito/man contact.

(4) *Kyasanur Forest Disease*

The virus of Kyasanur Forest disease has to date been found only in Mysore State, India. The disease occurs more frequently in the dry season and in persons working in the forest. The principal vector is the tick *Haemaphysalis spinigera*. Personal protection against the vector tick is the only practicable method of control.

Arboviruses: Group C

The group C viruses have only been isolated from Brazil, Trinidad, Panama and the USSR, while antibodies in man have been reported from Africa.

Other Viruses

Many other viruses, some grouped and others as yet ungrouped, are known to produce disease in man. The illness is usually mild and large segments of the population show neutralising antibodies to the various viruses resulting from subclinical infections.

(i) *Bunyamwera Group*

Bunyamwera virus was isolated from Uganda and neutralising antibodies have been detected from Uganda, Tanzania, Mozambique, Nigeria and other parts of Africa. No fatal cases have been reported.

(ii) *Phlebotomus Fever Group*

The diseases caused by viruses in this group are non-fatal. The vectors are various species of *Phlebotomus* and the distribution of the disease is limited between the latitudes 25° and 45°N. There are two types of viruses, the Sicilian and the Neapolitan. Sandfly fever appears epidemically over much of the tropics and subtropics, where it is transmitted by

Phlebotomus papatasii. Recovery from the disease is followed by a long-lasting immunity to the homologous strain of virus. Sandfly breeding can be controlled to some extent by clearing piles of rubbish and mending cracked and dilapidated walls. The insects are particularly susceptible to DDT, and have been drastically reduced in many places by residual house spraying employed for the control of mosquitoes.

(iii) *Simbum Group—Oporonche Virus*
Oporonche virus disease occurs in Trinidad and Brazil.

(iv) *Argentinian Haemorrhagic Fever*
Junin virus causes a severe and sometimes fatal disease characterised by fever, haemorrhagic manifestations and renal involvement. It occurs in Argentina and Bolivia and it is mainly a disease of adult male rural workers who seem to get infected at the time of the maize harvest in May. The mortality is greater in the older age-groups.

(v) *Rift Valley Fever Virus*
This virus causes a non-fatal disease in man, characterised by fever, myalgia, severe headache, epistaxis and occasionally ocular complications. It is widespread in Central and South Africa. The vectors are mosquitoes and the cycle is maintained through wild and domestic animals. Man is infected through contact with sick animals by inhalation of virus.

(vi) *Lassa Virus*
This virus has recently been isolated from patients suffering from Lassa fever, named after a village in Northern Nigeria. The incubation period is between 7 and 10 days and the disease presents with very high fever, a petechial skin rash, severe muscle pains, cardiac and renal failure. Although fatalities have occurred, Lassa fever probably includes a spectrum of illness, ranging from no symptoms or a mild disease to serious illness. No data yet exist to support the hypothesis that Lassa virus is an arthropod-borne virus.

Arbovirus Infections—Summary

	Yellow fever	Dengue fever	S.E. Asian haemorrhagic fever
(1) *Occurrence*	South America, Tropical Africa	Widely in tropics	S.E. Asia
(2) *Organisms*	Yellow fever virus	Dengue virus	Dengue virus
(3) *Reservoir of Infection*	Man, monkeys	Man	Man
(4) *Mode of transmission*	*Aëdes* spp. bites	*Aëdes* spp.	*Aëdes* spp.

| (5) *Control* | (i) Isolation of individual
(ii) Vector control
(iii) Immunisation | (i) Vector control | (i) Vector control |

The Rickettsial Diseases

The typhus fevers are caused by rickettsiae which are intracellular organisms living and multiplying in arthropod tissues such as those of the lice, fleas, ticks and mites. The rickettsial diseases of man can be divided into five main groups as shown in Table 6.3.

TABLE 6.3

Classification of rickettsial diseases

DISEASE	CAUSATIVE AGENT	VECTOR	ANIMAL RESERVOIR
A TYPHUS GROUP			
(i) Epidemic	*Rickettsia prowazekii*	*Pediculus humanus*	None
(ii) Brill-Zinsser disease	R. *prowazekii*	P. *humanus*	None
(iii) Murine	R. *mooseri*	*Xenopsylla cheopis*	Rat
B SPOTTED FEVER GROUP			
(i) American spotted fevers	R. *rickettsii*	Various species ticks	Many species of small mammals
(ii) African tick typhus	R. *rickettsii* var. *pijperi*		
(iii) Fièvre boutonneuse	R. *conori*		
(iv) Siberian tick typhus	R. *siberica*		
(v) Queensland tick typhus	R. *australis*		
(vi) Rickettsialpox	R. *akari*	Mite	
C SCRUB TYPHUS	R. *tsutsugamushi*	Trombiculid mites	Small mammals, mice and field rats
D TRENCH FEVER	R. *quintana*	P. *humanus*	None
E Q FEVER	*Coxiella burnetii*	None (ticks)	Cattle, sheep, goats and wild animals

Most of the rickettsial diseases have a world-wide distribution, and are not confined to the tropics.

The most important are epidemic louse-borne typhus, murine typhus, scrub typhus and, to a lesser extent, African tick typhus and Q fever.

(1) *Epidemic Louse-borne Typhus*

This acute disease is caused by R. *prowazekii* and is transmitted by the louse *Pediculus humanus*. The *incubation period* is about 10 days.

Medical geography

Epidemic typhus has a world-wide distribution but the incidence of the disease is generally low in tropical countries. Endemic foci exist in central Europe, Russia, China and North Africa. In the tropics it is common at high altitudes and in deserts.

Epidemiology

This disease is commoner in cold climates than in the tropics. Man is the main reservoir of infection although in Tunisia serological evidence has been obtained that the rat may also be a reservoir of epidemic typhus in that country. In Ethiopia it has lost its overwhelming dominance and epidemic typhus is now the least common of the rickettsial infections. The louse becomes infected by feeding on a person with the disease from 2 days before symptoms appear until the end of fever. The rickettsiae multiply in the cells of the louse midgut, and when these rupture the organisms are discharged in the faeces. Human infection follows contamination of breaches of the skin surface by infected louse faeces. The rickettsiae can remain viable for months on dried louse faeces, and may possibly cause infection through the conjunctiva or by inhalation, as well as percutaneously. Recovery is followed by immunity, which persists for several years. In some patients the infection appears to remain latent after symptoms have subsided and to relapse some years later (Brill's disease).

Laboratory diagnosis

This is established by the Weil-Felix reaction, in which B. *proteus* OX_{19} is agglutinated and also OX_2 to a lower titre, or more specifically by the complement-fixation test using suspensions or extracts of the specific organism.

Control

Delousing of the whole population with residual insecticidal powders is the principal control measure.

(a) *The individual*

Sporadic cases are isolated and deloused, but isolation of infected persons is not practicable in epidemics. On admission to hospital, the patient should be bathed with soap and water or a 1 per cent solution of lysol. The tetracyclines are highly specific and are given in a dosage of 10 mg per kg, four times daily. They must be continued for 3 days after the temperature is normal. Contacts should be deloused and kept under observation for 2 weeks. The patient's clothes and bedding should be sterilised and his house sprayed with residual insecticides.

(b) *The community*
Mass delousing of the entire population controls epidemic typhus. This is carried out by blowing insecticide (commonly 10 per cent insecticidal powder) with a dusting-gun under the clothes next to the skin over the whole body, the operation occupying only a few minutes. In some areas lice have become resistant to DDT, and other residual insecticides must be used, such as BHC.

(c) *Immunisation*
Vaccines containing attenuated strains of epidemic or murine rickettsiae will give some degree of protection for about 6 months and may be used in endemic areas before seasonal transmission starts. Dosage is 1 ml subcutaneously on two occasions at weekly intervals with booster doses every 6 months.

(2) *Murine Typhus*
The disease is caused by R. *mooseri* and transmitted by rat fleas. The *incubation period* is 10-12 days.

Epidemiology
Murine typhus has a world-wide distribution. Flea-borne (murine) typhus is widely distributed and occurs wherever the rat lives in close association with man, e.g. grain stores, irrespective of climate. In a recent serological survey carried out in the Ivory Coast, varieties of murine typhus had an overall frequency of 4·5 per cent but were more prevalent among adults (6 per cent) and also more frequent in the coastal regions (7 per cent). Converted old rat-infested farmhouses are sometimes foci of infection. Murine typhus is essentially a rodent infection which appears sporadically in man. It exists throughout the world, and the organism *Rickettsia mooseri* is conveyed to man by the faeces of infected rat-fleas of the genus *Xenopsylla* or the rat-mite *Bdellonyssus bacoti*. The Weil-Felix test gives the same reaction as in epidemic typhus.

Control
Control of murine typhus is rarely required, but if needed the anti-rat and anti-flea measures employed in plague will be effective. Individual patients should be treated with antibiotics as in epidemic typhus (see above).

(3) *Mite-borne Typhus*
Scrub typhus (tsutsugamushi disease; Japanese river or flood fever

tropical typhus; rural typhus) is an acute febrile disease characterised by fever, a cutaneous rash which appears on the 5th day, and an eschar at the site of attachment of the trombiculid mites which transmit the disease. The causative organism is *Rickettsia tsutsugamushi* (*R. orientalis*). The *incubation period* is about 12 days.

Medical geography
Mite-borne typhus occurs in Japan, Thailand, other countries in East and South-East Asia, some Pacific islands and Queensland in Australia. The distribution of scrub typhus is closely related to certain physical and ecological factors which produce 'scrub typhus country', resulting in a recurring cycle of passage of rickettsiae between rodents and mites with a spillover into man.

Epidemiology
'Scrub typhus' is enzootic in wild rodents and the two most important vectors are the larvae of *Trombicula akamushi* and *T. deliensis*. In Indonesia the rat flea is the vector. The reservoir of infection are rodents, and man becomes infected when the larval mites feed on blood. Only the larval mites feed on the vertebrate hosts' blood, and since the larva only feeds once, the rickettsiae persist through the nymph, adult and egg stages into the larval stages of the next generation, which are thus infective. Man contracts the disease by exposure, e.g. walking or resting in infected foci, particularly after slight rain or heavy dew.

The disease may be encountered in grassy fields, along the river banks, in abandoned rice-fields, in forest or jungles, and in the neglected shrubby fringes between field and forest. The different epidemiological patterns of the disease are related to the influence of climatic variations on the life cycle of the trombiculid mite vectors. The seasonal ocurrence of tsutsugamushi disease in Japan corresponds exactly with the time of appearance of each species of vector, *T. akamushi* in summer; *T. scutellaris* in autumn and winter; and *T. pallida* in winter and early spring. While the terrain of *T. akamushi* is limited to places along the rivers, other vectors seem to extend far beyond river banks. In Malaysia, scrub typhus occurs throughout the year. Man is only an accidental host, while field-mice, rats, possibly other small mammals, and ground-frequenting birds are the natural hosts responsible for the continuing transmission of *R. tsutsugamushi* from infected to uninfected mites. The mites function both as vector and reservoir since transovarial transmission of rickettsial infection occurs.

The presence of scrub-typhus infection in rodents or trombiculid mites in unusual habitats in West Pakistan—e.g. alpine terrain at 10 500 ft, semi-desert and desert 'oasis greenhouse'—has been reported.

Laboratory diagnosis

A diagnosis of scrub typhus can be made by recovering R. *tsutsu-gamushi* from the blood of a patient during the febrile period by culture in living-tissue culture media, or in the yolk-sac membrane of developing chick embryos. Intraperitoneal inoculation of blood or of tissue into white mice results in fatal illness, and on autopsy there is a white peritoneal exudate with numerous organisms in the peritoneal cells. The organism can also be recovered from human tissue taken at post-mortem.

The most widely used serological test for the diagnosis of scrub typhus is the Weil-Felix reaction. Agglutinins for Proteus OXK, but not for Proteus OX_{19} or OX_2 appear in the patient's serum about the 10th day of the disease reaching a maximum titre by the end of the third week, after which they rapidly decline. Serial examination reveals a four-fold or greater rise in titre. The complement-fixation test has also been used for diagnostic and sero-epidemiological surveys. Indirect immunofluorescence employing smears of rickettsiae as antigen can be used for the specific diagnosis of scrub typhus.

The results obtained by Weil-Felix tests from patients with various forms of typhus are summarised in Table 6.4.

TABLE 6.4

Weil-Felix reaction in typhus fevers

	STANDARD STRAINS		
TYPHUS FEVER	OX_{19}	OX_2	OXK
Mite-borne	−	−	+ + +
Tick-borne	− to + +	− to + +	−
Louse-borne	+ + + to −	+ + to −	−
Flea-borne			

In the majority of cases of louse-borne and flea-borne typhus OX_{19} is agglutinated to a high titre; while in tick-borne typhus OX_{19} and OX_2 are only agglutinated to a low titre.

Control

Control measures are based upon (i) control of the ecology, (ii) anti-mite measures and (iii) chemoprophylaxis and treatment of individual cases.

(i) *Control of the ecology*
The ecology of scrub typhus must be clarified in each area where it occurs before control measures can be successful. The ecology will

differ in different geographical areas, from the abandoned rubber plantations of Malaysia to the scrub typhus oases of Pakistan.

Known endemic areas which are often localised to small geographical sites should be avoided for the construction of camps and living-quarters. These areas are frequently second-degree growths in de-forested areas. Prospective camp sites may be prepared by cutting all vegetation level with the ground and burning it. After thorough clear-ing, the ground dries sufficiently in 2 or 3 weeks to kill the mites. If the site is required immediately, it should be sprayed with dieldrin or gamma Benzene hexachloride (0·25-1 kg per acre).

(ii) *Anti-mite measures*
Clothing must be rubbed or impregnated with dimethyl or dibutyl phthalate, benzyl benzoate or benzene hexachloride. These kill the mites on contact. Particular care should be given to those parts of the clothing that give access to the interior of the garment.

(iii) *Chemoprophylaxis*
Tetracyclines 3 g orally once weekly, will permit individuals to remain ambulatory even though rickettsiaemia will occur from time to time. The drug must be continued for 4 weeks after leaving the endemic area, otherwise clinical disease will occur within a week of withdrawal of the drug. Clinical cases respond to tetracyclines 3 g (loading dose) followed by 0·5 g 6-hourly until the temperature is normal.

(4) *African Tick Typhus*
This is found in Africa south of the Sahara, West Africa, East Africa (Kenya), South Africa, the Sudan, Somalia and Ethiopia.

The disease is contracted by man from ticks in the bush, where the reservoirs are wild rodents. Occasionally, the infection may be brought into suburban areas by dog ticks on domestic dogs. Transovarial transmission occurs in the tick. African tick typhus is a mild disease in man and deaths are almost unknown. A primary eschar is found at the site of the tick bite. Inapparent infections do not occur, although mild abortive attacks without a rash are not uncommon.

Control
No quarantine measures are necessary. Tetracyclines are specific in treatment as for scrub typhus. If antibiotic therapy is given at the time of appearance of the primary eschar, the attack will be aborted. Break-ing the tick/man contact is the most effective control measure. Known endemic areas should be avoided during the tick season when they are most active. When camping in these areas, individuals should sleep off the ground on camp beds. Where dogs act as tick carriers, then the animals, if they are household pets, should be regularly examined for ticks, which must be removed. Proper clothing should be worn, and

the shirt tucked inside the trousers. Socks and high boots should be worn outside the trousers. Since ticks rarely transmit the infection until they have fed for several hours, an important precaution is to remove the clothes and search both body and clothing twice daily, removing the ticks gently with a gloved hand or with forceps.

(5) Q Fever

This infection due to *Coxiella burnetii* has a world-wide distribution. The rickettsiae are distributed widely in nature in ticks, human body lice, small wild mammals, cattle, sheep, goats, birds and man. The epidemiology varies in different parts of the world, according to the local geographical and environmental factors present.

The infection is maintained in domestic animals, mainly by wild animals, ticks, domestic animal association, and man acquires the infection as an occupational hazard by direct contact with milk. Secondary cases are caused by the inhalation of infected dust or from human carriers, when the infection is transmitted from man-to-man, via the respiratory tract. Many mild and inapparent infections undoubtedly occur.

The epidemiology of Q fever is complex, but most human infections are acquired directly or indirectly from domestic animals (see p. 220).

Control

Control of the disease on a community basis rests upon control of the disease in domestic animals either by immunisation or by antibiotics. This requires a large economic effort. Milk from goats, sheep, and cows should be pasteurised. Calving and lambing processes in endemic areas should be confined to an enclosed area which can be decontaminated after the products of parturition have been disposed of. Immunisation is the most effective control measure from the individual point of view.

Vaccination will prevent infection with Q Fever amongst high-risk laboratory workers and in heavily exposed industrial groups, such as farm workers in endemic areas and workers handling farm products such as meat and milk. A standard vaccine Q-34, prepared by Cox's method from formolised *C. burnetii* and containing 10 complement fixing units per ml is given in 1 ml doses as 3-weekly subcutaneous injections. Preliminary skin testing with 0·1 ml of a 1/50 dilution of the vaccine should be performed to avoid reactions. Successful vaccination is shown by the development of a positive skin reaction after 40 days.

Typhus Fevers—Summary

	Louse-borne	Flea-borne	Mite-borne
(1) *Occurrence*	Central Europe, China, North Africa	World-wide	South-East Asia, Far East
(2) *Organisms*	R. *prowazekii*	R. *mooseri*	R. *orientalis*

(3) *Reservoir of infection*	Man	Rodents, man	Rodents
(4) *Mode of transmission*	Contamination by infected louse faeces	Contamination by infected rat faeces	Bites of mites
(5) *Control*	(i) Mass delousing (ii) Personal hygiene	(i) Anti-flea measures (ii) Anti-rat measures	(i) Control of ecology (ii) Anti-mite measures (iii) Chemoprophylaxis

The Bacterial Diseases

Plague

Plague is a rapidly fatal disease due to *Pasteurella pestis* which can manifest itself in a variety of ways—bubonic, pneumonic and septicaemic forms. The *incubation period* is 2-4 days.

Medical geography

Although the number of cases of plague have gradually declined, foci of the disease still exist in the Indian subcontinent, China, South-East Asia, Africa, South America and the Middle East. A noteworthy feature has been the continuing importance of the disease in Vietnam. The principal endemic foci are India, China, Manchuria, Mongolia, Burma, Vietnam, East Africa, Malagasy Republic, Brazil, Bolivia, Peru and Ecuador.

Bacteriology

The organisms are small, Gram-negative, ovoid bacilli showing bipolar staining. *Pasteurella pestis* is easily destroyed by disinfectants, heat and sunlight but in cold or freezing conditions it can survive for weeks or months.

Epidemiology

The reservoir of infection is rats and non-domestic rodents. The bubonic disease which is the commonest is transmitted by the bite of an infected rat flea *Xenopsylla cheopis* while pneumonic plague spreads from person to person by droplet infection.

(a) Bubonic Plague

The occurrence of plague in a human population is always preceded by an enzootic in the rat population and hence any unusual mortality among rats should be looked into promptly. Plague spreads rapidly wherever the human population is congested, living in insanitary conditions where rats are numerous and have access to food. When a flea ingests infected blood the plague bacilli multiply in its gut and may gradually block the flea's proventriculus. As a result, the flea cannot feed, becomes hungry and tries repeatedly to bite, regurgitating plague bacilli into the puncture at each attempt. These so-called 'blocked-fleas' are a very important factor in the dissemination of human disease. In temperate climates plague is common in the warmer months (i.e. summer), while in the tropics it appears in the colder months (i.e. winter). The efficiency of flea transmission declines with increasing temperatures. All ages and either sex may be infected. Plague spreads from region to region chiefly through rats in ships and strict surveillance is needed in busy seaports. Serological evidence indicates that there are a substantial number of asymptomatic plague infections.

Plague also occurs in non-domestic rodents—*wild rodent plague*—and epizootics affect many different species throughout the world. The infection is transferred to rats living in urban areas from wild rodents and thence to man. In rural areas man, e.g. hunters and trappers, can be infected in the field, bring the disease home, infect their own domestic rats and fleas and thereby their families.

(b) *Pneumonic Plague*

Pneumonic plague is transmitted from person to person by 'droplet infection' from patients suffering from primary pneumonic plague or from individuals with bubonic plague who develop terminal plague pneumonia—neither rats nor fleas play a part in the spread of the disease. Overcrowding favours dissemination of pneumonic plague. Recently in Vietnam, a mixed pneumonic bubonic plague outbreak occurred and *P. pestis* was recovered from the throats of asymptomatic healthy carriers.

Laboratory diagnosis

P. pestis may be detected in smears of material aspirated from buboes, from sputum, or even from the blood stained by Gram's method. Culture and animal inoculation should be performed. Smears from the spleen are positive at necropsy. Specimens of material aspirated from buboes, throat swabs and sputa can now be placed in a special holding medium which maintains the organisms in a viable condition during transport to distant laboratories. Fluorescent antibody, complement fixation, and haemagglutination techniques have also been used.

Control

Plague is a notifiable and quarantinable disease and the quarantine period laid down by the International Sanitary Regulations is 6 days.

(a) *The individual*

Cases of **bubonic** plague should be removed to hospital and isolated. Care should be taken in the nursing of such cases in case they develop pneumonia and hence masks and gowns should be worn by attendants. Contacts should be kept under surveillance for 6 days and dusted with DDT powder. All patients should be treated with streptomycin (2-4 g daily up to a total of 20 g) or the broad-spectrum antibiotics of the tetracycline series, (2-6 g daily up to a total of 40 g) as early as possible. The overall fatality rate of untreated bubonic plague is between 20 and 75 per cent while untreated pneumonic plague is almost invariably fatal. Prompt and adequate therapy reduces the overall mortality to less than 5 per cent.

Pneumonic plague is a highly infectious disease and immediate and strict isolation is vitally important. The patient, his clothing, his house and everything he has been in contact with must be disinfected. Medical and nursing staff attending such patients must wear protective clothing, including goggles. Strict surveillance of all contacts must be carried out daily and prompt isolation and treatment of infected cases carried out. While in hospital the strict 'current disinfection' must be done throughout the course of the disease.

All personnel engaged in flea or rat control during an epizootic must wear protective clothing impregnated with DDT, while dead rats should be sprinkled with DDT, and handled and disposed of carefully.

(b) *The community*

The immediate and widespread use of DDT in dusting rat-infested areas and thus eliminating the fleas is the most important single control measure that interrupts transmission. The elimination of fleas is coupled with the systemic destruction of rats which should commence on lines extending radially from the centre of infection in order to delimit the enzootic area. All rats caught should be examined for evidence of plague and any new foci infection found treated with DDT. The systemic rat trapping and destruction is followed by measures such as rat-proofing of houses and buildings, protection of food and sanitary disposal of refuse. Rat-proofing of ships and general maintenance of ship hygiene should be encouraged. Port health authorities are particularly responsible for supervising this and constant vigilance is required especially in busy ports such as Singapore.

(c) *Immunisation*

Personal protection is provided by the use of a dead vaccine or attenuated live vaccine of *P. pestis*. The latter is given in a single dose while two doses of the dead vaccine are required at weekly intervals. Protection commences a week after inoculation and lasts for about 10 months.

Most authorities also recommend *chemoprophylaxis* for all contacts of both forms of plague—tetracyclines 2 g daily for 1 week or sulpha-dimidine 3 g daily for 1 week.

Plague—Summary

(1) *Occurrence*—South-East Asia, South America, Middle East, Africa
(2) *Organisms*—*P. pestis*
(3) *Reservoir of infection*—Rats (bubonic), man (pneumonic)
(4) *Modes of transmission*—Flea bite (bubonic), droplet (pneumonic)
(5) *Control*— (i) Isolation
            (ii) DDT for elimination of fleas
            (iii) Rat destruction
            (iv) Raising standards of environmental hygiene

The Relapsing Fevers

Relapsing fever is due to infection of the blood by morphologically indistinguishable strains of spirochaetes which are transmitted by ticks resulting in endemic disease, and by body lice resulting usually in epidemic disease. The louse-borne spirochaete is known as *Borrelia recurrentis* while the tick-borne spirochaetes are often named according to their tick vector.

(1) *Tick-borne Relapsing Fever*

Non-epidemic relapsing fever is due to infection with *Borrelia duttoni* and is transmitted by a number of ticks, of which the African *Ornithodorus moubata* is one of the most important. The *incubation period* is 3-10 days, and recovery is followed by immunity lasting about a year.

Medical geography

The disease occurs in Central, East and South Africa as well as in North Africa, North, Central and South America, the Middle East and northern India.

Epidemiology

In most areas *B. duttoni* normally affects rodents and occurs only acci-dentally in man, while in central Africa it primarily affects man, in whom it is endemic. The vector in South America is *Ornithodorus rudis*. The other vector species are not domestic in habit, and they feed primarily on rodents and other small mammals. The disease, therefore, is highly endemic where the vector is domestic in habit and very spora-dic in areas where human contact with the tick is in open country or caves. The tick lives in the soil of the floor, or the mud-plaster walls of African huts; they are also found in caves and in the soil of bush or scrub country. The female lays batches of eggs each of which hatches to produce a larval tick with three pairs of legs. The larval forms pass through about five moults at intervals of 2 weeks. Larval forms and adults feed by sucking blood. A proportion of the offspring of infected female ticks are infected transovarially, thus the infection may persist through several generations. During feeding a saline fluid, called coxal fluid, is excreted from glands near the attachment of the legs.

It is generally believed that the infected fluid exuded by the coxal glands, saliva and bowel contaminates the wound made by the bite of the tick and spirochaetes enter the bloodstream.

Humans entering caves, working in bush country, living in infected African huts, or sleeping in rest houses in the vicinity of infected villages are liable to acquire the infection. It seems that babies and little children are very susceptible to the disease and it appears that immunity is acquired with increasing age by those living in endemic areas. There are several reports in the literature of newborn infants developing relapsing fever within the first 10 days after birth, but no case of congenital infection has been recorded. It has been suggested that infection is transmitted after birth during the process of suckling, possibly from cracks in nipples, to abrasions in the child's mouth. Although *B. duttoni* will infect lice, no large-scale change in vector has been proved to occur under natural conditions.

Control

(a) *The individual*
In areas where transmission is by non-domestic vectors control consists in wearing protective clothing, such a high-legged boots, or in using repellents.

(b) *The vector*
Domestic vectors can be controlled by treating the interiors of houses with benzene hexachloride or dieldrin. Spray treatments (usually suspensions) have been used in dosages ranging from 0·2 up to 6 g *gamma* BHC per square metre; the higher dosage will give protection up to a year or more.

(c) *The community*
The most satisfactory control results from rehousing the people in buildings which provide no harbourage for ticks.

(2) *Louse-borne Relapsing Fever*
This disease is usually epidemic and has a similar geographical distribution as epidemic typhus. The *incubation period* is usually from 2 to 10 days. In an attack of louse-borne relapsing fever there are only one or two, and never more than four relapses, and death, as opposed to tick-borne relapsing fever, is often in the first attack. Fever, headache, skeletal and abdominal pain, and the usual symptoms of acute infection are common. Tachypnoea, upper abdominal tenderness with a palpable

liver and spleen, jaundice and purpura occur. Hyperpyrexia, hypotension and cardiac failure can be fatal.

Medical geography
Louse-borne relapsing fever is more common in temperate than tropical climates, but outbreaks of epidemic louse-borne relapsing fever have occurred in parts of Africa, India and South America. The disease is endemic in Ethiopia.

Epidemiology
Like epidemic typhus fever, which it may accompany, it is associated with poor sanitation and personal hygiene, particularly overcrowding, undernutrition and lice-infested clothing. It is conveyed from one man to another by the human body louse *Pediculus humanus*, and the spirochaete responsible is *Borrelia recurrentis*. The blood of a patient suffering from relapsing fever contains spirochaetes only during the febrile periods and lice become infected at this time. Man is the only reservoir of louse-borne relapsing fever, and an endemic focus, as is present in Ethiopia, is capable of starting a widespread epidemic. African epidemics in the past seem to have occurred every 20 years, the last being in 1943. In contrast to ticks, no transovarial transmission in lice occurs. Infection is conveyed to human beings not by the bite of the louse, but by contamination of the wounds (made by biting or scratching) with the body fluids of the louse. Little is known of where relapsing fever lurks between epidemics and how it suddenly springs up after silent intervals of several years.

Laboratory diagnosis
Blood should be taken during the pyrexial period and examined either by dark-ground illumination or after staining with a Romanovsky stain. *B. duttoni* is about 15 μm long and made up of spiral turns occupying 2-3 μm. The numbers present in a blood film vary from case to case; at the height of the first pyrexial attack they are often numerous. Blood infection is less heavy in the tick-borne than in the louse-borne disease. The organisms may be recovered by culture or by intraperitoneal inoculation of blood into laboratory animals (e.g. mouse or rat). The Wasserman reaction may be positive.

Control
This essentially consists in mass delousing by residual insecticidal powders, as in epidemic typhus.

(a) *The individual*
The safest, most effective and economical method of treating louse-borne relapsing fever is one injection of 300 000 units of procaine

penicillin followed the next day by an oral dose of 250 mg tetracycline. Severe reactions of the Jarisch-Herxheimer type can occur.

(b) *The community*
The only effective measure is to control infestation with lice with DDT as has been described for epidemic typhus (p. 163).

Relapsing Fever—Summary

	Louse-borne	Tick-borne
(1) *Occurrence*	Ethiopia, parts of Africa, India, South America	Africa, South America, Middle East
(2) *Organisms*	*Borrelia recurrentis*	*B. duttoni*
(3) *Reservoir of infection*	Man	Rodents, man
(4) *Mode of transmission*	Contamination by infected louse body fluids	Contamination by infected tick body fluids
(5) *Control*	Mass delousing	(i) Individual protection (ii) Vector control (iii) Rehousing

Bartonellosis

Bartonellosis appears in two distinct forms: (*a*) Oroya fever and (*b*) Verruca peruviana.

Oroya fever is an acute, febrile illness associated with a rapidly developing anaemia and a high mortality.

Verruca peruviana is a non-fatal disease exemplified by generalised cutaneous lesions. It usually occurs following recovery from the Oroya fever stage although it occasionally arises apparently spontaneously.

The infection is limited to Bolivia, Peru, Colombia and Ecuador. The causative organism is *Bartonella bacilliformis*. Although known since 1905 it was first cultured in 1928 by Noguchi from an acute case of Oroya fever and the culture produced the nodules of verruga in monkeys. Oroya fever is also known as Carrion's disease since Carrion, a medical student, inoculated himself with material from a verruga lesion and died from Oroya fever 39 days later. The disease is transmitted from man to man by the bites of various species of sandflies *Phlebotomus*, which live at altitudes of 2000-8000 feet and bite only at night. The disease is most prevalent at the end of the rainy season when these insects are most numerous. When a susceptible person is bitten infection follows, usually in 3-4 weeks.

The organisms are pleomorphic Gram-negative coccobacilli and are found in blood smears, either free in the plasma or within red cells, in Oroya fever. They are sparse in the nodules in verruga and culture of material on serum agar is the most reliable method of isolation.

The principal cause of mortality is a particular susceptibility of patients with Oroya fever to septicaemic infections with Salmonella organisms, commonly *S. typhimurium*. Recovery confers some resistance to re-infection, so that in endemic areas the disease is most prevalent in children.

Control
The disease has been successfully controlled by applying residual insecticides to the interior of houses and outbuildings. Personal prophylaxis consists in the use of repellents and sandfly bed-nets. As soon as Oroya fever is diagnosed the patient should be given chloramphenicol in standard doses as for Salmonella infections.

The Protozoal Diseases

Malaria
Human malaria is a disease of wide distribution caused by sporozoa of the genus *Plasmodium*. There are four species of parasites that infect man: *P. falciparum*, *P. vivax*, *P. malariae* and *P. ovale*. The differentiation of the species depends on the morphology and staining of the parasites and associated changes in the containing cells. The most common and important infections are those caused by *P. falciparum* and *P. vivax*. Mixed infections occur.

The arthropod hosts are females of certain species of *Anopheles* mosquito. The predominant malaria vectors are *A. gambiae*, *A. funestus*, *A. darlingi* and *A. punctulatus*. Clinically malaria is characterised by fever, splenomegaly, varying degrees of anaemia, and various syndromes resulting from the involvement of individual organs.

Medical geography
Malaria is found in regions lying roughly between latitudes 60°N and 40°S. It is still commonly found throughout most of Africa, South America, South-East Asia, the Arabian peninsula and the Western Pacific.

Applied biology
The complete life cycle of the human malaria parasite embraces (1) a period of development within the mosquito, and (2) a period of infection in man.

After ingestion of human infected blood a period of development lasting 10–14 days occurs in the mosquito resulting in the production of sporozoites. A bite infects the human host with these forms which remain in the circulating blood for 30 minutes or less then enter tissue cells notably in the liver, where the *pre-erythrocytic* cycle takes place.

During the succeeding 7-9 days the sporozoites develop in the parenchymal cells of the liver. As in the short sporozoite phase no symptoms
of malaria are experienced during the pre-erythrocytic cycle. The libera-
tion of the merozoites from the liver cells and their entry into the
bloodstream initiates the *erythrocytic cycle*. The plasmodium first appears
in red cells as a small speck of chromatin surrounded by scanty cytoplasm, and soon becomes a ring-shaped trophozoite. As the parasite
develops, pigment particles appear in the cytoplasm, and the chromatin
is more prominent. Chromatin division then proceeds, and when
complete there is formed the mature schizont containing daughter
merozoites. The parasitised red blood cell now ruptures, releasing
merozoites the majority of which re-enter erythrocytes to re-initiate erythrocytic schizogony. In *P. falciparum* the erythrocytic cycle takes
36-48 hours (subtertian); in *P. vivax* and *P. ovale* infections 48 hours
(tertian); and *P. malariae* 72 hours (quartan). In response to some
unknown stimulus a number of the merozoites released after erythrocytic schizogony develop into male and female forms known as
gametocytes. Gametocytes are believed to be inert in man. They provide
the reservoir of infection enabling mosquitoes to perpetuate the malaria
cycle, and remain within the red cell for the duration of their survival,
i.e. up to 120 days.

A certain proportion of the merozoites liberated from the schizonts
of the pre-erythrocytic phase, do *not* enter the bloodstream but re-enter
the parenchymal cells of the liver and are responsible for the persistence
of the *exo-erythrocytic cycle* (EE). The reappearance of malaria after
clinical cure results from the parasite's ability to persist in the tissues
in this (EE) form. The eventual discharge of merozoites from these
EE forms into the bloodstream, results in reinvasion of red blood cells
so producing a relapse. The exo-erythrocytic cycle occurs in *P. vivax*,
P. ovale and *P. malariae* infections. *P. vivax* can usually produce relapses
up to 3 years after infection; while *P. malariae* has occasionally relapsed
10, 20 or even 30 years after infection. In *P. falciparum* malaria the liver
phase is said not to persist, it follows therefore that when adequate
treatment for the erythrocytic cycle is given relapses do not occur. It is
therefore rare for *P. falciparum* infections to relapse after 1 year of
freedom from exposure to infection, although a few authentic cases
with long intervals prior to relapse have been described.

Malaria pigment is derived from the haemoglobin of the invaded red
cell and is composed of haem plus denatured protein.

Epidemiology
The effect that malaria exerts on any population is largely governed
by its epidemiological pattern. In this respect two epidemiological
extremes are described—stable and unstable malaria. The salient differences are shown below.

Stable malaria	**Unstable malaria**
(1) Transmission occurs throughout the year. Fairly uniform intensity of transmission. Pattern repeats itself annually with astonishing regularity, showing little variation over several years.	Transmission seasonal—intensity of transmission variable. Liable to flare up into dramatic epidemics.
(2) Potent resistance in the community due to prevailing intense transmission.	General lack of immunity in the community due to the low level of transmission, which only occasionally becomes intense.
(3) Main impact of disease in young children.	Impact of disease on all age-groups.
(4) Difficult to eradicate.	Eradicated with greater ease than stable malaria.
(5) Classical areas where it occurs—West Africa, Lowlands of New Guinea.	Classical areas—high plateau of Ethiopia or Highlands of New Guinea.

Immunity to malaria is well developed among populations living in 'stable' malaria areas and can be considered under four main headings: (*a*) Cellular, (*b*) Humoral, (*c*) Inherited factors in the blood and (*d*) Racial.

Cellular Immunity

The response of phagocytic cells in malaria was shown in early histological studies and for many years resistance to the disease was considered to be exclusively cellular in nature. The reticulo-endothelial system undergoes intense proliferation during malarial infection and the macrophages of the spleen, liver and bone marrow have been shown to phagocytose parasitised and unparasitised erythrocytes, isolated parasites and malarial pigment. In areas of stable malaria, large amounts of this pigment are continuously being engulfed by the reticulo-endothelial system over periods of years, and the part that this possible 'blockade' plays in the immunological mechanism of the host, both in the fields of infection and malignancy, has still to be elucidated.

Humoral Immunity

Recent studies have demonstrated and stressed the importance of humoral immunity. Several workers have demonstrated that the concentration of gamma globulin in the serum of the newborn African infant is considerably higher than corresponding values reported from Europe. It was further shown that, in 'stable' areas, malarial infection contributes significantly to the maintenance of high γ-globulin levels in all subjects after the first year of life, and moreover that γ-globulin prepared from the sera of adults immune to malaria has a consistent therapeutic effect when administered to West African children suffering from heavy *P. falciparum* infection. Serum from the cord blood of infants born of immune mothers has a similar effect. It is now generally accepted that acquired malarial immunity is basically dependent upon the presence of circulating antibody which is associated with 7S γ-globulin fraction (IgG) of serum. It is probable that the two mechanisms of defence in malaria, the cellular (through the reticulo-endothelial system) and the humoral (through IgG immunoglobulin) are interdependent.

Inherited Factors in the Blood
It has been postulated that the following hereditary red cell traits protect against the lethal effects of malaria: (1) haemoglobin S, (2) haemoglobin C, (3) haemoglobin E, (4) thalassaemia, (5) glucose-6-phosphate dehydrogenase deficiency. The only convincing evidence to date concerns sickle-cell haemoglobin and G-6-Pd deficiency.

Racial Immunity
It has long been known that Negroes in the USA had a vivax infection rate lower than that of whites and that it was more difficult to infect them with this species in the course of malarial therapy. The most evident consequence of resistance to *P. vivax* in Negroes occurs in West Africa, where, in many regions, it cannot be found in the indigenous population; yet the parasite is common in the inhabitants of the Eastern Congo and East Africa.

Laboratory diagnosis
The certain diagnosis of malaria is parasitological and is made by examining thick blood films stained with Field or Giemsa stains. Although species diagnosis can be made on thick films it is usually made on thin films stained with Leishman or Giemsa stains. As a rule only ring forms and gametocytes are found in the peripheral blood in falciparum malaria unless the infection is severe, in which case, schizonts also appear. In cases of vivax, malariae and ovale malaria all forms of development of the asexual parasites are found.

Various more sophisticated techniques such as the fluorescent antibody test (FAT), immunoglobulin values and haemagglutination tests are valuable adjuncts to diagnosis, but do not supersede the direct microscopical identification of the parasite in stained blood smears.

Control
The control of malaria is either designed to protect particular individuals from infection or to prevent transmission and thereby protect the whole community. Control measures are therefore aimed at the individual, against the vector or to provide communal protection.

(a) *The individual*
Individual protective measures are best based on the regular use of a
prophylactic drug and of mosquito nets over the bed, to which may be
added, when there is a general mosquito nuisance, house-screening and
repellents such as dimethyl phthalate.

Synthetic antimalarial drugs have now completely superseded the
once popular quinine as prophylactics. Those in common use with the
appropriate dose for an adult are:

Proguanil	100-200 mg once daily
Pyrimethamine	25-50 mg once a week
Chloroquine or amodiaquine	
(4-aminoquinolines)	300-600 mg of base once a week

Proguanil and pyrimethamine have a considerable value as true prophylactics against *P. falciparum*, often completely aborting an infection
acquired while the dosage was being taken; none of the above drugs,
however, are reliable true prophylactics of infection with the other
species, which they usually suppress only for the period of administration of the drug. In these respects all of them are of comparable value,
and the choice between them often turns on secondary characteristics.
Proguanil carries the least risk of toxic side-effects, and its daily regimen
is easily remembered for personal administration, but it may be relatively
ineffective in a few parts of the world where parasites have developed
resistance to it. Pyrimethamine is tasteless and is readily taken by
children, but again resistance to it has been developed by parasites in
some limited localities. Chloroquine and amodiaquine are not quite so
free from risk of side-effects, but they are the most potent schizonti-
cides. Repository anti-malarials have been introduced, but their value
in the field has been disappointing. Similarly, combinations of sul-
phones with pyrimethamine, and sulphonamides with pyrimethamine,
are still undergoing field trials.

The drugs mentioned above must be taken as soon as one enters a
malarious area, they need not be taken a week before. They should
be continued for 4 weeks after leaving. Even then clinical malaria
is possible when the drug is stopped and the patient should be warned
of this.

Resistance to chloroquine and amodiaquine has been reported from
parts of South America and South-East Asia. A number of strains of
P. falciparum that are resistant to the 4-aminoquinolines also show
resistance to mepacrine, primaquine, quinine, proguanil and pyrimethamine. Resistance and sensitivity to chloroquine are not absolute,
and a system of grading has recently been devised—RI, RII and
RIII resistance.

RI = Clinical and parasitological response *but* recrudescence a few
     weeks after treatment.

RII = Clinical response but *no* parasitological response.

RIII = Neither clinical nor parasitological response.

There have been no reports of resistance to the 4-aminoquinolines in any species of human *Plasmodium* other than *P. falciparum*.

(b) *The vector*

The control of the mosquito has been attempted in two ways, (1) attack on the adult mosquito, i.e. imagicidal control. The choice of method depends on the nature of the terrain and on the habitats of the vector mosquito and (2) prevention of mosquito breeding by larval control.

Imagicidal control has been, in general, so effective that it has now virtually replaced control of breeding. Imagicidal attack is usually based on the application, every 6 months, of 2 g/m^2 of DDT as a suspension of a water-dispersible powder to the interior walls of all houses and animal shelters.

Larval control has, however, been used successfully to control malaria in Singapore and in urban areas of Malaysia. Control of breeding can be effected either by means of larvicides or more permanent measures such as subsoil drainage, depending on existing local conditions. Anopheline and other mosquito larvae may be killed by heavy oiling by antimalarial oil (with or without a little added insecticide) or by light spraying with kerosene containing high concentration of insecticide (e.g. 5 per cent DDT). The former treatment also kills weeds in irrigation ditches and seems to have a slightly residual action; the latter saves labour. Both liquids are intended to spread freely across water surface and must possess good spreading pressure to overcome natural contamination of pools. If drainage is used, it must be efficiently carried out and permanent drains must be kept unblocked and functional by regular supervision.

(c) *The community*

Mass treatment of the community is only feasible and important in the later stages of malaria eradication campaigns (see below). The antimalarials commonly used in these circumstances are either pyrimethamine or the 8-aminoquinolines, e.g. primaquine. The 8-aminoquinolines are effective gametocidal drugs while pyrimethamine prevents completion of the malaria cycle in the mosquito by arresting development at the oocyst stage.

(d) *Malaria eradication*

Wide malaria eradication programmes based on the use of insecticides have been sponsored for some years by the World Health Organisation.

The object of eradication is the total elimination of malaria first from countries, then from regions, and finally from the world (global eradication). Its phases, after a preliminary preparatory phase, are classified as attack, consolidation and maintenance. Attack is by the use of a residual insecticide, applied with complete uniformity inside all the houses of the malarious area of a country, over a period of 3 or more years with the objective of completely interrupting transmission, and it is estimated that if this is achieved the numbers of people with infections should decrease to 16 per cent of the original value in the course of each 12 months. After 3 years of successful interruption the remaining numbers should be very small. With some reasonable overlap of timing, the insecticidal attack is then replaced by a system of case finding and associated epidemiological study and treatment, called 'surveillance' in the consolidation phase. During this phase, which again should last at least 3 years, the objective is first to find and treat every remaining case and focus of infection, and then to prove by concentrated search the absence of any further local cases or foci in the absence of control measures. When this has been done, the detailed criteria of eradication can be met and the programme enters the final maintenance phase, in which activities are akin to epidemiological vigilance aimed at checking the absence of infection, finding and treating imported cases and the re-establishment of malaria. A marked geographical distribution of achievement has been reached, with very satisfactory results in some areas, e.g. parts of South America, and virtually no impact in others, e.g. West Africa.

A re-examination of the global strategy of malaria eradication is being undertaken, and WHO now stresses the crucial role of basic health services in such programmes (pre-eradication phase).

Malaria—Summary

(1) *Occurrence*—World-wide 60°N-40°S of equator
(2) *Organisms*—P. *falciparum*, P. *vivax*, P. *malariae*, P. *ovale*
(3) *Reservoir of infection*—Man
(4) *Mode of transmission*—Bite of Anopheles mosquitoes
(5) *Control*— (i) Chemoprophylaxis
         (ii) Vector control

The Trypanosomiases

The trypanosome species pathogenic for man can be classified into two groups: (1) those transmitted through the bite of a blood-sucking fly, i.e. *Trypanosoma gambiense* and *T. rhodesiense*, which cause African trypanosomiasis and (2) those transmitted by faecal contamination from an arthropod vector, e.g. *T. cruzi*, which causes South African trypanosomiasis (Chagas' disease).

(1) *African Trypanosomiasis*

African trypanosomiasis is caused by either *Trypanosoma gambiense* or *T. rhodesiense*, and the infection is conveyed to man by the bites of flies of the genus *Glossina*. The *incubation period* is usually between 2 and 3 weeks but can be very much longer (6 years).

Medical geography
African trypanosomiasis is confined to that part of Africa lying between latitudes 10°N and 25°S. *T. rhodesiense* infection is limited to Kenya, Tanzania, Uganda, Malawi, Zambia, Rhodesia, Mozambique, Northern Botswana and South-East Angola, while *T. gambiense* is more widespread, extending from West Africa through Central Africa to Uganda, Tanzania and Malawi. Recent epidemics of *T. rhodesiense* have been reported from Botswana, the Southern Sudan and Ethiopia.

Applied biology
In man, *T. gambiense* and *T. rhodesiense* are morphologically identical, varying in length from 10 μm to 30 μm with a pointed anterior end and blunt posterior. The cytoplasm stains blue with a Romanowsky stain, there is a large oval centrally placed nucleus, a small posteriorly placed kinetoplast, an undulating membrane projecting beyond the anterior end of the body. Other morphological forms in blood are also seen. *T. gambiense* and *T. rhodesiense* have a similar life cycle. When blood containing trypanosomes is ingested by a suitable species of *Glossina*, the trypanosomes reach the intestine of the fly and undergo cyclical development, eventually developing into infective metacyclic forms in the salivary glands. These are introduced when saliva is injected into the wound produced during the act of feeding. Multiplication of the trypanosomes occurs in the blood. The entire cycle of development in the fly, after feeding on blood containing trypanosomes, is about 3 weeks (extrinsic incubation period).

The main vectors of Gambian sleeping sickness are the riverine species of *Glossina*: *G. palpalis* and *G. tachinoides*; while the chief vectors of Rhodesian sleeping sickness are *G. morsitans*, *G. swynnertoni* and *G. pallipides*.

Epidemiology
The maintenance of human trypanosomiasis in Africa depends on the interrelations of three elements—the vertebrate host, the parasite and the vector responsible for transmission. Sleeping sickness is essentially a disease of rural populations and its prevalence is largely dependent on the degree of contact between man and tsetse, this is particularly so with Gambiense sleeping sickness. Thus at the height of the dry season, riverine species of fly are often restricted to isolated pools of water which are essential to the local human population for so many of their activities, e.g. collecting water and firewood, washing, fishing and cultivation. The sacred groves of some religions may also provide foci of intimate man/fly contact. Over recent years there has been an increasing incidence and dispersion of *T. rhodesiense* sleeping sickness on the north-east shores of Lake Victoria, associated with increased fishing

activity and increasing and irregular settlement of the tsetse-fly belt of south-east Uganda.

Each species of tsetse has particular requirements in regard to climate and vegetation, which determine its distribution. All of them tend to concentrate seasonally in habitats offering permanent shade and humidity. The distribution of the fly thus varies with the season, and in addition it advances and retreats spatially at intervals of years. Population density affects the incidence of the disease, which is sporadic at densities below 20 per square mile, and is liable to become epidemic at densities up to 200 or so per square mile, above which it disappears because testse habitats are eliminated.

In general, in endemic conditions, the incidence of sleeping sickness is greater in males. In contrast to this usual picture it has been reported that in the Gambia the women and older girls were most affected because they were exposed while working in the rice fields. In epidemic conditions no clear sex difference in incidence occurs and the proportion of children infected rises sharply. Adverse environmental climatic conditions can effect the mean period between emergence of the young fly (pupa) and the taking of the first blood meal as well as the period of development of trypanosomes in the vector; these factors can influence the chance of transmission of the disease. No animal reservoir for *T. gambiense* has yet been proved but *T. rhodesiense* has been isolated from a bush-buck, and so a reservoir in wild animals—long suspected—has now been proved. This wild animal reservoir plays an important role in the epidemiology of the human disease (Fig. 6.3).

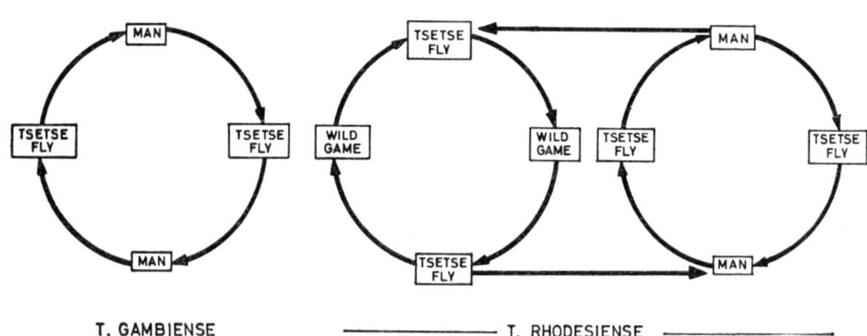

FIG. 6.3   Epidemiology of African Trypanosomiasis.

Laboratory diagnosis

Microscopical examination of blood, lymph fluid, serous fluids, or CSF with or without concentration techniques may reveal the organism in fresh or suitably stained preparations. *In vitro* culture of trypanosomes has proved sensitive and reliable, as has the complement-fixation test. A fluorescent antibody test for the serodiagnosis of African trypanosomiasis has been developed. A raised serum bilirubin level, excess urobilinogen and bilirubinuria is common in early acutely febrile *Rhodesiense* patients but these indices are not raised in the late stages of the disease. The bromsulphalein excretion test is also abnormal in the acutely febrile early-stage associated with a precipitous fall in the serum albumin. In the late stages of both *gambiense* and *rhodesiense* infections the total plasma proteins are high and the γ-globulin grossly increased, except in wasted patients in whom the total serum proteins and especially albumin are low. The lymphocytes and protein content of the CSF are invariably raised and sugar low when the central nervous system is involved. The fluorescent antibody test has been applied to the CSF of patients with sleeping sickness, antibodies were found in all the samples which showed pathological changes. The test is sensitive, specific and suitable for the early detection of involvement of the nervous system.

The serum levels of IgM, IgA and IgG are raised in both *T. gambiense* and *T. rhodesiense* infections. High levels of M-antiglobulins (rheumatoid-factor-like globulins) can occur in African trypanosomiasis. EEG sometimes shows a disturbed wave pattern, and air encephalography, dilatation of the ventricles when brain involvement has occurred.

Control
This is directed against the parasite in man and against the fly.

(a) *The individual*
The survey of infected communities and treatment of all those found infected rapidly lowers the incidence and reduces the reservoir of infection. Medical field units have been particularly successful using this approach both in West and East Africa.

Chemoprophylaxis, using pentamidine 200 mg in one single intramuscular injection, will give protection against *T. gambiense* for some 6 months in individuals or in circumscribed communities, e.g. labour force. It is generally felt that chemoprophylaxis against *T. rhodesiense* is not effective and possibly undesirable.

The wearing of long trousers and of long-sleeved shirts gives some protection against the bites of tsetse fly. Vehicles which have to pass through heavily tsetse-infected country should be fly-proofed with mosquito gauze. Individuals who are sensitive to insect bites may find repellents (dimethylphthalate or diethyl toluamide) useful quite apart from the protection which they may give against infection, for a severe local reaction to the tsetse bite is not uncommon.

The commonly used drugs for African trypanosomiasis are shown in Table 6.5.

G

TABLE 6.5

Drugs used in the treatment of African trypanosomiasis

Note: Adult dosage given

	T. gambiense	*T. rhodesiense*
Early stage (CNS not involved)	(1) Pentamidine 4 mg (base)/kg IM, daily for 10 days. (2) Suramin *Test dose:* 0·2 g IV. *Dosage* (if test negative): 20 mg/kg IV. Maximum single dose 1 g (patient of 50 kg or more). *Course advocated:* 20 mg/kg on days 1, 3, 7, 14 and 21 (i.e. 5 injections in 3 weeks). (3) Berenil (occasionally used) 2 mg/kg IM, daily for 7 days.	All cases should be treated as intermediate or late, since early invasion of the CNS occurs.
Intermediate and late stages (CNS involved)	(1) Melarsoprol (Mel B) 3·6% solution in propylene glycol. *Dosage:* 3-4 mg/kg IV. Maximum single dose 180 mg (5 ml) (patient of 50 kg or more). *Course advocated:* 180 mg (5 ml) on days 1, 2, 3. Repeat after an interval of 1 week. *Note:* Solution is very irritant and must be given slowly with a *dry* syringe and needle. (2) Melarsonyl potassium (Mel W) White powder made up in distilled water. *Dosage:* 3-4 mg/kg IM. Maximum single dose 200 mg (patient of 50 kg or more). *Course advocated:* 150-200 mg on days 1, 2, 3. Repeat after an interval of 1 week.	*Preliminary course:* Suramin *Test dose:* 0·2 g. *Dosage* (if no toxic reaction) Days 1, 3, 0·5 g; day 5, 1 g. *Follow-up course:* Melarsoprol *Course advocated:* Day 1, 0·5 ml (18 mg); day 2, 1·0 ml (36 mg); day 3, 1·5 ml (54 mg). 7 days rest. Days 11, 12, 13, 2·5 ml (90 mg). 7 days rest. Day 21, 3 ml (108 mg); day 22, 4 ml (144 mg); day 23, 5 ml (180 mg). *Note:* large doses of ascorbic acid (100 mg daily) may minimise toxic reactions.

(3) Melarsen (Melarsen sodium) 　20 mg/kg IV, weekly for 10 weeks. (4) Tryparsamide 　30 mg/kg IV, weekly for 6 weeks. Maximum single dose 2 g. 　*Note:* This course should be combined with a course of Suramin, 0·5 g IV, weekly for 6 weeks. Both drugs are given on the same day.	*Patients who fail to respond to Melarsoprol:* Nitrofurazone 　Yellow powder. 　*Test dose:* 0·5 g tablet daily for 2-3 days. 　*Dosage* (if no toxic reaction): 0·5 g tablet 3-4 times a day for 5-7 days. Repeat after an interval of a week. 　*Note:* Thiamin must be given at the same time. The course may be preceded by a short course of Suramin, in febrile patients.

(b) *The fly*

Control of the fly is effected most cheaply by concentrating the people to such a density that their normal agricultural and other activities eradicate the tsetse habitats. It is also possible to remove or alter the foci sheltering the fly during arid periods, and thus cause them to disappear; this must be done under the guidance of an entomologist who has studied the local vector species.

'Bush clearance' varies with the species of *Glossina*. *G. palpalis* at fords, bridges or watering and bathing places near villages can be kept at a distance by clearing stream banks for a distance of a quarter of a mile along each bank and 20 yards deep from the water's edge. A clearance of all trees and shrubs to a depth of a mile (*G. palpalis*) or two or more (*G. morsitans*) may be used to prevent extension of the range of the fly or to isolate a focus.

Game extermination has proved successful in eliminating certain species of fly which depend on them. Residual insecticides have in some circumstances proved effective against certain vectors when sprayed from the air, or at ground level on the trees and shrubs. Riverine species can be controlled or eliminated by a combination of insecticidal treatment of blocks of vegetation, applied at ground level, which are separated by cleared areas.

(c) *The community*

Pentamidine diisethionate in doses of 200-250 mg given to each labourer on engagement and thereafter at 4 to 6 months intervals is a very effective way of protecting labour forces working in trypanosomiasis-affected areas. This prophylactic measure should be applied to gangs of labourers working on road, railways or similar works in areas of high risk. Such controlled groups can be protected effectively and without difficulty.

Chemoprophylaxis for communities has been widely practised in most of the endemic areas of francophone West and Equatorial Africa, but nowhere has the hope of eradication been fulfilled and the dangers of 'cryptic infections'* are very real. The disadvantage of this control measure is that if it is used on recently infected persons who have not been diagnosed, the parasites are driven from the blood and may establish themselves in the central nervous system. It is mandatory, therefore, before using mass prophylaxis that every care must be taken to detect all infected persons.

African Trypanosomiases—Summary

(1) *Occurrence*—Africa 10°N-25°S of equator
(2) *Organisms*—T. gambiense, T. rhodesiense
(3) *Reservoir of infection*—Man
(4) *Mode of transmission*—Bite of tsetse fly
(5) *Control*— (i) Treatment of infected cases
     (ii) Chemoprophylaxis
     (iii) Reduction of man/fly contact

(2) American Trypanosomiasis

Chagas' disease may present as congenital, acute or chronic forms. The main impact of the infection especially in children is on the heart, enteromegaly is common in chronic Chagas' disease.

Medical geography

The infection is found in Central and South America, especially in Brazil, Venezuela, Colombia and northern Argentina.

Applied biology

The adult trypanosomes, which measure about 20 μm in length with a central nucleus and very large posterior kinetoplast, are found in the blood. When ingested by blood-sucking reduviid bugs, after a period of development in the invertebrate host's intestinal canal lasting 8-10 days, trypanosomes, known as 'metacyclic' forms reappear in the hind-gut and are passed with the faeces of the insect. Infection of man takes place when faecal matter is rubbed into scratch wounds and the wound caused by the bite of the insect. Certain trypanosomes leave the bloodstream and invade various organs, especially the myocardium. Here they assume a leishmanoid appearance and rapid multiplication by binary fission takes place forming nests of Leishman-Donovan bodies. At a later stage these leishmanoid forms elongate and are eventually transformed into trypanosomes, which make their way through the tissues and into the bloodstream.

---

* 'Cryptic infections' are characterised by gross abnormalities of the cerebrospinal fluid with no trypanosomes in the blood or glands.

Epidemiology
The reservoir of infection is man. The most important vector bugs belong to the genera *Triatoma, Panstrongylus* and *Rhodnius*. These reduviid bugs are largely disseminated throughout the rural areas of Latin America where the mud huts of the agricultural workers are their favourite habitats. The usual mode of transmission is by rubbing infected faeces into cuts of abrasions or into the intact skin or mucous membrane. Transmission occurs predominantly at night since reduviid bugs attack only in darkness. The disease is observed at any age, although children are mainly affected. Other unusual methods of infection are transplacental, by blood transfusion, and laboratory transmission from infected syringes or blood. Although an animal reservoir of infection has been established its role in the epidemiology of human disease is uncertain. Symptoms usually develop about 2 weeks after infective trypanosomes enter the skin.

Infections with another trypanosome, *T. rangeli*, have been found in various animals, and human infections with this trypanosome have occasionally also been reported. In contrast to *T. cruzi* the transmission of this disease is by the actual bite of the reduviid bug rather than through its excreta.

Laboratory diagnosis
Trypanosomes may be demonstrated in wet and stained thick blood films; in lymph gland juice, or in CSF and may be cultured on NNN medium. A complement-fixation test (Guenerio-Machado test)—employing antigen from flagellates cultivated *in vitro*—is widely used and is the most sensitive means of diagnosis. Immunofluorescence has been used in the diagnosis of Chagas' disease.

Control
Chagas' disease flourishes only where social and economic levels are low, and long-term control measures involve economic rehabilitation, in particular, better housing.

(a) *The individual*
Personal prophylaxis consists in avoiding sleeping in houses liable to harbour the vectors and in using bed nets. In endemic areas blood donors for transfusion should be carefully screened and rejected if infected.

(b) *The community*
Mud hovels with thatched roofs need to be replaced with houses of materials giving no harbourage to bugs. Residual insecticides, especially dieldrin (at $1 \cdot 6$ g/m²) or benzene hexachloride at ($0 \cdot 5$ g/m²), applied to floors, walls and thatch will eliminate most of the vectors, but re-infestation occurs in a few months.

American Trypanosomiases—Summary

(1) *Occurrence*—South America
(2) *Organism*—T. *cruzi*
(3) *Reservoir of infection*—Man
(4) *Mode of transmission*—Rubbing infected reduviid bugs' faeces into
                                                          skin
(5) *Control*— (i) Better housing
                       (ii) Using bed nets

The Leishmaniases

It is convenient (though not strictly justifiable) to subdivide the Leish-maniases into three clinical types: the visceral, the cutaneous and the muco-cutaneous (Table 6.6).

TABLE 6.6

Classification of leishmaniases

A Visceral	(1) Indian kala-azar	
	(2) Kala-azar predominantly associated with canine reservoir	
	(3) African kala-azar	*L. donovani**
B Cutaneous	(1) Oriental sore	*L. tropica*
	(2) Chiclero ulcer	*L. mexicana*
	(3) Uta	*L. peruviana*
	(4) Leishmaniasis tegumentaria diffusa	*L. pifanoi*
	(5) Ethiopian leishmaniasis	
	(6) Lupoid leishmaniasis	
C Muco-cutaneous		*L. braziliensis*

* Post-kala-azar dermal leishmaniasis is a sequel to visceral leishmaniasis following specific treatment.

Medical geography

The Leishmaniases occur over wide areas of the globe from China across Asia, India, Persia and Afghanistan, the Caucasus, the Middle and Near East, the Mediterranean basin, East and West Africa, the Sudan and South America.

Applied biology

There are two phases in the life cycle of Leishmania: an aflagellate (leishmanial) rounded form which occurs in man and in animal reservoir hosts; and a flagellate (leptomonad) form which is found in the vector sandfly and in culture media. The former is oval (2μm $\times 3\mu$m) and consists of cytoplasm, a round nucleus, and a small, more deeply staining, rod-shaped kinetoplast or rhizoplast and a vacuole. It is known as the Leishman-Donovan (L-D) body. In man leishmania multiply by binary fission. They are most commonly found in the large mono-nuclear cells of the reticulo-endothelial system, especially in the liver, spleen and bone marrow; leishmanial forms are also found in the leuco-cytes of the circulating blood.

When the appropriate sandfly feeds on an infected person, it ingests the parasites with the blood meal. These develop in its gut into the flagellate (leptomonad) forms: these migrate forwards, multiply and form a mass which may block the pharynx of the sandfly. When the sandfly next feeds, some of these leptomonads become dislodged and are injected into the new host in the process of feeding; they again assume the leishmanial form. They are phagocytosed by macrophages, multiply by simple division and cause the cells to rupture. They are then carried in the circulation to the sites already referred to where they give rise to the characteristic lesions. Following specific treatment in some cases they pass from their visceral habitat—liver, spleen, etc., back to the skin, giving rise to the condition described as *post-kala-azar dermal leishmaniasis*.

The above life-history applies to *L. donovani*, which is the causative organism of visceral leishmaniasis. In cutaneous and muco-cutaneous leishmaniasis, the multiplication of the leishmanial forms takes place in the skin and the appropriate sandfly vectors become infected by feeding on a cutaneous lesion.

Epidemiology
The epidemiology of the leishmaniases, whether visceral, cutaneous or muco-cutaneous, is in every case determined by a reservoir of infection (animal, man or both) from which local *Phlebotomine* sandflies, infect themselves by ingesting leishmanial forms from blood or infected tissues. The climatic conditions of the various foci of leishmaniasis range from arid to tropical humid and the terrain and altitude are equally variable. Modes of transmission other than by sandflies, e.g. marital, blood transfusion, and intra-uterine infection, are of little epidemiological significance. With the possible exception of Indian kala-azar it is increasingly being recognised that in most endemic foci the leishmaniases are zoonoses.

Visceral Leishmaniasis
There are three distinct types of visceral leishmaniasis: (*a*) Indian kala-azar, (*b*) kala-azar associated predominantly with a canine reservoir and (*c*) African kala-azar. Kala-azar is essentially a rural disease, and *L. donovani* is now accepted as the cause of all forms of kala-azar. Post-kala-azar dermal leishmaniasis occurs as a sequel of visceral leishmaniasis. The *incubation period* of visceral leishmaniasis ranges from 2 weeks to more than 1 year.

(a) *Indian kala-azar* is unique in so far as man is the only known natural host of the infection. The vector *P. argentipes* breeds in close proximity to human habitations and feeds readily on man. All age-groups are susceptible with a peak incidence at 10-20 years. Devastating epidemics may occur. The lesions of post-kala-azar dermal leishmaniasis are of epidemiological importance since they contain numerous L-D bodies in the dermis and are readily accessible to sandflies, they are a feature of Indian kala-azar but are also seen elsewhere.

(b) *Kala-azar predominantly associated with a canine reservoir.* In the Mediterranean basin, Portugal, North Africa, the Caucasus, China, Brazil and other parts of South America, the domestic dog, fox and jackal are very important reservoirs of human infection.

Visceral leishmaniasis associated with a canine reservoir is predominantly a disease of children under 10 years. The most important vector sandflies are *Phlebotomus chinensis* in China, *P. longipalpis* in Brazil, and *P. perniciosus* in the Mediterranean.

(c) *African kala-azar.* The epidemiology of the disease in the Sudan and Kenya presents unique features differing from those described above. There is a primary stage in the skin (leishmanoma) which lasts for some time before the symptoms of kala-azar develop, and this is of prime epidemiological importance; in this area rodents may form a reservoir of infection. There is a definite relationship between the proximity of homes to termite hills and the incidence of kala-azar. The most important vectors are *P. martini* in Kenya and *P. orientalis* in the Sudan where the disease attacks all age-groups but is commoner in adults than in children. Both these vectors are out-of-doors biters. The human distribution is affected by immunity as well as by relative exposure to infection.

Cutaneous Leishmaniasis
Several varieties of cutaneous leishmaniasis have been described from the Old and New World. These include (1) oriental sore, (2) chiclero ulcer, (3) uta, (4) leishmaniasis tegumentaria diffusa, (5) Ethiopian cutaneous leishmaniasis, (6) lupoid leishmaniasis.

(1) *Oriental Sore*
(tropical sore; bouton d'Orient; Aleppo, Baghdad or Delhi boil; Pendah sore).

Epidemiology
This cutaneous infection is widely distributed in the Indian subcontinent, the Middle East, Ethiopia, Southern Russia, the Mediterranean countries, Nigeria, China and the Sudan. The most important vectors are *P. papatasii* and *P. sergenti*. The disease is most commonly seen in children, and in highly endemic areas most of the adult population have been infected in childhood. The parasite responsible is *L. tropica*

of which two varieties are recognised on clinical and epidemiological grounds, *L. tropica* var. *major*, is an infection of rodents occasionally transmitted to man which produces a disease with a short incubation period, rapid course of under 6 months, much inflammatory reaction and the 'moist' lesion it produces contains few parasites; while *L. tropica minor* is an infection of dogs, only occasionally man, characterised by a 'dry' lesion containing many parasites with a long incubation period, course of over 1 year and a mild inflammatory reaction.

Immunity to *L. tropica* follows spontaneous cure and experimental attempt at reinfection very often (but not invariably) gives negative results; moreover, 98 per cent of cases of oriental sore show a delayed hypersensitivity test (Montenegro reaction) in response to the intradermal inoculation of dead and washed leptomonads.

(2) *Chiclero Ulcer*

The cutaneous leishmaniases of the New World—chiclero ulcer, uta, and leishmaniasis tegumentaria diffusa—are scattered in Central and South America over an area extending from 22°N to 30°S of the equator. They are characterised epidemiologically by the fact that they are (i) zoonoses and (ii) predominantly non-urban diseases, usually confined to the forest regions or jungles.

Epidemiology
L. mexicana is the cause of 'chiclero's ulcer' in Mexico and neighbouring countries. The infection is virtually restricted to people who habitually live and work in the forests with the result that women and children are rarely infected. It is an 'occupational disease' of the chicleros who spend a considerable time in the forests bleeding the *Sapodella* trees for chewing-gum latex. The disease is almost always limited to a single dermal lesion, usually in the ear. Forest rodents are the important animal reservoirs and man is an accidental host. Transmission of *L. mexicana* is by *Phlebotomus pessoanus* in British Honduras.

With *L. mexicana* a solid and long-lasting immunity is developed from the infection and the development of this immunity occurs very early in the course of the disease.

(3) *Uta*

L. peruviana causes cutaneous lesions on exposed sites such as the face, arm and leg—and the disease is known as uta in Peru. The infection occurs primarily in dogs which are the reservoir from which man acquires the disease. House-dwelling sandflies, e.g. *P. peruensis*, are the vectors of infection.

(4) *Leishmaniasis Tegumentaria Diffusa*

L. pifanoi causes a disseminated form of cutaneous leishmaniasis in

Bolivia and Venezuela. The leishmania intradermal test (Montenegro) is always negative.

(5) *Ethiopian Cutaneous Leishmaniasis*
This is an antimony-resistant cutaneous leishmaniasis which is endemic in Ethiopia and clinically is very similar to leprosy. The Montenegro test is negative in the 'pseudo-lepromatous' type of the disease and positive in the tuberculoid type.

(6) *Lupoid Leishmaniasis*
This is a relapsing form of cutaneous leishmaniasis which is common in the Middle East, and resembles lupus vulgaris. Leishmania are scarce in biopsies and the leishmania test is positive.

Muco-cutaneous Leishmaniasis (Espundia)
Espundia is widely distributed through South and Central America.

Epidemiology
Muco-cutaneous leishmaniasis is caused by *L. braziliensis* and the sand-flies *P. whitmani, P. passoai* and *P. migonei* are proven vectors of the disease. The most important animal reservoir of infection is the spiny rat. Espundia occurs mainly among men working in virgin forest. Human infections are acquired when new settlements are started in jungle areas and small clearings are made. At first, these settlements have an intimate contact with the forest, but after a time the wild rodents are driven away and the disease dies out. The infection is often confined to the skin but metastases to mucous membrane often occur through the bloodstream. The parasite has a predilection for the nasopharynx. It appears that clinical immunity to heterologous strains of leishmania does occur, an observation in keeping with the finding that although *L. braziliensis*, *L. tropica* and *L. mexicana* can easily be distinguished from each other serologically they share certain common antigens. It seems, moreover, that chiclero's ulcer, oriental sore and uta produce low levels of circulating antibody in the serum despite the fact that they result in life-long immunity in most patients, while patients suffering from muco-cutaneous leishmaniasis possess high levels of circulating antibody.

Laboratory diagnosis of the Leishmaniases
L. donovani can be demonstrated in Giemsa-stained smears from the peripheral blood (usually very scanty), spleen, liver, lymph nodes or bone marrow, and culture of material obtained from the above sources, or by inoculation into hamsters. Tests based on increase in serum gamma globulin are at best only indicative but not diagnostic of the disease (e.g. Napier, Chopra, etc.). The complement-fixation test is very useful in diagnosis of early cases. The indirect fluorescent antibody technique has been successfully used in the serodiagnosis

of kala-azar, negative results were reported from *L. tropica* patients.

The diagnosis of infection with *L. tropica* is made by examining microscopically material obtained by puncture of the undivided edge of the ulcer after appropriate staining. Culture of the material in NNN-type medium should also be done. Biopsy of skin under the edge of the ulcer can provide proof of infection. Histologically the organism may be confused with *H. capsulatum* which, however, stains well with methanamine silver and thus allows differentiation. The Montenegro (leishmanin) test is positive in 95 per cent of patients with *L. tropica*; in contrast it is negative in the active stages of Indian kala-azar.

L. mexicana can be demonstrated in material obtained from the initial ulcers, from the lesions in the mucous membrane, cultured material or NNN medium. The Montenegro skin test is positive in 92 per cent of patients but negative in the disseminated form of leishmaniasis due to *L. pifanoi*.

Control of the Leishmaniases

Control of visceral leishmaniasis consists in identifying and treating infected persons, including cases of dermal leishmaniasis; and in attacking the sandfly as well as the animal reservoir of infection.

(a) *The individual*

Pentostam is the drug of choice for visceral leishmaniasis. It is easy to administer and toxic effects are low. The dose for adults is 0·6 g intravenously or intramuscularly, daily for 6 days for Indian kala-azar; and for 30 days for all other forms of visceral leishmaniasis. Sandfly bites can be partially avoided by sleeping on the upper floors of houses and using repellents.

(b) *The vector*

The breeding places of sandflies in walls can be plastered over and the rubble of broken-down hoses cleared away. The indoor biting *Phlebotomus* species are very susceptible to DDT and residual spraying of dwellings eradicates the sandfly.

(c) *The animal reservoir of infection*

Infection in dogs can be controlled and eradicated by removing all infected dogs from the community. Mass diagnosis can be carried out using the complement-fixation test. A 10 per cent infection rate in the dog community implies a substantial reservoir for human infection and suspected dogs should be individually diagnosed and destroyed if sick. In endemic areas a licensing system should be instituted whereby dogs must be examined annually and destroyed if ill. Kala-azar can be eradicated from the community in this way. Wild canine and rodent reservoirs cannot of course be controlled in this way.

(d) *The community*

Villages should be sited away from ecological environments favourable to outdoor biting sandfly vectors. Thus, in Northern Kenya, houses should be sited more than 100 yards from termite hills, which can be destroyed or treated with DDT.

Mass surveys and treatment of the human population should be undertaken. Army and police personnel working in endemic areas should consist of leishman-positive vectors. When a large number of leishmaniasis-negative persons is introduced into endemic areas, epidemic of kala-azar can be expected. This is a particularly pertinent point to remember when populations are moved from one area to another as a result of the building of large dams, e.g. the Aswan dam.

Control of *cutaneous leishmaniasis* of the Old World (tropical sore) is achieved by breaking the man/sandfly contact, rodent destruction and immunisation.

Sandfly eradication by DDT spraying of houses and breeding places as above has markedly reduced the prevalence of cutaneous leishmaniasis. If this cannot be done, sleeping at night on the roof or the second floor of a house will reduce infection, since sandflies do not readily move above the ground floor. *Leishmania tropica major* mainly results from sandfly bites out of doors, and house spraying is not as effective as in *L. tropica minor*.

Since the main reservoir of infection in Asia is a communal rodent; rat destruction for a radius of 3 miles around villages should be carried out.

Since rodents cannot be eradicated from remote areas, travellers and nomads should be protected by immunisation. The immunity conferred by *L. tropica major* is virtually lifelong and protects also against *L. tropica minor*. A live culture on NNN of the gerbil leishmania is inoculated intradermally under the skin. A nodule forms which lasts 3-6 months and confers immunity to reinfection in the great majority of cases. The Montenegro test becomes positive.

Chiclero ulcer is difficult to control since both eradication of the rodent reservoir and spraying to destroy the sandflies in the forest canopy high above the ground, are both impracticable. Immunisation of gum collectors and forest workers is the only sensible remedy. Vaccination using a live culture of *L. mexicana* protects against the chronic disfiguring lesions found on the ears.

Uta can be eradicated by residual spraying of dwellings with DDT. Since little is known of the epidemiology of the diffuse cutaneous forms of leishmaniasis, control of this infection is not yet feasible.

Muco-cutaneous leishmaniasis being a sporadic jungle forest disease with an animal reservoir is extremely difficult to control. Dwellings in new settlements in the forest should be concentrated away from the forest edge so that a barrier of clear land is maintained between the village and the forest. Temporary spraying of the forest edges with insecticides can be carried out and travellers into forests should wear protective clothing and use repellents.

Leishmaniasis—Summary

	Visceral	Cutaneous	Muco-cutaneous
(1) *Occurrence*	India, Mediterranean, Middle East, Africa, South America	India, Mediterranean, Middle East, Africa, Central and South America	South and Central America
(2) *Organisms*	L. donovani	L. tropica, L. mexicana, L. peruviana	L. braziliensis
(3) *Reservoir of infection*	Man, dogs and rodents	Rodents, dogs	Rodents
(4) *Mode of Transmission*	Bite of sandfly (Phlebotomus spp.)	Phlebotomus spp.	Phlebotomus spp.
(5) *Control*	(i) Treatment of infected individuals (ii) Attacking animal reservoir of infection (iii) Attacking sandfly with insecticides		

The Helminthic Diseases

The Filariases

Under this generic title are grouped a variety of diseases which bear little relation to each other pathologically although they are produced by nematode worms all belonging to the superfamily Filarioidea. Man is the definitive host of several filarial nematodes. Their embryos (microfilariae) are taken up by insect vectors when feeding on man. They pass through a developmental cycle lasting about a fortnight, at the end of which infective larvae are present in the proboscis. When the insect next feeds, the larvae escape and pass through breaches of the skin surface into the tissues. The main differential characteristics of the various filarial infections are given in Table 6.7.

Filariasis (Bancroftian and Malayan)

Filariasis results from infection with the parasite nematodes *Wuchereria bancrofti* and *Brugia malayi*.

Applied biology
The features of the life cycles of these two filariae are practically identical. The adult worms live in the lymphatic system where the female worms, which are viviparous, produce sheathed microfilariae which

TABLE 6.7

General features of filarial worms infecting man.

<table>
<tr><th>Species</th><th colspan="2">Wuchereria bancrofti</th><th colspan="2">Brugia malayi</th><th>Loa loa</th><th>Onchocerca volvulus</th><th>Acanthocheilonema perstans</th><th>Acanthocheilonema streptocerca</th><th>Mansonella ozzardi</th></tr>
<tr><td>Geographical distribution</td><td>Africa America Asia Australia</td><td>Pacific Islands</td><td>Asia</td><td>Asia</td><td>West and Central Africa</td><td>Africa Central America</td><td>Africa South America</td><td>West Africa</td><td>West Indies South America</td></tr>
<tr><td>Site of adult worm</td><td colspan="2">Lymphatic system</td><td colspan="2">Lymphatic system</td><td>Subcutaneous tissues</td><td>Subcutaneous tissues</td><td>Body cavities, e.g. pleura, pericardium</td><td>Subcutaneous tissues</td><td>Visceral adipose tissue</td></tr>
<tr><td>Microfilaria: Periodicity</td><td>Nocturnal</td><td>Diurnally subperiodic</td><td>Nocturnal</td><td>Nocturnally subperiodic</td><td>Diurnal</td><td>Non-periodic</td><td>Non-periodic</td><td>Non-periodic</td><td>Non-periodic</td></tr>
<tr><td>Sheath</td><td>Sheathed</td><td>Sheathed</td><td>Sheathed</td><td>Sheathed</td><td>Sheathed</td><td>Unsheathed</td><td>Unsheathed</td><td>Unsheathed</td><td>Unsheathed</td></tr>
<tr><td>Site</td><td>Blood</td><td>Blood</td><td>Blood</td><td>Blood</td><td>Blood</td><td>Skin and tissues</td><td>Blood</td><td>Skin and tissues</td><td>Blood</td></tr>
<tr><td>Vectors</td><td>Culex fatigans Anopheles spp.</td><td>C. fatigans Aëdes spp.</td><td>Mansonia spp. Anopheles spp.</td><td>M. longipalpis M. annulatus</td><td>Chrysops spp.</td><td>Simulium spp.</td><td>Culicoides spp.</td><td>Culicoides spp.</td><td>Culicoides spp.</td></tr>
<tr><td>Animal reservoir</td><td colspan="2">None</td><td>Doubtful</td><td>Monkeys, rodents</td><td>None</td><td>None</td><td>None</td><td>None</td><td>None</td></tr>
<tr><td>Diagnosis</td><td>Blood film (night)</td><td>Blood film (afternoon)</td><td>Blood film (night)</td><td>Blood film (night)</td><td>Blood film (afternoon)</td><td>Skin snips or scarification</td><td>Blood film (day)</td><td>Skin snips</td><td>Blood film (day)</td></tr>
<tr><td>Clinical effects</td><td colspan="2">Lymphangitis, hydrocoele, elephantiasis of whole leg</td><td colspan="2">Lymphangitis, elephantiasis of lower legs (mainly below knee)</td><td>Subcutaneous swellings</td><td>Dermatitis, subcutaneous nodules, blindness</td><td>Ill defined, but occur</td><td>Ill defined, but occur</td><td>Ill defined, but occur</td></tr>
</table>

are about 200-300 μm long. The microfilariae make their way to and circulate in the bloodstream where they are ingested by a mosquito. After ingestion the microfilariae escape from the sheath, penetrate the gut wall of the insect and pass to the thoracic muscles where they undergo development. After 2 or more weeks the infective larvae reach the proboscis and enter another vertebrate host when the mosquito is biting. It is not certain how they reach the lymphatics after the insect bites. Many species of mosquitoes, belonging to the genera *Culex, Aëdes, Anopheles* and *Mansonioides*, can act as intermediate hosts of *W. bancrofti* and *B. malayi*.

The microfilariae of *B. malayi* can be distinguished from those of *W. bancrofti* on morphological grounds and by their staining reaction to Giemsa.

Microfilariae of both *W. bancrofti* and *B. malayi* appear in the peripheral blood at distinct times of the day—a characteristic referred to as periodicity. The controlling mechanism for this periodicity has never been satisfactorily explained. It does not appear to depend on the parasympathetic system, nor is the microfilaria count influenced by alteration in the corticosteroid level in the blood of man, or by a general anaesthetic.

Medical geography
The geographical distribution of the parasites is determined largely by climate and the distribution of their mosquito vectors.

Epidemiology
Whereas *W. bancrofti* has so far been found only in man, *B. malayi* is a parasite of both man and animals. The most consistent sign of infection is the appearance of microfilaria in the peripheral blood and many microfilaria carriers are apparently symptom-free and remain so for many years or for life.

Wucheria bancrofti
Two biologically different forms of *W. bancrofti* exist—the nocturnal periodic form, in which the microfilariae appear in the peripheral blood between 10 p.m. and 2 a.m., and is predominantly an infection of urban communities, transmitted by the domestic night-biting mosquito *Culex pipiens fatigans*. It has an almost world-wide distribution, occurring in Central and South America, West, Central and East Africa, Egypt and South-East Asia.

The other form, which is diurnally subperiodic, i.e. microfilariae are present in appreciable numbers throughout the 24 hours but show a consistent minor peak diurnally (usually sometime in the afternoon) is restricted to Polynesia and is transmitted mainly by day-biting mosquitoes.

Brugia malayi

Human infection with *B. malayi* has only been recognised in Asia, where it is predominantly an infection of rural populations, in contrast to the usual distribution of *W. bancrofti*.

There are two forms of *B. malayi*, the periodic in which the microfilariae show markedly nocturnal periodicity in the blood (10 p.m. to 2 a.m.), and which has a tendency to occur in small endemic foci in countries extending from the west coast of India to New Guinea, the Philippines and Japan; and the subperiodic form in which the microfilariae tend to be present throughout the 24 hours with a minor nocturnal peak from 10 p.m. to 6 a.m. This nocturnally subperiodic form has been found, to date, only in Malaysia, Borneo and Palawen Island in the Philippines. The nocturnal periodic form is transmitted by the *Mansonia* mosquitoes of open swamps, lakes and reservoirs which bite mainly at night, while the nocturnal subperiodic is transmitted by the *Mansonia* of swamp forest, mosquitoes which will bite in shade at any time. The periodic form is found mainly in man, and animal infections are rare. In contrast, the subperiodic form is found in many animals (primates, carnivores, rodents, etc.) as well as man (Fig. 6.4).

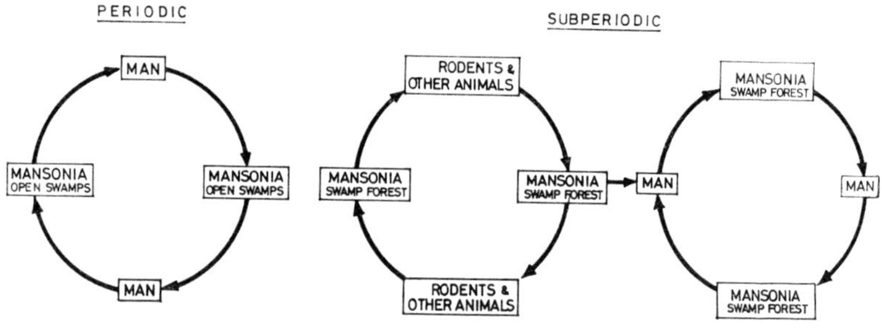

FIG. 6.4   Epidemiology of *Brugia malayi*.

Timor microfilaria

This new microfilaria was recently discovered in the Portuguese island of Timor. There is no animal reservoir and the vector is unknown. The periodicity and symptomatology are similar to that of the periodic form of *W. bancrofti*. Recently another new microfilaria has been discovered in Madagascar and named *W. bancrofti* var. *Vauceli*.

Symptoms attributable to filariasis can present many years after a relatively brief period of exposure to infection, although severe disabling symptoms or deformity are usually due to a long period of exposure and reinfection. Males are usually more frequently affected than females. This higher incidence of microfilaraemia in males is probably due to a greater chance of infection; it is possible, however, that a hormonal influence may be responsible. Most surveys for either form of *W. bancrofti* have shown low microfilaria rates in children below the age of 5 years, probably because *W. bancrofti* takes a long time to produce a patent microfilaraemia. In contrast it has been shown that high microfilariae rates occur in children under 5 years with both the periodic and the subperiodic form of *B. malayi*; thus a low infection rate among children under 5 years usually implies low transmission for *B. malayi* in the area surveyed.

Laboratory diagnosis

The finding of microfilariae in the blood provides the certain diagnosis of filarial infection. Thick blood films should be taken at the appropriate times (e.g. at night for microfilaria *bancrofti*) and fresh cover-slip preparations examined. Simultaneously, dried, stained specimens should be made and identification of the microfilariae made according to the diagnostic criteria given in Table 6.7. Microfilariae may also be found in fluids obtained from hydrocoeles, varices, pleura, joints and in ascitic fluid. Eosinophilia is usually present. It is important to realise that microfilariae may be absent in the very early or late stages of the infection—thus in only 4 per cent of patients with elephantiasis and 30 per cent with hydrocoeles are microfilariae found in the blood. Occasionally the adult filarial worms may be found in biopsy of lymph glands, or by X-ray when calcified.

Many techniques are available for concentrating blood microfilariae.

Serodiagnostic methods for the diagnosis of filariasis have been widely used. There is a range of variation in the results obtained and these variations derive partly from differences in technique of antigen preparation. These immunodiagnostic methods are group specific (i.e. positive in any filarial infection) and on the whole still unsatisfactory with the possible exception of the filarial complement-fixation test (FCFT).

Control

The filariases may be controlled by reducing the human reservoir or by attacking the vector mosquitoes. A combination of vector control and mass treatment with diethylcarbamazine offers the best hope of eventual eradication of bancroftian filariasis.

(a) Human reservoir

The human reservoir of infection may be reduced by treatment of the infected population with diethylcarbamazine (Hetrazan), which abolishes or greatly reduces circulating microfilariae and kills some of the adult worms. Sharp reactions may follow the use of this drug when microfilariae are numerous. Spaced doses over a long period, e.g. 4-6 mg/kg diethylcarbamazine citrate once weekly or once monthly for eight to twelve doses, have proved effective in South-East Asia against both forms of filariasis. These 'travelling treatment' teams have been particularly successful in Tahiti and West Malaysia. *B. malayi* seems more susceptible to diethylcarbamazine than is *W. bancrofti*. There are good reasons to believe that spaced doses of diethylcarbamazine given to a sufficient proportion of the population, and supplemented by follow-up surveys and treatment of those found infected, can bring about a long-lasting reduction in infection rates in areas of endemic filariasis due to *B. malayi*.

(b) *The vector*

Control measures may be taken against the aquatic stages of the mosquito by eliminating breeding places, using insecticides to kill aquatic forms, or in the case of *Mansonia* mosquitoes, destroying by herbicides or hand collection, the water vegetation on which the insect is dependent. Adult vectors may be controlled by residual insecticides applied to the inner walls of houses. *Culex fatigans*, a common vector, is naturally tolerant of DDT and strains resistant to benzene hexachloride and dieldrin have been reported. Organophosphorus insecticides (e.g. Fenthion) can be used against the larval stages, which often breed in septic pits and drains near houses.

Loiasis

This is an infection due to the filarial worm *Loa loa* and is characterised by transient subcutaneous swellings.

Applied biology

The adult worms live in the connective tissue of man and the females, which are about 70 mm long, produce microfilariae which pass into the bloodstream. The microfilariae are sheathed and about 300 μm in length, they appear in greatest numbers in the blood during the day. When the circulating microfilariae are taken up by suitable species of Chrysops, they pass from the stomach to the thoracic muscles and after a period of development, lasting about 12 days, present in the proboscis. When the fly next feeds on a human host the larvae penetrate the skin and migrate in the connective tissues, reaching maturity in about a year.

Medical geography

Loiasis is found in the equatorial rain-forest belt of Africa stretching from the Gulf of Guinea in the west to the Great Lakes in the east.

Epidemiology
Various species of *Chrysops* are the only known vectors of loiasis and
they breed in densely shaded, slow-moving streams and swamps. The
adults live in the tree tops, the females coming down to attack man at
ground level or to lay their eggs on the mud and decaying vegetation of
stagnant waters. The males do not feed on blood. *Chrysops* are attracted
by movement, light and smoke from wood fires, they bite in daylight
and seem to prefer dark to white skins. In man, all ages and both sexes
are affected, although overt infection in young children is uncommon,
probably due to the long incubation period of the filarial worm.

Laboratory diagnosis
Microfilariae may be found in the peripheral blood taken preferably
around midday and they can be differentiated on morphological
grounds from other sheathed microfilariae (see Table 6.7). Concentration techniques are useful to detect scanty infections. The adult
worms may be seen wriggling under the conjunctiva. A high eosinophilia (60-80 per cent) is usually present. The filarial complement-
fixation tests gives the highest incidence of positive results with
loiasis, and is particularly useful in early infections before microfilariae have appeared in the blood, or in unisexual infections when
microfilariae are absent. Intradermal tests are available but have the
same limitations in their use as in the other filarial infections.

Control
As in the case of Bancroft's filariasis, control measures are directed
against the parasite in man and against the vector fly. Diethylcarbamazine clears microfilariae from the blood and kills the adult worm in
recent infections, but it sometimes causes unpleasant reactions. The
drug can be used as a chemoprophylactic at an adult dosage of 200 mg
twice daily for three successive days once a month. The fly may be
controlled by clearing shade vegetation at breeding sites or by applying
residual insecticides to the mud in the breeding places. Personal protection against bites of *Chrysops* can be effected by screening of houses
and wearing long trousers.

Onchocerciasis
This infection is caused by the nematode *Onchocerca volvulus* and is
characterised by the development of skin changes, subcutaneous nodules and ocular lesions.

Applied biology
The adult worms are found in subcutaneous nodules and tissue spaces.
The females, which are ovoviviparous, measure about 50 cm in length
while the males are only 2-4 cm long. Worms of both sexes are found

coiled together in nodules and larvae are present in large numbers near the coiled gravid female. The developed larvae (microfilariae) vary greatly in size (150-350 μm) and are unsheathed.

Microfilariae are ingested when the vector—a *Simulium* fly—feeds on an infected individual. The microfilariae develop in the thoracic muscles of the fly after escaping from its stomach, and after a series of moults become infective larvae on reaching the proboscis. When the *Simulium* next bites an individual the larval forms of *Onchocerca* are injected under the skin. The development in the fly takes about 15 days and the common vectors are *S. damnosum* and *S. neavei* (in Africa), and *S. metallicum*, *S. callidium* and *S. ochraceum* (in Central America). The microfilariae introduced by the fly mature in the subcutaneous tissues. In some instances a fibrous tissue reaction around the adults causes the formation of nodules. After about a year the female worm produces microfilariae. The microfilariae remain in the skin and do not enter the peripheral blood. In Central America *O. volvulus* is called *O. caecutiens*, which is a morphologically similar nematode.

Medical geography
Onchocerciasis has a focal distribution in both African and tropical America. It is endemic in West Africa, in equatorial and East Africa, and in the Sudan. It occurs in Central America and in parts of Venezuela and Colombia.

Epidemiology
Although *O. volvulus* has been found in primates, in most endemic areas the infection is maintained by man-to-man transmission. *Simulium* can breed at high altitudes (2000 ft or more) and the larvae and pupae are found attached to submerged vegetation and stones in highly oxygenated waters. They are also found at sea-level along the banks of very large rivers such as the Niger. The larvae of *S. neavei* have been found adherent to the carapace of aquatic crabs. Though some species of *Simulium* have a long flight range, the infection is mainly concentrated near the breeding sites, and thus tends to be focal. Man is the only reservoir of infection.

The period of greatest transmission is in the rainy season coinciding, as might be expected, with the period of maximal *Simulium* breeding. The disease is widespread and males are infected more frequently than females, but this is probably an occupational hazard. The incidence of infection increases with age and in an endemic area 75 per cent of persons might be infected by middle age. No clear relationship is necessarily found between the number of microfilariae in the skin and the extent or degree of the lesions. Comparisons between African and Central American onchocerciasis reveal certain epidemiological and clinical differences. Thus in some parts of Africa there is tendency for the microfilariae to be most numerous in the most dependent parts of the body; while in Guatemala microfilariae are abundant in the upper parts of the body. A relationship seems to exist between the site of biting of the vector and the localisation of nodules. As would be expected, in Africa the majority of nodules are found in the lower parts of the body, whereas in Central America as many as 70 per cent are found on the head. Bony lesions of the occipital region of the skull produced by these nodules are found in 5 per cent of patients.

In Central America infection is acquired at an early age and in the Cheapas State of Mexico 50 per cent of children are infected by the age of 14 years. Both in Mexico and Guatemala 'erysipela de la costa' is found in children and young persons and 'mal morado' in the older age-groups. Both these syndromes are associated with high microfilaria densities. Moreover, in Guatemala very much more severe corneal and iris lesions are encountered than is usual in Africa.

In Africa, it is generally agreed that anterior segment lesions are due to *O. volvulus*. Considerable disagreement, however, exists as to whether choroidoretinal lesions are a direct complication of ocular onchocerciasis or not. The major cause of disagreement has been the demonstration that in the forest belt of Africa the incidence of ocular complications is low in contrast to the savannah regions where it is high, despite a high prevalence of onchocerciasis in both areas. It has been pointed out that there are distinct epidemiological differences between forest and savannah onchocerciasis. Thus in the savannah areas transmission is seasonal, man/fly contact probably more intimate, and the host resistance may be lower because of the shorter transmission season. There is no evidence that vitamin A is involved and though vitamin B-complex deficiency has been postulated, no proof has been produced that this plays any part in the onchocercal blindness of the savannah areas. The consensus of opinion is that the differences in the incidence of ocular onchocercal complications between the savannah and forest onchocerciasis in Africa are due to differences in intensity and duration of infection. Many believe that ocular lesions are invariably associated with onchocerciasis and that anterior and posterior lesions are part of a unified sequence of inflammatory processes. It has also been observed that high blindness rates are associated with communities in which infection is common in childhood and that a glance at the children's legs in a village could enable one to make a fairly close estimate of the local blindness rate. Onchocercal blindness is rare before the age of 30.

In contrast to the situation in Africa there is general agreement about the nature of the ocular complications in Central America which are predominantly found in the anterior segment of the eye, blindness being due to the end-results of onchocercal kerato-iridocyclitis with the typical occluded and down-drawn pupil described by Pacheco-Luna. In Guatemala more severe corneal and iris lesions are encountered than in Africa. In this context it is interesting to note that some workers believe that the Guatemalan and African strains of *O. volvulus* are different parasites and it is possible that they may possess different propensities for producing eye lesions. Not only the strain of parasite but the whole ecology of infection may differ from one area to another.

Little is known about immunity in onchocerciasis. It has been observed, however, that in Tanzania, microfilarial densities do not increase significantly beyond the age of 20 years. Whether this is due to the development of partial immunity or some other factor has yet to be determined.

Laboratory diagnosis

Microfilariae of *O. volvulus* are identified by examination of skin or conjunctival snips (see Table 6.7). They are most easily found in samples of skin taken from the region of the nodule. Alternatively, the skin snip is teased, immersed in saline, and the deposit examined after centrifugation. Excision of nodules for histological examination will reveal the adult worms, while aspiration of fluid from nodules will occasionally show microfilariae. Microfilariae may also be seen in the anterior chamber of the eye with an ophthalmoscope or slip lamp. A moderate eosinophilia is usually present.

Various serological tests have been used with variable success in the diagnosis of onchocerciasis—these include: complement fixation; intradermal; precipitin; immunofluorescence; and a haemagglutination reaction.

Control

Control is most commonly carried out by attacking the *Simulium* fly.

(a) The vector

When the volume of the stream is not too large, residual insecticides as emulsions or miscible oils may be added to the water above the highest breeding point in sufficient quantity to give a concentration below the lowest breeding sites of 0·5-1 part of DDT per million. This is lethal to the developing forms. Treatment should be repeated for half an hour every 10 days, for 3 months in order to cover the life-span of the adult fly. Insecticides may be sprayed from aircraft on the vegetation around breeding places on alternate days for a period of 3 weeks in order to kill the adult *Simulium*.

(b) The human reservoir

Removal of the subcutaneous nodules reduces the incidence of eye lesions, and mass treatment with diethylcarbamazine of all infected persons in the community kills the microfilariae and reduces transmission. This, however, is liable to cause sharp allergic reactions. Suramin kills the majority of adult worms, but the microfilariae disappear slowly.

A possibility, which has not yet been widely tested, is to use small weekly doses of diethylcarbamazine (50-200 mg) to reduce the microfilarial concentrations in the skin and to maintain this for long periods. For the first 3 to 4 weeks of this regime reactions of declining severity occur and, thereafter, once the main load of microfilariae has been eliminated, the weekly dose can be taken by most persons without inconvenience. Transmission of infection is reduced but the administrative and economic problems of such a campaign make this measure of control rather impracticable in endemic areas.

Ancanthocheilonema perstans

A. perstans has an extensive distribution throughout Africa, tropical America and the Caribbean. The adults have been reported in the liver, pleura, pericardium, mesentery, perirenal and retroperitoneal tissues. The microfilariae are non-periodic and are unsheathed (Table 6.7). The intermediate vectors are *Culicoides austini* and *C. grahami* in Africa. The detailed epidemiology has not been studied, but it is known that many individuals in some African villages may harbour the parasite.

Mansonella ozzardi

This filarial worm is confined to the New World and is found in South America and in certain foci in the Caribbean. The adult worms are embedded in visceral adipose tissue. The vectors are *Culicoides* spp.

Dirofilariasis

Various species of *Dirofilaria* have been reported from the Mediterranean basin, the Balkans, South America, Turkey, Africa and the United States. They include *D. conjunctivae, D. repens, D. magalhaesi* and *D. louisanensis*. The life cycle of these parasites in man is not fully known and it seems probable that mosquitoes or fleas are the natural intermediate hosts.

The adults do not develop normally in man.

Control

Control of *A. perstans, A. streptocerca* and *M. ozzardi*, which is dependent on controlling the vector species of *Culicoides*, has not been seriously attempted.

Insecticides in Public Health

Most of the insecticides manufactured are used in agriculture, many of them affect insects of public health importance and may cause poisoning in man.

Insecticides in public health are used either for a quick knock-down or for a residual effect.

(1) *Knock-down Insecticides*

Most knock-down insecticides contain pyrethrum (sometimes with addition of DDT to improve their efficiency). They are used, usually as a fine spray, to get rid of adult insects quickly, but the effect lasts for only a short time. They can be used when rapid control is required, as in an epidemic of an insect-borne disease, or to kill insects in aircraft. This quick knock-down can be achieved with insecticidal fogs, smoke and aerial spraying.

(2) *Residual Insecticides*

For long-continued effect (e.g. 6 months' duration) residual insecticides are used, DDT for example, applied to wall surfaces at a dose of 2 gm per m², will kill mosquitoes that rest indoors—providing they are still susceptible.

DDT the oldest, is probably still the best, certainly for malaria control. It is relatively non-toxic. **BHC** (HCH) is less long-lasting; **Dieldrin** is too toxic for general use without strict precautions.

Various organic phosphorus insecticides have been used in situations where DDT is not effective. These vary enormously in their toxicity, from parathion which is very dangerous indeed (it is used in agriculture but seldom in public health) to malathion which is only slightly more toxic than DDT. They are less long lasting and more expensive than DDT.

Methods of Application

The insecticides can be applied in many ways, depending on the objective to be achieved. Some of these formulations are:

(1) *Aerosols, fogs, vapours, smokes*

These are used where penetration is required but does not give a long-lasting residual effect.

(2) *Aerial spraying*

Spraying from low levels (up to 100 m) by slow-flying (150-200 mph) aeroplanes, or by helicopters, may be useful for treating large or inaccessible breeding grounds of some pests, such as mosquito larvae in large swamps, or tsetse flies in extensive bush. Air spraying can be done only during stable air conditions. In tropical countries ground heating during the day produces violent air convection, which restricts spraying to about an hour either just after sunrise and just before sunset. Aerial spraying is very useful in epidemic situations.

(3) *Larvicides*
These have been successfully used in the control of mosquitoes (see p. 181) especially when breeding sites are restricted or close to houses, e.g. *Aëdes aegypti* (see p. 158). They have also been successful in controlling *Simulium* (see p. 206).

The decision which insecticides and formulation should be used depends on the circumstances of the particular problem.

(4) *Water-dispersible powders (WDP)*
These are used for applying insecticides to wall surfaces. They are cheap but messy, leaving a white deposit of inert powder on the wall. Most malaria eradication campaigns use 5 per cent DDT (WDP).

(5) *Solutions, emulsions*
These have the same effect as water-dispersible powders. The solvent evaporates, leaving the insecticide on the wall. On some surfaces however, e.g. mud, soakage takes place and the insecticidal effect is markedly lessened.

Resistance
Insects of public health importance can have developed resistance to insecticides. House flies rapidly become resistant (therefore good sanitation is the control method of choice); anopheline mosquitoes are less liable to become resistant to DDT, than to dieldrin or BHC. The only measure to overcome resistance is to change the insecticide. The mechanisms of resistance are complex and beyond the scope of this book.

Toxicity
All the residual insecticides are toxic to man, but the degree varies enormously. DDT and BHC are only slightly toxic; parathion is extremely toxic.

Common-sense precautions, e.g. not eating when using insecticides, washing and changing clothes at the end of the day's work, avoiding contact with concentrated insecticides especially when in solution or emulsion, must be taken by everyone involved in spraying operations. Special precautions must be taken when anything more toxic than DDT or BHC is being applied.

Other Effects of Insecticides
There is a world-wide controversy about the relative damage caused by residual insecticides to wild-life and the benefits they give by increasing food production. The decision as to the choice of insecticides, timing of application, dosage and formulation demands a careful study of each situation. Unless this is done money may be wasted and the desired result may not be achieved.

Chapter Seven

Airborne Infections

Infections of the respiratory tract are acquired mainly by the inhalation of pathogenic organisms.

Infective Agents
The infective agents which cause respiratory infections include viruses, bacteria, rickettsiae and fungi (Table 7.1). The spread of infection from

TABLE 7.1

Examples of pathogens which cause airborne infection

VIRUSES of	RICKETTSIAE	BACTERIA	FUNGI
Smallpox*	*Rickettsia burnetti*	*Mycobacterium tuberculosis*	*Histoplasma capsulatum*
Chickenpox*		*Streptococcus pneumoniae*	
Measles		*Neisseria meningitidis*	
Rubella			
Mumps		*Streptococcus pyogenes*	
Psittacosis		*Haemophilus pertussis*	
Atypical pneumonia		*Corynebacteria diphtheriae*	
Influenza		*Haemophilus influenzae*	
'Common Cold'		*Pasteurella pestis* (Pneumonic plague)	

* See Chapter 5.

the respiratory tract may lead to the invasion of other organs of the body. Bacterial meningitis is often secondary to a primary focus in the respiratory tract, e.g. infections due to *Streptococcus pneumoniae, Haemophilus influenzae* or *Mycobacterium tuberculosis*. In the case of meningococcal infection, there are usually no local symptoms from the primary focus of infection in the nasopharynx.

These pathogens vary in their ability to survive in the environment. Some are capable of surviving for long periods in dust, especially in a dark, warm, moist environment, protected from the lethal effects of ultraviolet rays of sunshine. For example, *M. tuberculosis* can survive for long periods in dried sputum.

Man is the reservoir of most of these infections but some have a reservoir in lower animals, e.g. plague in rodents. Carriers play an important role in the epidemiology of some of these infections, e.g. in meningococcal infection carriers represent the major part of the reservoir.

Mode of Transmission

There are three main mechanisms for the transmission of airborne infections—droplets, droplet nuclei and dust.

Droplets

These are particles which are ejected by coughing, talking, sneezing, laughing and spitting. They may contain food debris and micro-organisms enveloped in saliva or secretions of the upper respiratory tract. Being heavy, droplets tend to settle rapidly. The transmission of infection by this route can only take place over a very short distance. Because of the relatively large size, droplets are not readily inhaled into the lower respiratory tract.

Droplet nuclei

These are produced by the evaporation of droplets before they settle. The small dried nuclei are buoyant and are rapidly dispersed. The droplet nuclei are also usually small enough to pass through the bronchioles into the alveoli of the lungs.

Dust

Dust-borne infections are important in relation to organisms which persist in dust for long periods and dust can act as the reservoir for some of them. The organisms may be derived from sputum, or from settled droplets. Streptococci or staphylococci may also be derived from skin and infected wounds.

Host

A number of non-specific factors protect the respiratory tract of man. These include mechanical factors such as the mucous membrane which traps small particles on its sticky secretions and cleans them out by the action of its ciliated epithelium. In addition, the respiratory tract is also guarded by various reflex acts such as coughing and sneezing which are provoked by foreign bodies or accumulated secretions. Mucoid secretions which contain lysozyme and some biochemical constituents of tissues have anti-microbial action.

Specific immunity may be acquired by previous spontaneous infection or by artificial immunisation. For some of the infections, a single attack confers life-long immunity (e.g. measles) but in other cases, because there are many different antigenic strains of the pathogen, repeated attacks may occur, e.g. influenza.

Control of Airborne Infections

The main principles involved in the control of respiratory infections are outlined under three headings—infective agent, the mode of transmission and host factors.

A. *Infective Agent*
(1) Elimination of human and animal reservoirs.
(2) Disinfection of floors and the elimination of dust.

B. *Mode of Transmission*
(1) *Air hygiene* through good ventilation and in special cases, air disinfection with ultraviolet light.
(2) *Avoid overcrowding*—in bedrooms of dwelling-houses, and in public halls.
(3) *Personal hygiene*—avoid coughing, sneezing, spitting or talking directly at the face of other persons. Face masks should be worn by persons with respiratory infections to limit contamination of the environment.

C. *Host*
(1) *Specific immunisation*, e.g. (a) *Active immunisation* against measles, whooping cough, influenza, etc.; (b) *Passive immunisation* in special cases, e.g. gamma globulin for the prevention of measles.
(2) *Chemoprophylaxis*, e.g. Isoniazid in selected cases for the prevention of tuberculosis.

Measles

Measles is an acute communicable disease which presents with fever, signs of inflammation of the respiratory tract (coryza, cough), and a characteristic skin rash. The presence of punctate lesions (Koplik spots) on the buccal mucosa may assist diagnosis in the early prodromal phase. Deaths occur mainly from complications such as secondary bacterial infection, with bronchopneumonia and skin sepsis. Post-measles encephalitis occurs in a few cases.

The *incubation period* is usually about 10 days, at which stage the patient presents with the prodromal features of fever and coryza. The skin rash usually appears three to four days after the onset of symptoms.

Geographical distribution
Measles is a familiar childhood infection in most parts of the world.

Until recent years there were a few isolated communities in which the infection was unknown, but the disease is endemic in virtually all parts of the world.

Virology
The aetiological agent is the virus of measles.

Epidemiology
Man is the reservoir of infection. Transmission is by droplets or by contact with sick children or with freshly contaminated articles such as toys or handkerchiefs. The outcome of measles infection is largely determined by host factors, in particular the state of nutrition of the child. Measles tends to be a severe killing disease in malnourished children; the infection not infrequently precipitates severe protein-calorie malnutrition ('kwashiorkor'). One attack of measles confers lifelong immunity. Babies are usually immune during the first few months of life through the transplacental transmission of passive immunity from immune mothers.

The disease tends to occur in epidemic waves; in some areas, large epidemics occur on alternate years in densely populated urban areas but at longer intervals in sparsely populated rural areas. The explosive outbreaks seem to occur only when there has been a sufficient accumulation of these susceptible children.

Control
Isolation of children who have measles is of limited value in the control of the infection because the disease is highly infectious in the prodromal coryzal phase before the characteristic rash appears. Thus often by the time a diagnosis of measles is made or even suspected, a number of contacts would have been exposed to infection.

Active immunisation can be induced by the use of a live vaccine. The 'further attenuated' live vaccine is much better tolerated than the attenuated live vaccine. The reactions to the vaccine include fever, and rarely convulsions. Some children develop modified measles with a skin rash and Koplik spots. The frequency and severity of the reactions, can be reduced by giving a dose of gamma globulin (0·05 ml per kg) at the same time that the attenuated live vaccine is given.

Measles infection may be prevented or modified by artificial passive immunisation using immune gamma globulin. If the gamma globulin (0·25 ml/kg) is given early, within 3 days of exposure, the infection will be prevented; if a smaller dose (0·05 ml/kg) is given 4 to 6 days after exposure, the infection may be modified, the child presenting with a mild infection which confers lasting immunity. Since passive immunity by itself given only transient protection, it is more desirable to achieve a modified attack rather than complete suppression of the infection unless the presence of some other serious condition in the child absolutely contraindicates even a mild attack.

Measles—Summary

(1) *Occurrence*—World-wide
(2) *Organism*—Measles virus
(3) *Reservoir of infection*—Man
(4) *Modes of transmission*—Droplets, airborne, contact
(5) *Control*— (i) Active immunisation with further attenuated live virus
       (ii) Improvement in the nutrition of the children

Rubella ('German Measles')

Rubella or German measles is an acute viral infection which presents with fever, mild upper respiratory symptoms, a morbiliform or scarlatiniform rash and lymphadenopathy usually affecting post-auricular, post-cervical and suboccipital lymph nodes. The illness is almost always mild, but infection with rubella during the first trimester is associated with a high risk (up to 20 per cent) of congenital abnormalities in the baby.

The *incubation period* is 2 or 3 weeks.

Geographical distribution
World-wide.

Virology
The aetiological agent is the rubella virus.

Laboratory diagnosis
Clinical differentiation from other mild exanthematous fever may be difficult or impossible. The rubella virus can be isolated from culture of the throat washings in the catarrhal phase.

Epidemiology
Man is the reservoir of infection and the infection is spread from person to person by droplets or by contact, direct or through contamination of fomites. Infection results in lifelong immunity. Infection during early pregnancy may cause such abnormalities as cataract, deaf mutism and congenital heart disease in the baby.

Control

The main interest is to prevent the infection of women who are in the early stages of pregnancy. One practical approach is the deliberate exposure of pre-pubertal girls to infection with rubella. Pregnant women should avoid exposure to rubella, especially during the first 4 months of pregnancy; those who have been in contact with such infections should be protected with gamma globulin.

Some progress has been made with artificial immunisation but the vaccine is not yet widely available.

Mumps
This is an acute viral infection which typically affects salivary glands, especially the parotids but may also involve submandibular or the sublingual salivary glands. Pancreatitis, orchitis, inflammation of the ovaries or meningo-encephalitis may complicate the infection; some of the complications occasionally occur in the absence of obvious clinical symptoms or signs of the salivary glands.

The *incubation period* varies from 2 to 4 weeks; usually it is about $2\frac{1}{2}$ weeks.

Geographical distribution
World-wide

Virology
The infectious agent is the mumps virus.

Epidemiology
Man is the reservoir of infection. The virus is present in the saliva of infected persons; it may be isolated as early as 1 week before clinical signs occur, and it may persist for 9 days after the onset of signs. Healthy carriers, who remain asymptomatic throughout the infection, may also transmit the infection. The source of infection therefore, includes sick patients, incubatory ('precocious') carriers and healthy carriers.

The infection is transmitted by droplets or by contact, directly or indirectly, through fomites.

One infection, whether clinical or subclinical, confers lifelong immunity. Artificial active immunisation with live or inactivated vaccine provides protection for a limited period of a few years.

Laboratory diagnosis
The typical case can be identified clinically but confirmation of diagnosis may be required in atypical cases. Serological tests; haemagglutination, neutralisation and complement-fixation tests are available; the organism may be cultured from saliva, blood or cerebrospinal fluid.

Control
The sick patient should be isolated, if possible, during the infectious phase; strict hygienic measures should be observed in the cleansing of spoons, cups and other utensils handled by the patient, and also in the disposal of his soiled handkerchiefs and other linen.

Routine vaccination of the general public is not recommended but this measure may be of value in protecting susceptible young persons in residential institutions in which epidemics occur frequently.

Mumps—Summary

(1) *Occurrence*—World-wide
(2) *Organism*—Mumps virus
(3) *Reservoir of infection*—Man
(4) *Modes of transmission*—Droplets and contact
(5) *Control*—Isolation of cases and active immunisation

Psittacosis

This may present as an acute severe pneumonia which may prove fatal but mild, subclinical infections do occur.

The *incubation period* is about 4 to 14 days.

Medical geography

The distribution of the disease in man is determined by infection in parrots, budgerigars and other psittacine birds. These birds are found in Australia, Africa and South America, but may be imported as pets to other parts of the world.

Virology

The causative agent is a large virus of the psittacosis-lymphogranuloma venereum group.

Laboratory diagnosis

The organism may be isolated on culture of sputum, blood or vomitus on yolk sacs of embryonated eggs or by inoculation into mice.

Serological tests on paired sera may show rising titres in complement fixing, neutralisation or agglutination tests.

Epidemiology

Psittacosis is basically a zoonotic infection of birds. The affected birds excrete the organisms in their faeces, and through the respiratory tract. Man acquires the infection by inhalation of the infective agent from bird faeces; those who own and handle such birds are at high risk. Person-to-person spread may occur in close contacts.

Control

The importation of these birds should be strictly controlled. They can be held in quarantine to ensure that they are free from infection; infected birds can also be detected on serological tests. Broad-spectrum antibiotics, e.g. tetracycline, can be used to eliminate the carrier state. In case of human infection, the source of infection should be traced and the bird destroyed.

Psittacosis—Summary

(1) *Occurrence*—World-wide
(2) *Organism*—Psittacosis virus
(3) *Reservoir of infection*—Birds, e.g. parrots
(4) *Modes of transmission*—Airborne, contact
(5) *Control*— (i) Quarantine of imported birds
　　　　　　(ii) Antibiotic therapy to eliminate carriers
　　　　　　(iii) Destruction of infected birds

Influenza

This is an acute respiratory infection which is characterised by systemic manifestation—fever, rigors, headache, malaise and muscle pains, and by local manifestations of coryza, sore throat and cough. Secondary bacterial pneumonia is an important complication. The case fatality rate is low but deaths tend to occur in debilitated persons, those with underlying cardiac, respiratory or renal disease, and in the elderly.

The *incubation period* is usually 1 to 3 days.

Virology

There are three main types of the influenza virus—Influenza A, B and C; A and B types consist of several serological strains. An important feature of the epidemiology of influenza is the periodic emergence of new antigenically distinct strains which account for massive pandemics.

Laboratory diagnosis

The virus can be isolated on culture of throat washings. Serological tests include complement-fixation and haemagglutination tests; these can be performed on acute and convalescent sera of patients to show the rising titre of antibodies.

Epidemiology

Man is the reservoir of infection of human strains of the influenza virus. The infection is transmitted by droplets, and also by contact both direct and indirect through the handling of contaminated articles.

All age-groups are susceptible, but if the particular strain causing an epidemic is antigenically related to the cause of an earlier epidemic, the older age-group with persisting antibodies may be less liable.

Deaths occur mostly in cases with some underlying debilitating disease.

Massive epidemics of influenza periodically sweep throughout the world with attack rates as high as 50 per cent in some countries. The pandemic may first appear in a specific focus ('Asiatic 'flu', 'Hong Kong 'flu') from which it spreads from continent to continent. Rapid air travel has facilitated the global dissemination of this infection.

H

Control
Active immunisation with inactivated influenza virus protects against infection with that specific strain. Polyvalent vaccines are also available but they are only effective if they contain the antigens of the particular strain causing the epidemic. Sometimes, it may be possible to prepare vaccine from strains which are isolated early in the epidemic for use in other areas or countries which have not been affected.

Influenza—Summary
(1) *Occurrence*—World-wide; local endemic/epidemic picture; massive pandemics
(2) *Organism*—Influenza virus
(3) *Reservoir of infection*—Man
(4) *Modes of transmission*—Airborne, contact
(5) *Control*—Killed vaccine, identical antigenic strain

Acute Upper Respiratory Infection
Acute infection of the upper respiratory tract is a common but mainly benign disease. The most typical manifestation, 'the common cold', presents with coryza, irritation of the throat, lacrimation and mild constitutional upset. Local complications may occur with secondary bacterial infection and involvement of the para-nasal sinuses and the middle ear. Infection may spread to the larynx, trachea and bronchi.

The *incubation period* is from 1 to 3 days.

Medical geography
The distribution is world-wide.

Microbiology
These symptoms can be induced by infection with various viral agents, including the rhinoviruses, certain enteroviruses, influenza, para-influenza, adeno-viruses, reoviruses and the respiratory syncitial virus. Superinfection with various bacteria may determine the clinical picture in the later stages of the illness.

Laboratory diagnosis
Some of the viruses can be isolated from the throat washings or stool but this diagnostic test is not routinely done.

Epidemiology
Man is the reservoir of these infections. Transmission is by airborne infection, or by contact both direct and indirect (contaminated toys, handkerchiefs, etc.). All age-groups are liable but the manifestations and complications tend to be severe in young children. Repeated attacks are very common.

Epidemics occur commonly in households, offices, schools and in other groups having close contact.

Control

No specific control measures are available. Infected persons should avoid contact with others. The exposure of young persons to infected persons should be avoided if possible.

Acute Upper Respiratory Infection—Summary

(1) *Distribution*—World-wide
(2) *Organisms*—Rhinoviruses, reoviruses, some enteroviruses, etc.
(3) *Reservoir of infection*—Man
(4) *Modes of transmission*—Airborne, contact
(5) *Control*—Avoid exposure of young children to infected persons

Infectious Mononucleosis

This is an acute febrile illness which is characterised by lymphadenopathy ('glandular fever'), splenomegaly, sore throat and lymphocytosis. A skin rash and small mucosal lesions may be present. Occasionally jaundice and rarely meningo-encephalitis may occur.

The *incubation period* is from about 4 days to 2 weeks.

Medical geography

Isolated cases and epidemics of the disease have been reported from most parts of the world.

Virology

The causative agent is probably a virus, but it has not been definitely identified.

Laboratory diagnosis

In the acute phase, there is marked leucocytosis mainly due to an increase in monocytes and large lymphocytes. Heterophile antibodies to sheep red cells can also be demonstrated.

Epidemiology

Man is presumed to be the reservoir of infection, with the sputum being regarded as the most likely source of infection. Transmission may be airborne or by person-to-person occurring in closed institutions for young adults, there is some suggestion that kissing may be an important route. Infection occurs mostly in children and young adults.

Control

No satisfactory control measures are available.

Infectious Mononucleosis—Summary
(1) *Distribution*—World-wide
(2) *Organism*—Unknown virus
(3) *Reservoir of infection*—Probably man
(4) *Modes of transmission*—Airborne, contact
(5) *Control*—No effective measures are available

Q Fever
This is usually present as an acute febrile illness with chest symptoms but minimal clinical signs; involvement of the lungs occurs in the form of atypical pneumonia.

The *incubation period* is from about 14 to 21 days.

Medical geography
It is probably endemic in most parts of the world, but it is likely that its frequency has been underestimated in areas with poor laboratory facilities.

Microbiology
The causative agent is *Rickettsia burnetii (Coxiella burnetii)*. The organism survives adverse physical conditions, e.g. drying; pasteurisation at 60°C for 30 minutes.

Laboratory diagnosis
The organism can be recovered on culture in eggs or animal inoculation of blood taken soon after the onset of the illness. Serological tests may show rising titre of antibodies in the complement-fixation test using yolk-sac antigen. The Weil-Felix reaction using strains of proteins is negative in Q fever.

Epidemiology
The reservoir of infection is in birds, goats, sheep and cattle. Transmission is mainly by airborne infection, but infection may occur from ingestion of milk. The soil may be contaminated from the excrement of infected sheep. The pregnant uterus and the products of conception are also important sources of infection. Most infected persons will recover spontaneously, and with antibiotic chemotherapy (tetracycline or chloramphenicol), death is rare.

Control
Susceptible persons who are at risk can be protected by immunisation with inactivated vaccine. Pasteurisation of milk at high temperature (62·9°C for 30 minutes or 71·7°C for 15 seconds) will destroy the rickettsiae. The infection should also be controlled in animals by vaccination (see p. 168).

Q Fever—Summary
(1) *Distribution*—World-wide
(2) *Organism*—*Rickettsia burnetii*
(3) *Reservoir of infection*—Domestic animals, ticks
(4) *Modes of transmission*—Airborne, milk
(5) *Control*— (i) Immunisation of man and animals
          (ii) Pasteurisation of milk at high temperature

Tuberculosis

Tuberculosis remains one of the major health problems in many tropical countries; in some countries the situation is being aggravated by dense overcrowding in urban slums. Tuberculosis presents a wide variety of clinical forms, but pulmonary involvement is common and is most important epidemiologically, as it is mostly responsible for the transmission of the infection. On first infection, the patient develops the primary complex which consists of a small parenchymal lesion and involvement of the regional lymph node; in the lungs, this constitutes the classical Ghon focus, with a small lung lesion and invasion of the mediastinal lymph node. In most cases the primary complex heals spontaneously, with fibrosis and calcification of the lesions, but the organisms may persist for many years within this focus. In a small proportion of cases the primary complex progresses to produce more severe manifestations locally (e.g. caseous pneumonia) or there may be haematogenous dissemination to other parts of the body. Thus within a few years of the primary infection, especially during the first 6 months, there is the danger of haematogenous spread either focal (e.g. bone and joint lesions) or disseminated in the form of miliary tuberculosis and tuberculous meningitis. Apart from the primary complex and its early complications, the 'adult' pulmonary form of tuberculosis may occur either as a result of the re-activation of an existing lesion or by re-infection. Destruction of the lung parenchyma, with fibrosis and cavitation are important features of this adult form. Clinically, it may present with cough, haemoptysis and chest pain, with general constitutional symptoms—fever, loss of weight and malaise; often it remains virtually asymptomatic especially in the early stages.

The *incubation period* is from 4 to 6 weeks.

Medical geography
Tuberculosis has a world-wide distribution. Until recently, it was absent from a few isolated communities where the local populations are now showing widespread infections with severe manifestations on first contact with tuberculosis.

Medical bacteriology
The causative agent is *Mycobacterium tuberculosis*, the tubercle bacillus.

The human type produces most of the pulmonary lesions, also some extrapulmonary lesions; the bovine strain of the organism mainly accounts for extrapulmonary lesions. Other types of *M. tuberculosis*, avian and atypical strains, rarely cause disease in man, but infection with these strains may produce immunological changes in man with non-specific tuberculin skin reaction.

Tubercle bacilli survive for long periods in dried sputum and dust.

Laboratory diagnosis

The organism may be identified on examination of sputum and other pathological specimens (cerebrospinal fluid, urine, pleural fluid or gastric washings). The tubercle bacillus is Gram-positive, but because of its waxy coat it does not stain with the standard procedure. It is usually demonstrated by the Ziehl-Neelsen method, using hot carbol-fuchsin stain; the tubercle bacillus like other mycobacteria resists decolourisation with acid ('acid fast bacilli') but unlike the others it is also not decolourised by alcohol ('acid and alcohol fast').

The organism can be isolated on culture using special media, or by inoculation into guinea-pigs.

Tuberculin test

With the first infection with *M. tuberculosis*, the host develops hypersensitivity to the organism; this hypersensitivity is the basis of various tuberculin skin tests. The material used may be a concentrated filtrate of broth in which tubercle bacilli have been grown for 6 weeks ('Old tuberculin') or a chemical fraction, the purified protein derivative (PPD). The skin reaction to tuberculin is of the delayed hypersensitivity type, and the result of tuberculin test is usually read in 48 or 72 hours. In the Mantoux test, the material is injected intradermally, a positive reaction being denoted by an induration of 10 mm diameter or larger in response to five tuberculin units. The tuberculin test can also be performed using the Heaf gun.

The tuberculin test usually becomes positive 4 to 6 weeks after primary infection with tubercle bacilli; other mycobacteria may produce cross-sensitivity. A negative reaction usually indicates that the patient has had no previous exposure to tubercle bacilli but occasionally the test is negative in patients with overwhelming infection or in certain conditions which suppress allergic response, e.g. measles, sarcoidosis.

The tuberculin test can be used in various ways:

(a) *Clinical diagnosis*—the tuberculin test is usually positive in infected persons, and tends to be strongly positive in cases of active disease.

(b) *Identifying susceptible groups*—a negative reaction usually indicates that the person has had no previous exposure to tuberculous infection and therefore, no acquired immunity.

(c) *Epidemiological surveys*—to determine the pattern of infection and immunity in the community.

Epidemiology
Man is the reservoir of the human strain and patients with pulmonary infection constitute the main source of infection. The reservoir of the bovine strain is in cattle, with infected milk and meat being the main sources of infection. Transmission of infection is mainly airborne by droplets, droplet nuclei and dust; thus it is enhanced by overcrowding in poorly ventilated accommodation. Infection may also occur by ingestion, especially of contaminated milk and infected meat.

The host response is an important factor in the epidemiology of tuberculosis. A primary infection may heal with the host acquiring immunity in the process. In some cases the primary lesion progresses to produce extensive disease locally or infection may disseminate to produce metastatic or miliary lesions. Lesions that are apparently healed may subsequently break down with reactivation of disease. Certain factors such as malnutrition, measles infection, use of corticosteroids and other debilitating conditions predispose to progression and reactivation of the disease.

Control
In planning a programme for the control of tuberculosis, the entire population can be conveniently considered as falling into four groups:

(1) Those who have had no previous exposure to tubercle bacilli. They would require protection from infection.

(2) Those with healed primary infection. They have some immunity but must be protected from re-activation of disease and re-infection.

(3) Those who are known to have active disease. They must have effective treatment and remain under supervision until they have recovered fully.

(4) Those who have active disease but are as yet undiagnosed. Without treatment the disease may progress with further irreversible damage and also as potential sources of infection, they constitute a danger to the community.

The control of tuberculosis can be considered at the five levels of prevention:

(1) *General health promotion*
Improvement in housing (good ventilation, avoidance of overcrowding) will reduce the chances of airborne infections. Health education

should be directed at producing better personal habits with regard to spitting and coughing. Good nutrition enhances host immunity.

(2) *Specific protection*

Three measures are available: (a) active immunisation with BCG (Bacille Calmette Guerin), (b) chemoprophylaxis, (c) control of animal tuberculosis.

(a) *BCG vaccination*

This vaccine contains live attenuated tubercle bacilli of the bovine strain. It may be administered intradermally by syringe and needle or by the multiple-puncture technique. It confers significant but not absolute immunity; in particular, it protects against the disseminated miliary lesions of tuberculosis. BCG vaccination may be used selectively in tuberculin-negative persons who are at high risk, e.g. close contacts, doctors, nurses and hospital ward attendants. A strain of BCG which is resistant to isoniazid has been developed; this can be used in vaccinating tuberculosis contacts who require immediate protection with isoniazid.

BCG may also be used more widely in immunising tuberculin-negative persons, especially children, in the community. In some developing countries where preliminary tuberculin testing may significantly reduce coverage, BCG may be administered in mass campaigns without tuberculin tests. The disadvantage of this method of 'direct BCG vaccination' is that those who are tuberculin-positive are likely to show more severe local reactions at the site of vaccination.

Various complications have been encountered in the use of BCG. These may be:
- (i) *Local*—chronic ulceration, discharge, abscess formation and keloids.
- (ii) *Regional*—adenitis which may or not suppurate or form sinuses.
- (iii) *Disseminated*—a rare complication.

One disadvantage of BCG vaccination is the loss of the tuberculin test as a diagnostic and epidemiological tool.

(b) *Chemoprophylaxis*

Isoniazid has proved an effective prophylatic agent in preventing infection and preventing progression of infection to severe disease. Treatment with isoniazid for one year is recommended for the following groups:
- (i) Close contacts of patients.
- (ii) Persons who have converted from tuberculin-negative to tuberculin-positive in the previous year.

(iii) Children under 3 years who are tuberculin-positive from naturally acquired infection. The tuberculin-negative person may be
protected by BCG or INH; the decision as to which method to
use would depend on local factors, the acceptability of regular
drug therapy and the availability of effective supervision.

(c) *Control of bovine tuberculosis*
The ideal is to maintain herds that are free of tuberculosis. Infected
animals can be identified by the tuberculin skin test and eliminated.
Milk, especially from herds that are not certified tuberculosis free,
should be pasteurised. Carcasses of cattle should be examined after
slaughter looking for signs of tuberculosis. Such infected meat should
be condemned.

(3) *Early diagnosis and treatment*
Case-finding operations should aim at identifying active cases at an
early stage of the disease. This would depend on maintaining a high
index of suspicion in clinical practice and also by carrying out routine
screening, especially of high-risk groups. Screening methods include
tuberculin testing, sputum and chest X-ray examination. The interpretation of the tuberculin test would depend on local epidemiological
factors; microscopic examination of Ziehl-Neelsen stained smears of
sputum is a simple cheap screening technique which is particularly useful in rural areas of developing countries where resources are limited.
Mass miniature radiography (MMR) has been widely applied and has
been particularly valuable in detecting pre-symptomatic disease, but it
is relatively expensive to establish and run, it requires highly trained
personnel and it has little specificity, showing many lesions which are
definitely non-tuberculous or of doubtful origin.

High risk and special groups that should be screened include:
(*a*) Contacts of tuberculous patients both household contacts and
workmates
(*b*) Persons who have cough persisting for 3 weeks or more
(*c*) Workers in hospitals and sanatoria
(*d*) Teachers, food handlers and other persons who come into contact with the public.

Drug treatment
Drug therapy usually commences with three drugs, Streptomycin,
para-amino salicyclic acid PAS (or thiacetazone) and isoniazid (INH).
After 3 months (when the sensitivity of the organism to these drugs
may be known) the patient may be maintained on two oral drugs,
PAS (or thiacetazone) and INH, if the organism is sensitive. Second-
line drugs such as viomycin and cycloserine are available for dealing
with resistant strains, but these drugs are very expensive and are more
toxic than the standard drugs.

Treatment must be maintained 1 year or more. Surgery may be indicated for dealing with destructive lesions of bones or the lungs.

Ambulant treatment has proved successful; in-patient care is required for only a few special cases. It is important to have adequate supervision by home visitors of out-patient treatment.

(4) *Limitation of disability*

Apart from early diagnosis and effective drug treatment, steps should be taken to limit the physical, mental and social disability associated with the disease. The physical aspect may require active physiotherapy, e.g. breathing exercises, appropriate exercises and support for diseased bones and joints. The mental disability may be limited by suitable diversional or occupational therapy and by simple reassurance or more expert psychotherapy.

(5) *Rehabilitation*

This should, as always, commence from the beginning of the treatment of the patient. Most patients recover sufficiently well to return to their former occupation. Where chronic physical disability is unavoidable, the patient can be re-trained for alternative employment.

Careful health education of relatives and the community by breaking down prejudices will assist the rehabilitation of patients.

Surveillance of Tuberculosis

For effective control of tuberculosis, there should be a surveillance system to collect, evaluate and analyse all pertinent data, and use such knowledge to plan and evaluate the control programme. The sources of data will include:

(a) Notification of cases
(b) Investigation of contacts
(c) Post-mortem reports
(d) Special surveys—tuberculin, sputum, chest X-ray
(e) Laboratory reports on isolation of organisms including the pattern of drug sensitivity
(f) Records of BCG immunisation—routine and mass programmes
(g) Housing, especially data about overcrowding
(h) Data about tuberculosis in cattle
(i) Utilisation of anti-tuberculous drugs.

Usually these data are co-ordinated by one central tuberculosis authority which has the overall responsibility for the control of the disease.

Tuberculosis—Summary

(1) *Occurrence*—World-wide
(2) *Organism*—*Mycobacterium tuberculosis* (human and bovine strains)
(3) *Reservoir of infection*—Man, cattle

(4) *Modes of transmission*—Airborne, droplets, droplets nuclei and dust. Milk and infected meat

(5) *Control*— (i) General improvement in housing, nutrition and personal hygiene
(ii) Immunisation with BCG
(iii) Chemoprophylaxis
(iv) Case finding and treatment

Pneumonias

A variety of organisms may cause acute infection of the lungs. The non-tuberculous pneumonias are usually classified into three groups:

(*a*) Pneumococcal
(*b*) Other bacterial
(*c*) Atypical.

(a) Pneumococcal Pneumonia

Pneumococcal infection of the lungs characteristically produces lobar consolidation but bronchopneumonia may occur. Typically the untreated case resolves by crisis, but with antibiotic treatment there is usually a rapid response. Metastatic lesions may occur in the meninges, brain, heart valves, pericardium or joints.

The *incubation period* is 1 to 3 days. The disease is usually notifiable.

Geographical distribution

The aetiological agent is *Streptococcus pneumoniae*, a Gram-positive lancet-shaped diplococcal organism. It is enveloped in a polysaccharide capsule. There are 75 or more antigenic types of pneumococcus, the typing being done by the effect of the specific serum on the capsule.

Epidemiology

Man is the reservoir of infection; these include sick patients as well as carriers. Transmission is by airborne infection and droplets, by direct contact or through contaminated articles. It may persist in the dust for some time.

All ages are susceptible, but the clinical manifestations are most severe at the extremes of age. Negroes seem to be more susceptible than Caucasians.

Pneumonia may complicate viral infection of the respiratory tract. Exposure, fatigue, alcohol and pregnancy apparently lower resistance to this infection. On recovery, there is some immunity to the homologous type.

Epidemics of pneumococcal pneumonia occur in prisons, barracks and work camps.

Laboratory diagnosis
The organism may be recovered on culture of the sputum, throat swab and, less commonly, the blood. The specific type can be identified by direct serological testing of the sputum or, later, the organisms isolated on culture.

Control

The general measures for the prevention of respiratory infections apply—avoidance of overcrowding, good ventilation and improved personal hygiene with regard to coughing and spitting. Prompt treatment of cases with antibiotics would prevent complications. Chemoprophylaxis with sulphonamide is indicated in cases of outbreaks in institutions.

Pneumococcal Pneumonia—Summary

(1) *Occurrence*—World-wide; epidemics occur in work camps, prisons
(2) *Aetiology*—Streptococcus pneumoniae
(3) *Reservoir of infection*—Man
(4) *Modes of transmission*—Droplets, dusts, airborne contact, fomites
(5) *Control*—   (i) Avoid overcrowding
           (ii) Good ventilation
           (iii) Improve personal hygiene (spitting, coughing)
           (iv) Chemoprophylaxis to control institutional outbreaks

(b) Other Bacterial Pneumonias

The other bacteria which can cause pneumonia include *Streptococcus pyogenes* (Group B beta paemolytieus): *Staphylococcus aureus*; *Klebsiella pneumoniae*; *Haemophilus influenzae*.

Geographical distribution
World-wide

Bacteriology and laboratory diagnosis
Although in some cases one particular organism predominates, it is not unusual to encounter mixed infections especially in persons with chronic lung disorders. The organisms can be isolated on culture of the sputum or occasionally from blood.

Epidemiology
These infections often complicate influenza, measles and other viral infections of the respiratory tract. These organisms are commonly found in man and in his environment, the occurrence of infection is largely determined by host factors, such as the presence of debilitating illness such as diabetes or chronic renal failure. Patients suffering from chronic bronchitis are also particularly liable. Transmission is by droplets, airborne infection and contact.

Control

The frequency of these bacterial pneumonias can be diminished by the:

(*a*) Prevention of predisposing viral infection, e.g. by vaccination against measles and influenza.

(*b*) Prompt treatment of upper respiratory infection especially in children and in the elderly.

(*c*) Prevention and treatment of chronic disease of the lungs.

(*d*) Improvement in housing conditions.

Other Bacterial Pneumonias—Summary

(1) *Occurrence*—World-wide

(2) *Aetiology*—S. pyogenes, S. aureus, K. pneumoniae, H. influenzae

(3) *Reservoir of infection*—Man

(4) *Modes of transmission*—Airborne, contact

(5) *Control*— (i) Prevention of predisposing viral infections

(ii) Prompt treatment of upper respiratory infection in children and elderly people

(iii) Prevention and treatment of chronic respiratory diseases

(c) Atypical Pneumonia

This is an acute febrile illness usually starting with signs of an upper respiratory infection, later spreading to the bronchi and lungs. Radiological examination of the lungs shows lazy patchy infiltration.

The *incubation period* is usually about 12 days, ranging from 7 to 21 days.

Geographical distribution
World-wide

Infective agent
The infective agent is *Mycoplasma pneumoniae* (pleuro-pneumonia-like organism).

Epidemiology
Man is the reservoir of infection. It is transmitted from sick patients as well as from persons with subclinical infection. Transmission is by droplet infection and by contact. Only a small proportion of infected persons (1 to 30) show signs of illness. After recovery, the patient is immune for an indefinite period.

Laboratory diagnosis
The diagnosis can be established by showing a rising titre of antibodies to *M. pneumoniae*. The organism can also be identified by collecting throat swabs or washings at an early stage of the infection. During the convalescence, patients usually develop cold agglutinins and agglutinins for Streptococcus M.G.

Control

General measures for the control of respiratory diseases are advocated. Treatment with tetracycline is advocated in cases of pneumonia.

Atypical Pneumonia—Summary

(1) *Occurrence*—World-wide
(2) *Aetiology*—Mycoplasma pneumoniae
(3) *Reservoir of infection*—Man
(4) *Modes of transmission*—Droplets, contact
(5) *Control*— (i) General measures for controlling respiratory infection
       (ii) Treatment of patients with tetracycline

Meningococcal Infection

A variety of clinical manifestations may be produced when human beings are infected with *Neisseria meningitidis*; the typical clinical picture is of acute pyogenic meningitis with fever, headache, nausea and vomiting, neck stiffness, loss of consciousness and a characteristic petechial rash is often present. There is a wide spectrum of clinical manifestations ranging from fulminating disease with shock and circulatory collapse to relatively mild meningococcaemia without meningitis presenting as a febrile illness with a rash. The carrier state is common.

The *incubation period* is usually 3 to 4 days, but may be 2 to 10 days.

Medical geography

There is a world-wide distribution of this infection. Sporadic cases and small epidemics occur in most parts of the world, including the developed countries of the temperate zone. Massive epidemics occur periodically in the so-called 'meningitis belt' of tropical Africa, a zone lying 5-15°N of the equator and characterised by annual rainfall between 300 and 1100 mm. In this zone, the epidemic comes in waves followed by periods of respite.

Bacteriology

N. meningitidis (Meningococcus) is a Gram-negative, bean-shaped, diplococcal organism. It is differentiated from other Neisserial organisms, including the commensal *N. catarrhalis*, by fermentation reactions. Six major antigenic strains, A, B, C, D, X and Y, have been identified on serological testing. In the 'meningitis belt' of Africa, type A is the causative agent of epidemics.

Epidemiology

Man is the reservoir of infection. The carrier state may be 5 to 20 per cent or even higher, during epidemics. Transmission is by airborne droplets or by direct contact. It is a delicate organism; it dies rapidly on cooling or drying, and thus indirect transmission is not an important route.

Children and young adults are most susceptible, but in epidemics all age-groups may be affected. In institutions such as military barracks, new entrants and recruits usually have higher attack rates than those who have been in long residence.

In the epidemic zone of tropical Africa, the outbreaks usually begin in the dry season, reaching a peak at the end of the dry season, and end sharply at the onset of the rains.

Laboratory diagnosis

The organism can be recovered from bacteriological examination of nasopharyngeal swabs, blood and cerebrospinal fluid. The cerebrospinal fluid will, in addition, show the typical changes of pyogenic meningitis (cloudy fluid, numerous pus cells, raised protein content, low or absent glucose).

Control

There are three basic approaches to the control of meningococcal infections:

(*a*) The management of sick patients and their contacts
(*b*) Environmental control designed to reduce airborne infections
(*c*) Immunisation.

(a) *Sick patients and their contacts*

Where the problem of drug resistance has not emerged, sulphonamides remain the drug of choice for the treatment of cases of meningitis; it is most conveniently adminstered as injections of long-acting sulphonamides, e.g. sulphormethoxine ('Fanasil'). Where resistant strains of the organism are present, chloramphenicol should be given by intramuscular injection, in addition to or in place of sulphonamides.

The isolation of patients is of no value in controlling epidemics of meningococcal meningitis because healthy carriers always far outnumber the sick patients.

In closed communities, prophylactic treatment may be used to prevent disease among contacts; sulphonamides proved valuable for this purpose. Because of the emergence of resistant strains, it is probably not advisable to use sulphonamides for chemoprophylaxis; if indicated, other antibiotics may be used for such preventive treatment. Similarly, mass chemoprophylaxis, which was widely practised, is no longer recommended as such indiscriminate use of sulphonamides may prove ineffective and may accelerate the emergence of resistant strains.

(b) *Environmental control*

Overcrowding should be avoided in institutions such as schools boarding-houses and military barracks; the dormitories should be spacious and well-ventilated. In areas where people tend to live in cramped overcrowded accommodation, they should be advised to sleep out of doors so as to limit the risk of transmission of infection.

(c) *Immunisation*

Effective protection against type C meningococcal infection has been achieved using a polysaccharide extract of the organism. Vaccines, for protection against type A are currently being tested.

A number of practical problems have to be solved in dealing with outbreaks of meningitis in rural Africa. The cases tend to overwhelm the local health services and they are usually supplemented by mobile teams which can be organised and rapidly deployed to deal with the emergency. In the most peripheral units, the management of cases may have to rely mainly on auxiliary personnel.

For the effective control of this disease, a system of epidemiological surveillance must be established. Data derived from treatment centres, hospitals, laboratories and special surveys must be collated, evaluated, analysed and disseminated to those who have to take action in the field. National data on epidemics should be made available to neighbouring states and co-ordinated through the World Health Organisation.

Meningococcal Infection—Summary

(1) *Occurrence*—World-wide; massive epidemics occur in a zone of tropical Africa—'the meningitis belt'; epidemics among recruits in military barracks
(2) *Organism*—*Neisseria meningitidis*
(3) *Reservoir of infection*—Man
(4) *Modes of transmission*—Airborne, droplets, direct contact
(5) *Control*— (i) Avoid overcrowding
　　　　　　 (ii) Sulphonamide prophylaxis

Streptococcal Infections

Streptococcus pyogenes, Group A haemolytic streptococci can invade various tissues of man—skin and subcutaneous tissues, mucous membranes, blood and some deep tissues. Some strains produce an erythrogenic toxin which is responsible for the characteristic erythematous rash of scarlet fever. Rheumatic fever and acute glomerulonephritis result from allergic reactions to streptococcal infections. The common clinical manifestations of streptococcal infection include streptococcal sore throat, erysipelas, scarlet fever, and puerperal fever.

Geographical distribution

Streptococcal infections have a world-wide occurrence, but the pattern of the distribution of streptococcal diseases varies from area to area.

Bacteriology
There are at least 40 serologically distinct types of Group A streptococci; some of these specific serological types tend to be associated
with particular forms of streptococcal disease, e.g. Type 12, Group A
is frequently associated with glomerulonephritis. Apart from Group A,
other groups of streptococci, B, C, D and G, have been identified.

Epidemiology
Man is the reservoir of infection; this includes acutely ill and convalescent patients, as well as carriers, especially nasal carriers. The sources
of infection are the infected discharges of sick patients, droplets, dust
and fomites. The infection may be airborne, through droplets, droplet
nuclei or dust. It may be spread by contact or through contaminated
milk. Although all age-groups are liable to infection, children are
particularly susceptible. Repeated attacks of tonsillitis and streptococcal
sore throat are common but immunity is acquired to the erythrogenic
toxin and thus it is rare to have a second attack of scarlet fever with the
scalartinous rash.

Laboratory diagnosis
The organism can be isolated by culture of bacteriological swabs
taken from the throat, nose or pus. The particular group and serological type can be identified from cultures grown on blood agar.
Organisms can also be isolated from blood culture. A rising titre of
the anti-streptolysin O antibody is also evidence of current streptococcal infection.

Control
The general measures for the control of airborne infections are applicable. In addition, such measures as the pasteurisation of milk and
aseptic obstetric techniques are of value. Specific chemoprophylaxis
with penicillin is indicated for persons who have had rheumatic fever
and for those who are liable to recurrent streptococcal skin infections.
The penicillin can be given orally in the form of daily doses of penicillin
V or by monthly injections of long-acting benzathine penicillin.
Sulphonamides can be used in place of penicillin, but they are less effective in preventing recurrences of rheumatic fever.

Streptococcal Infections—Summary

(1) *Occurrence*—World-wide; varying pattern from area to area
(2) *Organism*—*Streptococcus pyogenes*, Group A
(3) *Reservoir of infection*—Man
(4) *Modes of transmission*—Airborne, contact or milk-borne
(5) *Control*— (i) As for other airborne infections
        (ii) Pasteurisation of milk
        (iii) Penicillin or sulphonamide prophylaxis

Rheumatic Fever

Rheumatic fever is a complication of infection with Group A haemolytic streptococci. The initial infection may present as a sore throat or may be subclinical; the onset of rheumatic fever is usually 2 to 3 weeks after the beginning of the throat infection. Apart from fever, the patient may develop pancarditis, arthritis, chorea, subcutaneous nodules and erythema marginatum. Residual damage in the form of chronic valvular heart disease may complicate clinical or subclinical cases of rheumatic fever, the complication is more liable to occur after repeated attacks of rheumatic fever.

Geographical distribution

The disease has a world-wide occurrence. Although there is a falling incidence of the disease in the developed countries of the temperate zone, it is becoming a more prominent problem in the overcrowded urban areas of some tropical and subtropical countries, e.g. in South-East Asia.

Bacteriology and laboratory diagnosis

Group A haemolytic streptococci may be isolated from the bacteriological swab of the throats of some of these patients but not from the heart or the joints which are not directly invaded by the organism. A rising titre of anti-streptolysin antibody may also be demonstrated.

Epidemiology

Rheumatic fever represents an allergic response in a small proportion of persons who have streptococcal sore throat. The factors which determine this sensitivity reaction in a small proportion are not known.

Control

The control of rheumatic fever involves the control of streptococcal infections in the community generally and the prevention of recurrences by chemoprophylaxis after recovery from an attack of rheumatic fever.

Rheumatic Fever—Summary

(1) *Occurrence*—World-wide, declining in developed countries but increasing prominence in some tropical developing countries

(2) *Aetiology*—Complication of streptococcal infection of the throat

(3) *Reservoir of infection*—Man

(4) *Mode of transmission*—See 'Streptococcal infections'

(5) *Control*— (i) Control of streptococcal infections

(ii) Long-term chemoprophylaxis to prevent recurrences

Pertussis

Infection with *Bordetella pertussis* leads to inflammation of the lower respiratory tract from the trachea to the bronchioles. Clinically, the infection is characterised by paroxysmal attacks of violent cough; a rapid succession of coughs typically end with a characteristic loud, high-pitched inspiratory crowing sound—the so-called 'whoop'.

The *incubation period* is usually 7 to 10 days but may be as long as 3 weeks.

Geographical distribution

The disease has a world-wide distribution but there is falling morbidity and mortality following immunisation programmes.

Bacteriology

The pertussis organism is a Gram-negative rod which can be cultured on blood-enriched media. It can be differentiated by immunological tests from *B. parapertussis*, the aetiology of a similar but milder disease.

Epidemiology

Man is the reservoir of infection. Transmission of infection may be airborne or by contact with freshly soiled articles. Children under 1 year old are highly susceptible and most deaths occur in young infants.

Laboratory diagnosis

The organism can be recovered from infected patients during the early stages of the infection, from nasopharyngeal swabs or from cough plates, followed by culture on special media.

Control

The sick children should be kept away from susceptible children during the catarrhal phase of the whooping cough; isolation need not be continued beyond 3 weeks because the patient is no longer highly infectious even though the whoop persists.

Routine active immunisation with killed vaccine is highly recommended for all infants. The pertussis vaccine is usually incorporated as a constituent of the triple antigen (Diphtheria-Pertussis-Tetanus) which is used for the immunisation of children starting from 2 to 3 months.

Pertussis—Summary

(1) *Occurrence*—World-wide
(2) *Organism*—Bordetella pertussis
(3) *Reservoir of infection*—Man
(4) *Mode of transmission*—Airborne
(5) *Control*—Active immunisation with killed vaccine

Diphtheria

This disease is caused by infection with *Corynebacteria diphtheriae* (Klebs-Loeffler bacillus). There may be acute infection of the mucous membranes of the tonsils, pharynx, larynx or nose; skin infections may also occur and are of particular importance in tropical countries. Much faucial swelling may be produced by the local inflammatory reaction and the membranous exudate in the larynx may cause respiratory obstruction. The exotoxin which is produced by the organism may cause nerve palsies or myocarditis.

The *incubation period* is 2 to 5 days. It is usually included in the list of diseases which are notifiable nationally.

Medical geography

Although there is a world-wide occurrence of the disease and it was a common epidemic disease in childhood, it is now well controlled in most developed countries by routine immunisation of infants.

There is evidence to suggest that in some parts of the tropics a high proportion of the community acquires immunity through subclinical infections, mainly in the form of cutaneous lesions.

Bacteriology

C. diphtheriae is a Gram-positive rod, with a characteristic bipolar metachromatic staining. Virulent strains produce a soluble exotoxin which is responsible for the systemic manifestations and the sequelae of the disease. Three major types, *gravis*, *intermedius* and *mitis*, have been differentiated being associated with severe, moderately severe and mild clinical manifestations respectively.

Epidemiology

Man is the reservoir of infection; this includes clinical cases and also carriers. The infective agents may be discharged from the nose and throat or from skin lesions. The transmission of the infection may be by:

(*a*) Airborne infection
(*b*) Direct contact
(*c*) Indirect contact through fomites
(*d*) Ingestion of contaminated raw milk.

All persons are liable to infection but susceptibility to infection may be modified by previous natural exposure to infection and immunisation.

The newborn baby may be protected for up to 6 months through the transplacental transmission of antibodies from an immune mother.

The most severe illness is associated with faucial or laryngeal infection in children; nasal infections tend to be more chronic and less severe; and the cutaneous lesions which are often not recognised produced immunisation of the host with low morbidity.

Susceptibility to infection may be tested by means of the *Schick test*: a test dose of 0·2 ml of diluted toxin is injected intradermally into one forearm, with a similar injection of toxin, destroyed by heat, into the other forearm to serve as a control. A positive *Schick test*, consists of an area of redness 1-2 cm diameter at the site of the test dose, reaching its maximum size in 3-4 days, later fading into a brown stain. This positive reaction is confirmed by the absence of reaction at the site of the control injection. Redness at both sites is recorded as a pseudo-reaction, and probably represents non-specific sensitivity to some of the protein substances in the injection. A negative Schick test is recorded when there is no redness at either injection site. Both the pseudo-reaction and the negative Schick test are accepted as indicating resistance to diphtheria infection.

Laboratory diagnosis
Clinical diagnosis can be confirmed by bacteriological examination of swabs of the nose and throat or of skin lesions.

Control

(a) *The individual*
Active immunisation with diphtheria toxoid has proved a reliable measure for the control of this infection. It is usually administered in combination with pertussis vaccine and tetanus toxoid (DPT or triple antigen) for the immunisation of infants, starting from the 2 to 3 months old. A booster dose of diphtheria toxoid is recommended at school entry and this may be given in combination with typhoid vaccine.

In case of an outbreak of infection, anti-toxin should be given promptly on making the clinical diagnosis and without awaiting laboratory confirmation. Treatment with penicillin or other antibiotics may be given in addition to, but not instead of, serum. The patient should be isolated until throat cultures cease to yield toxigenic strains.

Non-immune young children who have been in direct contact with the patient should be protected by passive immunisation with anti-toxic serum and at the same time, active immunisation with toxoid is commenced. Susceptible (Schick-positive) adult contacts should be protected with active immunisation and a booster dose can be given to immune (Schick-negative) persons.

(b) *The community*
The search for carriers and their treatment with antibiotics may be indicated in the special circumstances of an outbreak in a closed community such as a boarding school, but the major approach to the control of this infection is routine active immunisation of the susceptible population.

Diphtheria—Summary

(1) *Occurrence*—World-wide, but now largely controlled in developed countries
(2) *Organism*—*Corynebacteria diphtheriae*
(3) *Reservoir of infection*—Man
(4) *Modes of transmission*—Airborne, contact—direct and indirect, contaminated milk
(5) *Control*—Vaccination with toxoid

Histoplasmosis (Histoplasma capsulatum infection)

The classical form of histoplasmosis due to *Histoplasma capsulatum* presents a variety of clinical manifestations. Infection is mostly asymptomatic, being detected only on immunological tests. On first exposure there may be an acute benign respiratory illness, which tends to be self-limiting, healing with or without calcification. Progressive disseminated lesions may occur with widespread involvement of the reticulo-endothelial system; without treatment this form may have a fatal outcome.

The *incubation period* is from 1 to $2\frac{1}{2}$ weeks.

Medical geography

The infection is endemic in certain parts of North, Central and South America, Africa and parts of the Far East.

Mycology

The causative agent is *H. capsulatum*, a dimorphic organism (both yeast phase and mycelial phase occur). In the host tissues, only the yeast phase is found. Spores can survive in the soil for long periods. They flourish particularly well in soil that is manured by bird or bat droppings, especially in caves.

Laboratory diagnosis

The organism can be isolated on culture of pathological specimens—sputum, or biopsy material—by culture on selective media, e.g. enriched Sabouraud's medium. The skin test with histoplasmin is useful epidemiologically to detect inapparent infections, including old infections. Serological tests (e.g. complement fixation) are also positive on infection, a rising titre may indicate recent exposure or current disease.

Epidemiology

The reservoir is in soil especially chicken coops, bat caves and areas polluted with pigeon droppings. The infection is acquired by inhalation of the spores. Person-to-person transmission is rare. It is not clear why in some patients the infection progresses to severe disease.

Control

The main measure is to avoid exposure to contaminated soil and caves. Infected patients with significant disease can be treated with Amphotericin B.

Histoplasmosis—Summary

(1) *Distribution*—Parts of America, Africa, Asia and the Pacific
(2) *Organism*—Histoplasma capsulatum
(3) *Reservoir of infection*—Soil, especially those contaminated with bird droppings
(4) *Mode of transmission*—Airborne from spores in soil
(5) *Control*—Avoid exposure to infected areas

Chapter Eight

The Epidemiology and Control of Nutritional Diseases

Introduction
The problem of feeding the populations of the world, and therefore maintaining an adequate status of nutritional health, is a serious one. Its magnitude and severity have only recently received attention, and there is no completely reliable assessment in quantitative terms. Hunger, as manifest through famines or chronic undernutrition, has been recognised from prehistoric times. However, the problems related to the absence of specific nutrients have been understood only very recently.

In a chapter of this nature it is impossible to deal with the specific epidemiological aspects of each individual nutrient whose absence may lead to a disease. For such information the reader is referred to large texts on nutrition and small monographs for specific deficiency diseases. The international organisations, especially WHO, FAO and UNICEF, have drawn universal attention to the fact that the food and nutrition problems of the world are among the most important threats to world peace that there is. In the last few years, through the efforts of the Economic and Social Council of the United Nations, as well as the United Nations General Assembly, world-wide awareness of the threat of protein deficiency to the levels of living of millions of people have also received great attention. Action on a world-wide scale is slowly gathering momentum.

Incidence and Prevalence
As may be expected from a disease group including such diverse aetiological agents and backgrounds, no completely reliable international figures are available, and even at the national level, very few countries have any but the most rudimentary of statistics. The United Nations Agencies have reckoned that about a third of the world's population goes to bed hungry every day. The term 'Hunger', here, includes both the quantitative deficiency in the food as well as the qualitative defects. This one-third is to be found largely in the countries of Asia, Africa and Latin America: in other words, those countries which are

in the warmer parts of the world, which are less advanced, and which have very grave problems of development.

In these countries, however grave the nutritional problems, there are certain groups among whom higher rates of occurrence obtain, and these groups are usually described as the 'vulnerable' groups. For the world as a whole, and taking the total nutritional problems, the infant, the pre-school child, and pregnant and nursing mothers constitute the most vulnerable groups if protein-calorie malnutrition were to be used as an example. Protein-calorie malnutrition is the name accepted now for a disease syndrome which includes kwashiorkor, believed to be largely due to protein deficiency, and nutritional marasmus which is due to a general deficiency of all nutrients, especially calories. The experts no longer separate these diseases because one can merge into the other in the same child, and in the community one sees cases ranging from one extreme to the other. In actual practice it is almost impossible in the human to have pure protein deficiency without some calorie deficiency, and vice versa.

In Africa, this group of conditions occurs mainly in the infant after about 6 months of age and the pre-school child up to about 4 or 5. There is some evidence that pregnant and nursing mothers also suffer from protein-calorie malnutrition, although overt signs are very difficult to find in these. In tropical Africa, it has been estimated that 2 to 9 per cent of all children aged 0-4 at any given time have overt signs of protein-calorie malnutrition, and if weight loss as the most important sign is the only one used, then some 40 to 50 per cent of all African children in the tropical parts can be considered as being malnourished. Among adults, acute periods of undernutrition may occur in large populations because of failure of food crops or catastrophes of one kind or another: floods, earthquakes, wars and failure of the rains. In sub-Sahara Africa, weight loss of significant levels occurs in the total population regularly every year in the period known as the 'hungry season', and in some years this is very severe and prolonged. Protein-calorie malnutrition is easily the most important nutrition problem of the whole world, though deficiencies due to vitamins A, B and D are also quite common.

The background of nutritional deficiency conditions is very wide, and can be seen to be more dependent on the socio-economic level of the society than practically any other disease. It is the deficiency in total quantity or quality of foods consumed that leads to poor nutrition, and therefore the epidemiology must be dependent on the chain of food production, processing, distribution, preparation and consumption.

(1) *Food Production and Distribution*
The major developed areas of the world have solved their food production problems, and by and large are now exporters of food, or

TABLE 8.1

Nutritive value of the main whole cereal grains
(Values per 100 g)

	Calories	Protein	Fat	Calcium	Iron	Thiamine	Niacin	Riboflavin	Vitamin A	Ascorbic acid
		g	g	mg	mg	mg	mg	mg	i.u.	mg
Wheat (wholemeal)	334	12·2	2·3	30	3·5	0·40	5·0	0·17	Trace	0
Rice (husked)	357	7·5	1·8	15	2·8	0·25	4·0	0·12	Trace	0
Maize (wholemeal)	356	9·5	4·3	12	5·0	0·33	1·5	0·13	0–400	0
Millet (Sorghum)	343	10·1	3·3	30	6·2	0·40	3·5	0·12	Trace	0
Oats (rolled)	385	13·0	7·5	60	3·8	0·50	1·3	0·14	Trace	0
Rye	319	11·0	1·9	50	3·5	0·27	1·2	0·10	Trace	0

else have such strong economies that they can afford to pay for food without necessarily running into any difficulties. The food availability in the developed areas is, therefore, *per capita*, far ahead of availability in the less-developed parts of the world.

In the tropics, food production is still dependent on very primitive methods of agriculture. Some 60 to 90 per cent of the population of most countries is engaged in agriculture, and much of this is peasant farming. Barely enough food is produced for the needs of the family and what is left over is exchanged for other requirements. Climatic conditions, such as rainfall, winds and soil erosion, determine the outcome of agriculture. Production per acre is very low. Recently, cash

TABLE 8.2*

Starchy roots—Potato, sweet potato, cassava, yams, taro
(composition in terms of the retail weight, as purchased)

	Range	Selected value	Notes
Moisture, per cent	65-85	...	...
Calories/100 mg	50-125	80·0	...
Carbohydrate, g/100 g	10-25	18·0	...
Protein, g/100 g	0·7-2·5	1·5	Tapioca and sago as sold in Europe, 0·3-0·4
Fat, g/100 g	Trace	0	...
Calcium, mg/100 g	10-30	20·0	...
Iron, mg/100 g	0·5-2·0	0·8	...
Vitamin A, i.u./100 g	0	0	Sweet potato: most varieties 500; deep yellow and red up to 7000
Ascorbic acid, mg/100 g	5-25	15·0	...
Thiamine, mg/100 g	0·05-0·10	0·075	...
Riboflavin, mg/100 g	0·03-0·08	0·05	...
Niacin, mg/100 g	0·5-1·5	1·0	...

* Taken from *Human Nutrition and Dietetics*. Davidson and Passmore.

crops have been successfully produced in many parts of the world; but the concentration of farm effort on cash crops under the guidance of governments, and the incentives given have tended to depress food production in some very needy countries.

The internal or external migration of able-bodied workers into industrial areas and towns has also tended to drain the rural areas of hands for farm work. The types of staple food produced have a very important role to play in the nutrition problems. The cereals are, by and large, better foods than the root crops (see Tables 8.1 and 8.2).

Cereals are, weight for weight, richer in calories as well as proteins.

Their storage and transportation do not pose the same extreme problems as are posed by the root crops, because of bulk and easy deterioration of the latter. The root crops, by and large, can therefore not set a good basis for a meal, and wherever the people are dependent on root crops and starchy fruits, the nutritional problems, especially protein-calorie malnutrition, will be great.

In many parts of the developing world, transport and communications are very poor. The developing countries, by and large, are able to produce 90 per cent or more of their calorie requirements, yet it is a fact that this average hides serious regional and local differences, and even differences created by food distribution and consumption within families.

Although the total region may have a hundred per cent or more of its estimated calorie requirements available, yet poor feeder roads, poor trunk roads and absence of marketing and distribution facilities may make for a situation where part of this food may be rotting in one place while there is actual starvation in another. A similar situation often exists within individual families. In many instances, in spite of the fact that enough food is going into the family pot, the male adults often receive a high proportion of their calorie and protein requirements while the children do not.

(2) *Food Storage and Processing*
Quite apart from severe losses in the field which may be due to locusts, nematodes and climatic conditions, post-harvest losses of food range from 10 to 30 per cent of all harvested grains, and for the starchy roots and vegetables this may be an underestimate. Such losses are due to poor storage and transportation facilities and the lack of processing. Food technology has yet to make an extensive impact on the food situation of developing countries.

(3) *Demographic Problems related to Food*
In most of the developing countries, the rate of increase of the population is over 2 per cent and yet the rate of increase of food production, except in some very special areas, has not kept up with this population increase. There is, therefore, a continuing gap between the population and its food resources. In these same areas, 45 to 50 per cent of the population is under 15 years of age, and with increasing scholarisation, this young population is being more and more taken out of the food production group and they are becoming almost entirely consumers.

Towns and cities are growing at a very high rate, and many young men are moving into towns, again creating a situation where large proportions of the population are no longer food producers but are buyers. By and large, the structures of the towns themselves are such that no real food production activity can be undertaken in or near them. Urbanisation increases the food problems in another way. So attractive is the pull of the ready market of the larger towns that transportation of food usually by-passes many smaller towns and villages, and may help to create a town glut with relative shortage in the countryside. Within the town itself, cash is the major determinant of the level of feeding, and it is not surprising to find that casual labourers and the urban poor and their families are among groups whose nutrition is unsatisfactory.

(4) *Education and Socio-cultural Factors*

Education is a very important factor in the choice of food. It operates indirectly by the fact that the more educated a person is, the better is his chances of a good job and, therefore, a higher level of living. But it also has a direct influence in that nutrition knowledge, making for a better choice of food as well as for better practices within the family, is significantly related to education. In analysing the epidemiological aspects of protein-calorie malnutrition in Accra, it was found that some 97 per cent of mothers whose children had overt protein-calorie malnutrition have had no education at all. Lack of formal education also appears to hinder good nutrition practices in another way, and that is to create insecurity about choosing new and not too well-known foods. Family budgeting is another characteristic which is directly related to education, food choice and nutrition. The less educated adhere most strictly to food taboos and practices, some of which may be completely injurious to health. Jeliffe has gone into the question of food practices in relation to child feeding and classified them under good, neutral or bad. In each area there is the need to find out which practices make for good nutrition and which do not. The latter are to be discouraged.

(5) *Food Preparation and Consumption*

Food choice is dependent, therefore, on availability, on education and on accepted preferences and principles. Methods of preparation sometimes improve the quality of the food, sometimes there is an adverse effect, e.g. fermentation of cereals increases the availability of the group of vitamins, exposure of chopped-up vegetables and fruits make for cooking losses of the vitamin C group; overwashing of cereals, or at the industrial level, over-milling makes for a poorer quality food. In the home, there are certain foods which are not considered good food for certain physiological groups, yet these same foods may be nutritionally just what the groups require. Meat, fish and eggs, in many parts of Africa, are not considered as good food for children. In some parts, eggs and groundnuts are forbidden to pregnant women. Quite apart from these, the pecking order at individual foods and at the meal generally, is usually the men folk first, the older boys next, and then women and young children last.

In fact, the idea that, for its size, the child requires more of everything than the adult is not yet accepted in many populations of the developed areas. The child is in a special category from birth. The breast milk is his major food; and whilst this is available, the child develops well till about 4 to 6 months. Supplementary foods are then required and yet at this time most of the developing countries do not seem to have a satisfactory supplementary food. There is also an unfortunate increase in the number of women who either do not breast feed or do so only for a very short time. The tendency of town mothers to be in salaried employment away from home also makes it necessary for breast feeding to stop early.

At the present time, the problems of protein-calorie malnutrition in urban areas are quire severe. There is no satisfactory weaning food, and children are weaned with starchy gruels and paps, very poor in protein and, therefore, unsatisfactory for the maintenance of growth and health. The highest incidence of protein-calorie malnutrition occurs in the post-weaning child.

(6) *The Role of Infection*

The exact role that infections play in the actual precipitation or degree of seriousness of nutritional diseases has been subject to some argument. Much of the statements made in the past have been based on animal experiments extrapolated to the human. There is, however, enough reason to accept that infection may contribute to the nutritional status of an individual through two possible avenues. One is indirect and the other direct.

Direct. When a person suffers from an infection, there is loss of appetite, which means that his intake is reduced and where his previous nutritional state has been unsatisfactory and the infection rather prolonged, such as typhoid, tuberculosis or even malaria, weight loss will result. Diarrhoea and vomiting are usually accompaniments of the acute childhood infections in the tropics, and these may be severe enough to be significant in nutrition.

As soon as the child falls ill, changes may be made in its diet. More often than not, it is solids with the higher protein content that get removed. Most ill children, if they were having milk already, may have these withdrawn. In some cases, even the breast has been known to be stopped for a very young child who is ill. Finally, certain therapeutic practices, such as enemas and purgatives, are resorted to, and all of these combined may help to drain a sick child of valuable nutrients and lay the foundation for nutritional-deficiency conditions.

Indirect. Practically all infections lead to a negative nitrogen balance, and if this is maintained for any length of time, the patient's protein stores may be sufficiently depleted. There are, however, specific interactions between the infectious illness and the nutritional state of the individual. The infectious process may precipitate or aggravate the nutritional condition, or alternatively the nutritional condition may make an ordinary infection much worse. Scrimshaw, Gordon and others have used the terms 'Synergism' and 'Antagonism' to describe the types of relationship. By 'Synergism' is meant the situation whereby the infection or infectious process tends to help precipitate or aggravate the poor nutritional status of the individual. Acute and chronic bacterial infections, as well as helminths, are known to behave in this way. By antagonism is meant the poor nutritional state preventing the establishment of an infection. Some viral diseases such as chickenpox are known to be unable to get established properly in a malnourished child.

Whether the individual infection has a synergistic or antagonistic effect, no infection has proven to be useful to an individual in a poorly nourished state. Frequently, the poorly nourished individual may have a disease subsequent to infection by organisms considered harmless in the well-nourished. Children in the tropics have very high mortality and rather severe morbidity from common childhood illnesses which are considered rather mild in Europe and America. The mortality and morbidity from measles is given as some 5 to 10 per cent, similar to what it was in Europe in the eighteenth and nineteenth centuries.

The regularity with which kwashiorkor and marasmus get precipitated by an attack of measles has been commented upon by several writers. Some infections create nutritional problems because of the partition of nutrients between the host and the infecting organism, or because of a high cellular turnover which may mop up nutrients. The fish tapeworm which absorbs vitamin B_{12} and leaves the host with megaloblastic anaemia is the classic example of the former. The large-scale destruction and consequent rapid turnover of the erythrocytes in malaria consumes folates and may lead to folic-acid deficiency anaemia. The hookworm causes its anaemia by simply leading to blood loss into the faeces. It will, therefore, appear that irrespective of the laboratory and experimental findings, infections might have to be controlled if nutritional conditions are to be permanently warded off.

Control
The measures required for controlling any nutritional disease might be *specific* or *general*.

Specific Measures
The specific measures will be directed to special individual diseases or groups, essentially or actually at risk, and measures which are largely within the province of the doctor and other members of the health team. Such measures would include the identification of the nutrition problems and the major groups that are affected. Those actually requiring treatment have to be treated, and the occasion of their treatment used

for educating them as to the origin of their sickness and what is to be done about it.

(i) *Treatment*
This usually requires special dietetic measures to be followed by prolonged rehabilitation.

(ii) *Supplementary feeding programmes*
These may be undertaken to anticipate the needs of the at-risk group. Such programmes may be entirely local or be supported from international aid. Skimmed milk, corn, soya and milk preparations, as well as ordinary cereal and pulses of various kinds, may be used in these programmes. The success of supplementary feeding programmes has not been very good, since the pre-school child who is most vulnerable in this respect, is hard to reach. Secondly, by their very nature, supplementary feeding programmes are dependent on foods which may not be too readily available locally, and, therefore, their continuity is often in doubt. These are very good, however, in times of special catastrophes, such as during floods, famines, drought, earthquake or wars. Special feeding programmes for schools and industrial workers may also help ward off malnutrition in these groups. Programmes for industrial workers, however, are usually not very popular and the food co-operatives may be more satisfactory from point of view of whole family feeding than the industrial canteen.

(iii) *Nutrition education*
As part of general health education programmes nutrition education needs to be emphasised. This should be undertaken through all avenues such as in the clinic with women's clubs, with school children and even through the markets and other places where people gather. The aims and objectives should be determined by local requirements. By and large, emphasis would be required on (*a*) encouraging breast feeding, (*b*) emphasising the points for satisfactory weaning, and (*c*) teaching better nutrition for pregnant and nursing women.

The doctor's leadership is very necessary for success of nutrition education programmes, and it is important for him to understand this and try to learn as much as possible of the local nutritional requirements and the foods available for meeting the real needs of the community.

(iv) *Control of infection*
There is no clear-cut experimental evidence that simply by controlling infections the nutritional state of the population will improve. However, efforts to improve nutrition without doing anything about infections have not proved satisfactory. It would, therefore, appear that any effort to control infections, especially the acute febrile illnesses of

childhood and the pneumonia-diarrhoea group of diseases, can only help the nutritional status. There is some non-quantified evidence that the control of measles in a community brings down the hospitalisation rate for protein-calorie malnutrition. There is also evidence that malnourished children who do not have an infection, whether subsequent to the malnutrition or antedating it, are on the whole less ill and have the most favourable prognosis.

General Measures

The most important requirements for adequate feeding of any population are the production of foods in the right quantity and quality required, at a price that is within reach of the general population and which are available to the population.

(i) *Improvement in agriculture, especially food production*

This is the first essential and can be achieved by better land use, better farm practices, and better seed selection. Recent experiments helping to produce high-yielding cereals, e.g. lysine maize and high protein or high lysine cereals, are a step in the right direction. However, some of these newer varieties may lead to trouble because of qualities that may make them not too well acceptable. The opaque corn, for instance, is more floury than the natural corn, and it is therefore not as well accepted by Latin Americans for their tortilla. The high-yielding STRC rice has taste which is not very well liked in Asia.

The better storage of agricultural produce, especially of cereals, will help to cut down food losses by a substantial percentage and thereby lead to an increase in the available food supplies. Strategically located silos, as well as village storage of cereals and root crops, will provide some measure of incentive for greater food production effort.

The problems of marketing and distribution of foods have to be tackled nationally by price incentives of various kinds, and better organised collection and handling of food from producer to consumer will bring down prices sufficiently for a better distribution of foods. The current trend in most developing countries is a fall in the *per capita* availability of pulses and legumes which are the high-protein foods. Governmental and local effort needs to be directed to reverse this trend.

Food technology has not yet come into its own in developing countries. It has a big contribution to make by assisting in the processing of known foods and the creation of new preparations which may be more readily available and acceptable. Village-level preparation of foods should also be undertaken. So far, food technology has been in the field of enrichment with vitamins, minerals and amino acids and the preparation of special foods. Special foods aimed at particular groups must accord with available resources, the food practices, and the behaviour of the general population.

I

(ii) *Education and training*
There is a need for formal education and training of nutrition workers
at all levels. These will include research level scientists both in food
technology, food science and nutrition, and for educators of the public.
The workers supposed to be educators of the public should have multi-
disciplinary subject-matter content, including basic nutrition science,
sociology and psychology. Education of the public as to what constitutes good nutrition should be based on what is good and available
and the realities of the economic situation.

(iii) *Food policy*
All of the above control measures can only take place satisfactorily if
there is a national food policy which has been evolved after the
integration and co-ordination of the views and experiences of national
specialists in nutrition, agriculture, health, economics and sociology.
For most countries in the developing areas, the policy should have
objectives in the fields of food production, food storage, processing,
marketing, imports and exports, pricing, distribution, consumption,
food legislation and health protection and promotion by means of
education as well as control of disease. It must also make provision for
the training of personnel for home management, extension education
and perhaps include, where necessary, provision for special feeding
programmes.
   Needless to say, such a policy can only be based on adequate information both of the needs and resources, and it is unlikely that any
developing country can satisfactorily formulate such an all-embracing
policy at the present time. It is necessary, however, for each country to
identify its principal problem area and formulate a policy to do something about it. A major role of the doctor is to use his status to bring
to the attention of policy makers, the actual needs of his community in
this respect.

Further Reading

FAO/WHO (1965). Protein requirements: report of a joint FAO/WHO
   expert group (Geneva, 1963). *Tech. Rep. Ser. Wld Hlth Org.,* **301.**

DAVIDSON, Sir STANLEY, PASSMORE, R. and BROCK, J. (1972). *Human
   Nutrition and Dietetics,* 5th edition. Edinburgh and London:
   Livingstone.

NICHOLLS, L. (1972). *Tropical Nutrition and Dietetics,* 4th edition, rev.
   H. M. Sinclair and D. B. Jeliffe. London: Baillière, Tindall and
   Cox.

JELIFFE, D. B. (1966). The assessment of the nutritional status of the
   community. *World Health Organisation Monograph Ser.,* **53.**

Chapter Nine

Family Health

The concept of the family as the unit of care in Preventive and Social Medicine, Community Medicine and Community Health, is rightly gaining wider and wider acceptance. There can be no doubt that, as far as our present knowledge goes, this concept is a most rational and promising one. The idea of providing services for the mother and her child, at the same time, at the same place; of including everything that either may need and of going beyond that and making provisions for the future welfare of each particular unit of family, makes sense. It makes sense at community and national levels.

To meet the challenge of providing adequate, even if minimal, services for the promotion, the maintenance, the protection and the restoration of the health of the mother and her child, the further concept of Family Health Care comprising **Maternal Care, Infant and Child Care** and **Family Planning** as an item of health services has assumed considerable importance. These three subdivisions can provide all the essential requirements for the care of women and children which is the prime preoccupation of Family Health.

The division of Family Health into its three components is purely arbitrary. The three subdivisions are so interrelated and interdependent that they should not be regarded as separate activities but as phases of the same activity. The care of the child today promotes the health of the mother tomorrow. The care of the pregnant woman ensures the health of the unborn child, and effective family planning undoubtedly protects the health of the child-bearing woman and may prevent the birth of an unwanted child, or avert an incipient kwashiorkor.

Maternal Care

The objectives of the maternal care component of family health care (in so far as it can be separated from the other components) are:

  (i) The preservation of the health of the mother
  (ii) The reduction of the risks and damaging sequelae of pregnancy and child birth
  (iii) The reduction of post-natal morbidity and mortality
  (iv) The prevention and treatment of sub-fertility and sterility.

Within this component, provision must be made for the education of women, especially the young adolescent female and those in the child-bearing age-range, to enable them to manipulate the physical, biological, social and emotional environment in which they live and grow. Education should be directed at enabling them to:

(1) Improve and maintain their personal hygiene
(2) Improve and maintain their nutritional level
(3) Undertake those measures that will protect them from diseases (especially those that are preventable)
(4) Cure everyday common ills, as well as those peculiar to the special groups
(5) Use rehabilitative services when the need arises.

Public health care should include competent obstetric services, to take care of the pregnancy and delivery periods, and of the puerperium. The woman must be taught to cope with the immediate post-natal period as well as the pre-pregnancy period. The concept of family health enables the services for the mother to be integrated with the services for the child and with family planning services.

In countries where a sizeable proportion of the population is rural, new approaches to take the services to the people will be required. In urban situations, where communication is easier and quicker, obstetric practice, in theory, could be hospital-based and deliveries might be shared between hospital and the home. But when this pattern of service has been tried in developing countries the coverage is usually poor and the service inefficient, besides being extremely expensive. In rural situations some other way of providing delivery facilities, other than conventional or specialised hospitals and away from the home, needs to be found. For example, simple inexpensive delivery centres can be designed attached to family health clinics, to provide an integrated service for the mother and child. These will include family planning services and be organised in such a way that at every contact with the service, the woman, or her child, is provided with whatever is needed, be it educational, protective or curative.

From such a base, women can be supervised during the puerperium, in their own homes. The same team can undertake follow-up visits in the child-care programme, and even provide domiciliary family planning consultation, service and follow-up. The actual delivery should be undertaken at the centre, and the mother returned to her home very soon afterwards, if everything has gone according to plan. This ensures a standard environment within which the midwives and other staff can function and to which it will always be easy to summon urgent help. Local health workers, trained, adequately supervised and realistically provided with drugs and other items, would form the base of the teams providing such services with the public health nurse as the leader and pivot.

Factors that affect Maternal Health
The factors which influence maternal health can be grouped under three main headings:

(1) *Personal*
(*a*) General health, and all the factors that contribute to it, including nutritional status. The immunisations received and the facilities that are available for maintaining, protecting and restoring general health.
(*b*) Educational and socio-economic status of the mother and of her relatives. These determine the degree of acceptance and use of available facilities.
(*c*) The traditions, customs, beliefs and practices of the group to which the mother belongs. These factors determine behaviour and practices in hygiene as in other relevant matters.

(2) *Environmental*
(*a*) Housing and the degree of overcrowding. These factors affect the degree and the kind of hazards to which the mother is exposed.
(*b*) The sanitation of the area in which she lives and the availability of safe water in adequate quantities.

(3) *Maternal Health Service Provisions*
(*a*) The training, skill and experience of midwives, doctors and other health workers decides the quality, and effectiveness of any service that is provided.
(*b*) The availability, quality and quantity of facilities, drugs and equipment bear a direct relationship to maternal health.

The factors that tend to jeopardise maternal survival can be further divided as avoidable or unavoidable. One factor needs special mention because it is often overlooked and can be critical. This is the co-operation between the patient (and her relatives) and the health workers. This will affect the mother's willingness to accept advice and treatment and the facility with which she comprehends what is going on around her. Lack of sensitivity or lack of awareness of the difficulties caused by language differences, will often jeopardise maternal health.

Unavoidable Factors
These include:
  (1) genetic factors
  (2) congenital abnormalities (which may or may not be the result of an avoidable failure of previous maternal care)
  (3) the poor understanding of the causes of toxaemia of pregnancy, hypertension, diabetes and mental illness, etc.
  (4) The intrusion of tradition, culture, beliefs, prejudices and local practices.

Prophylactic Measures

Some routine prophylactic personal measures can be advocated for most antenatal clinics in the tropics, though these will naturally vary from country to country. Thus, in areas where neonatal tetanus is a problem, tetanus toxoid vaccination of pregnant mothers is mandatory (see p. 135). Similarly, in malarious areas, prophylactic antimalarials should be administered throughout pregnancy, since this measure significantly lowers the incidence of pregnancy anaemia. Iron and folic acid supplements are often required by pregnant women in many tropical countries, while routine medical antenatal examinations are implicit in the concept of personal maternal health.

Child Care

The concept of Family Health which we are considering presupposes an integrated care service for the woman and her child. Within such a service, the objectives of child care must be to bring the child safely into the world with a reasonable assurance that he will survive to be an adult and will be equipped with such physical and mental potentials that will permit normal social, cultural and educational activities. It involves the protection of the woman during the early part of pregnancy when the foetus is particularly vulnerable. It includes the reduction of peri- and neonatal deaths. The risk of death is greater during the perinatal period than at any other time before the age of 50 in developing countries (65 in the more advanced countries). Child care also includes all measures designed to overcome genetic and other factors which tend to operate detrimentally in the early foetal and perinatal periods.

Child care also aims to ensure that the child, once born, grows satisfactorily through infant, pre-school, school and adolescent periods to full healthy adulthood. It seeks to provide all the services necessary for the promotion, maintenance, protection and restoration of health. In other words, it aims to provide for the total care of the child, continuously through each of its developmental periods, attempting to ensure, by regular medical supervision, that the child is not prevented from taking full advantage of its educational opportunities by reason of any physical or mental defect.

The period of life from birth to 1 year is a time of exceptionally rapid growth. At birth, many organs have not attained their full potential for physiological and biochemical functions, but within the first year considerable maturity takes place.

After the first birthday, the risk of death in a child begins to drop, but it increases again, in developing countries, as the child's mobility increases and it is brought into closer and wider contact with a physical environment that favours pathogens and contains hazards that cause injury and threaten life. After the fifth year the risk begins to drop again.

During this time, both physical and psychological growth proceed at an incredibly rapid rate. The period offers special opportunities for laying the foundations on which to build a long, productive and healthy life. At the same time, injuries which at a later age may be trivial can at this period be devastating and cause permanent damage or even death.

The health needs of a child can be considered under the headings environmental, physical and emotional.

(1) *Environmental needs*
A clean, comfortable and safe environment; the provision of safe water and food; protection from disease-carrying insects, harmful toxins, other disease agents and accident hazards.

(2) *Physical needs*
Adequate nutrition, education of the mother to ensure satisfactory personal hygiene for the child, adequate medical supervision including immunisation against the prevalent diseases as soon as the child's immune mechanism can respond. As soon as possible, a schedule of immunisations against diseases such as tuberculosis, tetanus, diphtheria, whooping cough, smallpox, measles and poliomyelitis must be begun. The timing and the order in which they are administered will be dictated by local circumstances (see Table 9.1). Chemoprophylaxis against malaria must also be considered and weighed against the desirability of the child developing its own resistance in those areas where this is relevant.

(3) *Emotional needs*
The basic needs such as understanding love, adequate human contact and stimulation are usually fully met in the early infant stages. When the child moves into the toddler stage, such factors as socio-economic status, education, culture of the parents, or the advent of another pregnancy may interfere with the fulfilment of some of its needs. The way in which the emotional needs of the child are met will depend on the traditions, culture, beliefs and practices of the particular community.

The development of a child from an organism with unco-ordinated reflexes to a well co-ordinated, informed and social animal is a remarkable process. It advances simultaneously with another series of developmental changes: those which lead to acquiring an individual personality. Those who are involved with the care and supervision of children during their development must remember that neither of these developmental processes can be forced. If the physical and emotional environments provide suitable stimuli and opportunities for a child with the potential, the pace at which the developmental milestones are reached and passed can increase.

TABLE 9.1

A guide to immunisation in childhood in the tropics
(After R. G. Hendrickse)

Vaccine	Recommended age of administration	Method of administration	Special problems associated with use	Other comments
BCG	(i) Neonatal period as a routine. (ii) Tuberculin-negative subjects of any age exposed to mycobacterial infections.	Intradermal injection may also be given by multiple-puncture technique using modified 'Heaf Gun'.	Vaccine light and heat sensitive—risk of inactivation in unskilled hands.	(i) INH Resistant BCG may be used in special circumstances. (ii) Multiple-puncture technique recommended for use by semi-skilled personnel.
Triple antigen (combined tetanus and diphtheria toxoids and pertussis vaccine)	Start at 2 months. Give 3 shots at monthly intervals. Booster at 12-18 months.	Subcutaneous or IM injection.	None of note. Rarely encephalitis due to pertussis component of vaccine.	Where high risk of pertussis can start at age of 1 month.
Poliomyelitis vaccine (*a*) killed (Salk) type	Start at 2 months and monthly × 3.	Subcutaneous or IMI.	None.	May be simultaneously administered with Triple antigen in *separate* syringe unless combined vaccine used. Best for small local clinics.

(b) live (Sabin) type (Trivalent)	Start at 2 months and monthly × 3.	Oral.	Cool storage required. May get poor antibody response when used on small groups in tropics.	Most effective when mass vaccination campaigns undertaken.
Smallpox	Under 6 months.	Multipuncture by bifurcated needle. Jet injection (intradermal).	None of note.	Contra-indicated if patient has eczema or some other generalised skin eruption.
Measles. Further attenuated vaccine	8 months.	Subcutaneous injection. Jet injection for mass immunisation campaigns.	Refrigerated storage and maintenance of 'cold chain' before use.	Expensive. Indications that reduced dosage (to $\frac{1}{5}$ recommended dose) may be effective.

Notes: (1) *Cholera* epidemics—Cholera vaccine is given subcutaneously or intramuscularly ideally in two doses of 0·5 ml and 1·0 ml 7 to 28 days apart—one injection of 1·0 ml is usually used in *mass* immunisation campaigns.

(2) *Yellow fever* epidemics—Mass immunisation is done by using a dose of 0·5 ml given subcutaneously—infants under 1 year of age should not be vaccinated.

(3) *Tetanus*—In areas of the tropics where tetanus is prevalent, tetanus toxoid should be given to as many adults as possible who have not been immunised in childhood and to all pregnant women in order to protect the infant from neonatal tetanus.

Child care services, particularly in countries with minimal medical resources, should endeavour to provide everything the child needs at each contact it makes with the service. It is unjustifiably prodigal to persist with the historical pattern of separating well child services from those that are intended to provide for the sick child. The advantages of having an integrated service are many:

(1) More children will receive attention
(2) More children can be provided for with the same outlay of scant resources
(3) A single scheme makes more sense to uneducated parents
(4) Caring for the sick reinforces the commitment of auxiliary staff and provides more job-satisfaction for them
(5) Only one set of supporting administrative staff is needed.

One important disadvantage is the likelihood of a well child being exposed to a serious communicable disease. Whilst this is a real danger, its importance is unduly magnified since simple common-sense precautions are demonstrably effective in providing safeguards, even against the most infective communicable disease. The exposure need not be greater than in the community at large.

Family health implies, of course, a good deal more than merely the care of mother and child. It encompasses the well-being of fathers, brothers and sisters within the general concept of 'community health'.

Family Planning
Family planning is the third leg of the tripod on which Family Health rests. Its main theme is 'Babies by choice and not by chance'. All the measures that enable a couple to have the number of children they desire, including provisions for the sub-fertile, contribute to the strength, the stability, the growth and the survival of the family as a unit of society. Birth limitation therefore, as well as all other activities related to reproduction, becomes the concern of Community Health or Preventive Medicine.

Physicians in this area of medicine are facing a cruel paradox. They have, on the one hand, exciting and exotic new tools and techniques for combating diseases and preventing premature death, new drugs to aid in preventing and treating diseases, and the ability to provide for their communities positive health experience embracing rehabilitation of the handicapped. On the other hand, they are frustrated by their inability to make even minimal health care available and accessible to the majority of their peoples. They share the anxiety, of world-wide dimensions, over what is perhaps the most fundamental issue facing mankind today: the question of the true implications of unrestrained rapid population growth. Upon them, and allied medical professions has devolved the urgent need for determining the amount and kind of responsibility they should accept in the relationship between development and population growth and individual community health and well-being. Ironically, the worst of the ills of development is rapid population growth due to saving more children whilst too many are being born.

The causes of the high mortality and morbidity rates of the developing areas of the world are infective, communicable, insect-borne diseases, and malnutrition. All these ills are preventable, either by specific measures which are known and are being applied, or by general measures which enhance a person's resistance in a non-specific way. Success in the application of these measures depends to a great extent on improvements in the environment, which in turn is dependent on available resources. Such improvements very rapidly reduce the mortality rate, especially of children, without decreasing birth rates.

Family planning may or may not affect population growth significantly. It does however help the public health doctor break the vicious circle of over-fertility causing poverty, which causes disease, which in turn perpetuates the poverty and causes more disease.

Evidence that birth limitation enhances family health is accumulating, although, as yet, there are no conclusive data which relate family size and birth spacing to favourable health outcomes. However, the circumstantial evidence is striking and it would seem reasonable to adopt the hypothesis that family size limitation and birth spacing will yield substantial benefits to family health.

In a British study involving 13 000 births occurring in a 1-week period, it was noted that mothers were less likely to have low birth weight babies when the interval between babies was between 2 and 6 years. Many medical studies have shown that there is a substantially higher than average incidence of infant mortality, maternal mortality, prematurity, mental retardation, congenital malformation and brain damage when number of children exceeds four. Perinatal mortality indices are closely related to maternal age and parity. Foetal mortality is extremely high amongst very young mothers (under 17 years of age); it is at its lowest between 20 and 29 years and then begins to rise again until at above 40 it is several times the rate at 20.

In the USA in 1967 over 30 per cent of the babies born were to poor parents, and nearly 50 per cent of that nation's poor children live in families of five or more children. Because America is a land of opportunities not all the poor children remain poor as adults but, significantly, most of those who escape poverty come from one- and two-child families.

No figures are available for tropical communities, but it is not unreasonable to expect a similar pattern since the amount of education a child receives is likely to decide his earning capability and the number of years he can devote to education is likely to be influenced by how many children his parents have to educate.

For many women, pregnancy can be far removed from the conventional 'joy of motherhood' and be an extremely serious problem. It may damage a woman's health or endanger her life. In many tropical countries, the risk of dying as a result of pregnancy may be 10 to 20 times greater than in developed countries.

Birth Limitation

Births can be prevented by one of two ways: by preventing pregnancy or, conception having occurred, by abortion, i.e. preventing the foetus from developing.

Abortion, performed primarily for the purpose of limiting birth, is philosophically unacceptable to the preventive medicine physician for obvious reasons. However, the concept that acceptance of the principle of contraception must also entail an acceptance of abortion, as a final safeguard against an unwanted pregnancy, deserves support. This is different from abortion as a method of first resort.

Pregnancy can be prevented either by sterilisation or by contraception, if abstinence is not practicable.

Sterilisation

This can be of the man or the woman, and when competently performed is the most absolute form of birth limitation. In the female, tubal ligation/resection is the most satisfactory. Until recently, with the introduction of laparoscopic and culdoscopic techniques. it involved a major operation. Vasectomy, the male form of sterilisation, has been gaining popularity. It is a relatively simple operation which is now regularly performed on out-patient basis. In the last decade over $1\frac{1}{2}$ million vasectomies have been performed in India and in the first 6 months of 1968 some 21 000 were done in Pakistan. Neither of these processes affect a person's coital ability or libido. They only render the subject incapable of producing children. If family planning is the only consideration, vasectomy is the only procedure that has relevance, especially in countries where illegitimacy has little significance.

Sterilisation is a once-for-all activity. It needs no maintenance and does not require repeated motivation. It is important to bear in mind that vasectomy does not immediately render a man sterile. About 3 months must elapse to ensure that all the sperm cells already in the seminal vesicles and in the vas past the point of division are all disposed of. Usually two test seminal fluid analyses at the end of the 2nd and 3rd months after operation are required for confirmation.

Contraception

This is the process by which the chain of events leading to conception is interrupted. This interruption can be effected at any of several points, either by interfering with the functioning of the organs and tissue of reproduction or by erecting barriers which will effectively prevent the fertilisation of the ovum by the sperm-cell.

A good contraceptive must meet the following criteria. It must be safe, effective, devoid of side-effects, reversible, easy to use, cheap and if possible, independent of coitus. No single method, so far, meets all these criteria, although several meet many of them.

For a family health clinic, before a method is recommended, it must be safe and free from serious side-effects over short- and long-term use, and must be completely reversible.

It must be acceptable to the patient so that it will be used consistently and conscientiously. Factors like education, mentality, psychological make-up, availability of privacy and the basic attitudes and practices of the husband and wife, will affect acceptability and influence the effectiveness of the method. Whichever method is used, it must prevent pregnancy at all times. Very few methods are 100 per cent safe. Failures may be due to the method or the user. It is often not possible to distinguish which. An ideal method is one that eliminates failure irrespective of cause.

Methods of Contraception

Until the introduction of the oral contraceptives and the intra-uterine devices, the principle on which contraceptives was based was simply that of preventing a healthy normal male sperm from meeting and uniting with a healthy normal female egg. This was achieved in one of four ways: (1) avoiding ejaculation into the vagina (coitus interruptus); (2) placing a barrier between the ejaculate and the egg cell (condoms, diaphragms and cervical caps); (3) using chemical substances to kill the sperms or otherwise incapacitate them (the chemical contraceptives, foam, jellies, creams); (4) having intercourse only when no ovum is available to be fertilised (rhythm, safe-period).

(1) *Coitus interruptus*

Coitus interruptus is a very ancient method of contraception. It is mentioned in the Bible, in the Book of Genesis. It consists of the withdrawal of the penis just in time to prevent ejaculation into the vagina. It is an unreliable method as it is possible for a few spermatozoa to escape from the penis before orgasm occurs. It is also unsatisfactory as it puts a very great psychological strain on the man and is frustrating to both partners. It costs nothing and calls for no special preparation.

(2) *Barrier methods*

Of the barrier methods the *condom* is the commonest and possibly the most used of all contraceptives. It has the fringe benefit that it protects both parties from possible exposure to venereal disease as well as preventing pregnancy. It is reasonably effective, cheap and easy to use.

However, it has the disadvantage that it may interfere with sensation and it is not always possible to tell if it is defective. Its effectiveness is enhanced by the use of a spermicidal cream which also acts as a lubricant.

The *diaphragm* and the *cervical cap* act by occluding the cervix and so prevent sperms from entering the uterus. Properly fitted, used and cared for, they have high effectiveness among intelligent and highly motivated persons. They have the disadvantage that they have first to be correctly fitted as to size, and the user taught how to insert and remove them correctly (they should be retained in place at least 8 hours after intercourse). They must be used with spermicidal cream or jelly, and washed and stored carefully after use.

A number of *chemical substances* can be used to prevent pregnancy. They act by immobilising and subsequently killing the sperm cells, and must be able to do so when diluted by the ejaculate and vaginal secretion. They must be non-toxic if absorbed and non-irritant to the vaginal mucosa. They are prepared in the form of creams, jellies, tablets, vaginal foam and foaming tablets.

Usually, they must be introduced high into the vagina not less than 5 minutes and not more than 1 hour before coitus, and a fresh dose must be used before each coitus. Douching is prohibited for at least 6 hours after use.

The vaginal foam is the most effective of this group, followed by the jellies and creams, with tablets and suppositories the least effective. Used alone, they are much less effective than the barriers, especially when those are used with cream or jelly.

(3) *The rhythm or safe-period*
The rhythm or safe-period method is based on the principle of avoiding coitus during the period when an ovum is available for fertilisation. This period is believed to be 72 hours made up of 24 hours, the life-span of an ovum plus the 48 hours it is believed the sperm can survive in the uterus without deterioration in its potential to fertilise an ovum. Unfortunately the time of ovulation can only be determined, with consistent accuracy when the 1st day of the subsequent period is known, even for the most regular cycles. Therefore the safe-period has to be estimated by counting 14 back from the expected date of the next period and adding 3 or 4 days on either side of this date to give a total of about 8 days on which coitus must be avoided. Standard charts have been prepared for reading off safe days based on the lengths of the shortest and longest cycles of the woman.

A more precise method of determining the date of ovulation is the recording of daily anal temperature and watching for the slight rise in temperature when ovulation occurs. The possibilities for errors are great and this makes the method unreliable. One side-effect which may arise from this method is the result of an accidental conception involving an ageing ovum or a deteriorating sperm with its higher incidence of embryonic abnormalities.

(4) *Chemical contraceptives*

Chemical contraceptives consisting of synthetic hormones, progesterones, and small amounts of oestrogen have been found to prevent pregnancy by suppressing ovulation, causing alteration in tubal factors, accelerating endometrial development, producing a hostile cervical mucus, or by a combination of two more of these means. These substances, oral contraceptives, are widely known as the 'Pill' and are available, generally as:

(i) *Combined preparations*—tablets which are taken in cycles of 21 days after a 7-day rest during which bleeding usually occurs.

(ii) *Sequential preparations*—tablets containing oestrogen, taken for 14 or 16 days followed by tablets containing both progesterone and oestrogen taken for 5 or 7 days.

(iii) *Continuous dose preparations*—also called 'mini-pills', are taken every day and they prevent pregnancy without suppressing ovulation.

Similar substances are available which can be given by injection. They are so prepared that they release their active principles slowly over 1, 3 or 6 months, depending on dosage.

These are the most effective methods of contraceptives presently available. They have the added advantage of not being associated with the act of coitus or the sexual organs which enhances their acceptability. When used properly they provide, for all practical purposes 100 per cent protection.

The use of oral contraceptives has been associated with side-effects which include nausea, breast discomfort, weight gain and spotting, usually slight, of short duration and easily controlled by changing the preparation. A more disturbing complication is the association of the pill with thrombo-embolism. Studies have now shown that women on the 'Pill' have a slightly higher incidence of thrombo-embolism than others, but serious consequences are rare, and research has shown that the risk of dying as a result of pregnancy, especially in developing countries where maternal mortality is relatively high, is greater than the risk of dying of a blood clot due to the 'Pill'.

(5) *Intra-uterine devices (IUD)*

The knowledge that a foreign body inserted into the uterus prevents pregnancy has been known for many years. The accidental discovery that the stem pessary, originally used to correct retroversion, protected against pregnancy, led to the discovery that an intra-uterine device possessed contraceptive efficacy. With the development of plastics and the realisation of their inert features, the widespread use of intra-uterine devices became possible. These devices are made from polythene in various shapes and forms. Nearly a dozen types, not including sizes, are known and have been tested. Their mode of action has not been convincingly explained, but evidence is available that, like the 'Pill', they may act on more than one point in the reproductive chain of events.

For an IUD to be satisfactory, it must be easy to insert, difficult to expel, but relatively easy to remove. It must also be effective in preventing pregnancy and cause no discomfort when *in situ.*

An introducer is always required to push the device past the internal os of the uterus. For an introducer to be satisfactory, it must be easily sterilisable, pliant, at least in the portion that enters the cervical canal, and it must possess a guard to prevent it passing too far into the uterus.

This method has the distinct advantage that it is cheap, convenient and, when adopted, does not need re-inforcing motivation. It also provides effective protection as only between one and five women out of a hundred using an IUD will become pregnant within a year.

Side-effects attendant upon this method include irregular, sometimes very heavy and prolonged bleeding, backache, cramps and pains in the pelvic region. Most of these, in most women disappear after the first few months. Expulsion of the device, spontaneously without the user being aware, is relatively common. Usually changing the size or the type is effective in controlling this, and those devices with strings for which the user can feel provide a safeguard and reassurance.

Perforation, usually begun at the time of insertion, has occurred with the IUD, but it is uncommon and does not give rise to any serious complication.

Pelvic inflammatory disease may develop or be aggravated by the IUD. Experience suggests that care in assessing the condition of the patient before insertion, and a meticulous attention to asepsis in the procedures of inserting the device reduce the incidence to negligible limits. Only devices carefully sterilised should be used.

Pregnancy has occurred with the IUD *in situ,* but is extremely rare. Since the device is related to the maternal and not the foetal tissues, pregnancy may proceed to term unaffected. Usually the device is removed as soon as pregnancy is confirmed. These pregnancies have a high spontaneous abortion rate.

Sub-fertility

The capacity of a man, a woman or a couple to participate in the production of a live child is known as fertility. When this capacity is below normal the person, or the couple, is said to be sub-fertile. If it is absolute, then the word infertile is used. As a general rule, a couple is considered sub-fertile if, in the absence of contraception, the woman fails to become pregnant after 1 year of normal married life.

About 15 per cent of married couples in countries for which figures are available, provided that the woman is in the child-bearing age-range, find it difficult or impossible to produce children, without some help. Thirty to forty per cent of these never succeed in becoming parents. The factors which affect the probability of a couple producing children, in the absence of contraception and sterilisation of one of the partners, are:

(i) The age of the woman (optimum for conception 22-24 years)
(ii) The age of the man (optimum for conception 24-26 years)
(iii) The frequency of coitus, that is exposure to pregnancy (two to three times a week for conception) and
(iv) The length of exposure (optimum for conception 0-4 years of marriage).

For pregnancy to occur, coitus or its equivalent must take place at or very near the time of ovulation; it must be efficient; the ejaculate must be adequate; the cervical condition must be receptive to the sperm cell and the fallopian tubes must be patent. For the pregnancy to be maintained to full term, the woman must be relatively normal in her hormonal production, the ovum transport unimpeded, the uterine mucosa suitable and the cervix competent. Normal ovulation occurs once in a month, and only if efficient intercourse takes place around this time, within no more than 48 hours on either side of its occurrence, can pregnancy occur. In the male, spermatogenesis goes on all the time making it theoretically possible for a fertile male to father a child each time he has intercourse.

Causes of Sub-fertility

Difficulty in producing a child may be due to either one or both parents.   The factors which contribute to sub-fertility may be:

(a) *General*—including diet, anxiety and anaemia in the female and fatigue, excesses (smoking, alcohol, sexual activities) and anxiety in the male.

(b) *Developmental*—congenital defects including malformation and absence of any part of the reproductive system in either the man or the woman.

(c) *Endocrinal*—deficiencies, inadequacies and diseases affecting the endocrine systems of either sex.

(d) *Diseases of the genital organs*—infection, obstructions, new growths on either side.

Sub-fertility may be attributable to the couple. Such factors as marital maladjustment, incompetent coitus, bad timing, false beliefs and, rarely, immunologic incompatibility.

Management of the infertile couple calls for empathy and patience. A careful history must be taken, followed by general examination as well as examination of the sexual organs of both parties. This should be followed by detailed discussion of the reproductive process explaining and stressing the fertile period, and the need for the woman keeping meticulous record of her menstrual periods for three or four cycles. This makes it possible to determine her probable ovulation period which is the optimal time for undertaking a post-coital test (PCT). This test is the pivot of sub-fertility investigations. A positive PCT provides information that (*a*) coitus is efficient, (*b*) the woman is probably ovulating, (*c*) the man is fertile, (*d*) provided no abnormality exists, pregnancy is likely. On the other hand, pregnancy is practically impossible, if the test is negative, until the problem is put right.

The test consists of examining a specimen of seminal fluid sucked up from the vaginal pool and the cervical canal of the uterus. The presence of many, freely motile, healthy looking sperms constitutes a successful test. The man should have abstained from intercourse for 2 days prior to the test and specimens must be taken between 6 and 12 hours after coitus.

The two other investigations that affect the female are (i) tests for tubal patency and for confirming that ovulation takes place. Insufflation with CO_2, especially if the equipment can produce a graphic record, is adequate to determine patency in most cases. Doubtful cases can be resolved in hysterosalpingography.

(ii) For determining ovulation, several features provide presumptive evidence. These include recording of basal temperature, exactly as it is done to identify the safe period but for the opposite reason. Examination of cervical secretion, vaginal cytology and endometrial biopsy also contribute to the evidence.

In some 30 per cent of cases (Western world figures) the sub-fertility is due to the male partner. Difficulties arise since the male of the species tends to assume that the fault is with his spouse. He equates potency or copulating ability with fecundity. The physical examination of the male and his past medical history may or may not provide clues to the situation. If after three tries, at least 1 month apart, no sperms or very few motile sperms are seen in the PCT a seminal fluid analysis (SFA) is indicated. Semen is collected, after 2 days' abstinence, either by masturbation or coitus interruptus. The specimen must, ideally, be examined within 2 hours of collection or stored in a well-regulated refrigerator. The colour, volume, sperm count and percentage motility of the cells are examined and evaluated, and treatment undertaken as indicated.

The sub-fertile couple, individually and together, feel inadequate and ashamed. Often each blames the other and the tensions invariably aggravate the situation. Sub-fertility in man or woman is not normal. It is wrong for a doctor to cover up his ignorance and inability to determine what is wrong by insisting, with or without petulance, that 'there is nothing wrong with you . . . .'.

Conclusion

Patterns of medical service are changing everywhere. The countries from which most tropical areas receive their directions are already changing, yet such is the strength of the feeling of insecurity in the developing countries that they are timorous and reluctant to grasp their opportunity to make innovations.

The family must be the unit of care in preventive medicine. Family Health stands on three legs: maternal care, child care and family planning. There can no longer be any justification for perpetuating the dichotomy which separates health care into curative and preventive services.

Further Reading

WHO Tech. Rep. Series. No. 476. *Family Planning in Health Services.*

Chapter Ten

The Child at School

It is universally recognised that the health of schoolchildren deserves special attention. In order to derive the maximum benefit from the educational programme, the child must be healthy physically, mentally and emotionally. It is also well known that children at school are exposed to a variety of hazards—physical injury, infection and emotional problems. School age is a period during which the child is undergoing rapid physical and mental development; a healthy environment is required to provide the child with the best opportunity of making the appropriate adjustments that are required during this critical period. The school provides a unique opportunity for health education; a means of establishing a firm foundation for the healthy habits of the future adult population. By safeguarding the health of the schoolchildren of today, one is ensuring the health of the adults of tomorrow. In many developing countries the need for good school health programmes is particularly critical. Apart from the universal reasons for having a special programme for schoolchildren, there is the additional factor that in many developing countries, the schoolchildren are the survivors of a high childhood mortality. Many of them still bear the sequelae of the diseases which were responsible for the deaths of the other children and most of them are still subject to the environmental conditions which predisposed to the high morbidity and mortality of pre-school age.

The overall objective of the school health programme is to ensure that every child is as healthy as possible so that he can obtain the full benefit from his education.

The Elements of a School Health Programme
Although the detailed organisation of a school health programme varies from place to place, the following elements are usually represented:

(1) *Medical Inspection of the Children*
Routine, periodic medical examination is designed to detect defects which require medical attention. The medical examination also provides the opportunity of discussing with parents and teachers the health problems and needs of the children. It includes screening for defects of

hearing and sight. The school examination will ascertain whether the child is fit to take part in school activities, including sports.

(2) *Assessment of Handicapped Children*
The school health programme must include some mechanism for finding children who are physically or mentally handicapped, assessing them, supervising them and placing them in the most appropriate institution if special care is indicated. The main categories of handicapped children are:

(*a*) Blind and partially sighted
(*b*) Those with defective hearing and/or speech
(*c*) Epileptic
(*d*) Educationally sub-normal
(*e*) Maladjusted and psychotic
(*f*) Physically handicapped or delicate.

(3) *Health Education*
The objective of the health education programme at school is to make the children value health as a desirable asset, and to know what the individual and the community can do to maintain and promote health. The course of instruction would include basic information about the normal structure and function of the human body, the agents of disease, and the role of the environment in maintaining good health. At the appropriate age-group, various aspects of sex education can be incorporated into the syllabus. All fit children should participate in a well-designed programme of physical education.

(4) *Environmental Sanitation*
It is necessary to ensure that the school environment is maintained at a high standard in order to safeguard the health of the children and to provide them with a practical example of healthy living. The school environment must reinforce the theoretical lessons learnt in the classes on health education. The school should be sited in a safe place, in an area free from excessive noise and other nuisances such as smoke or soot. The building should be well constructed so as to minimise accidents. The classrooms should be of adequate size, well lighted and ventilated. Sanitary facilities for the disposal of wastes should be provided, and there should be an adequate supply of safe water for drinking and washing. There should be adequate facilities for recreation.

(5) *Control of Infection*
Going to school represents for many children the first opportunity to mix with children other than close relatives and immediate neighbours. Hence, schooling often represents their first contacts with infections to which they are susceptible. The control of infection includes the exclusion of sick children from school and the protection of susceptible

children against such infections as smallpox, diphtheria and typhoid by immunisation. Parents should be urged not to send sick children to school and teachers should, in the course of daily inspection of the children, note any sign of illness. The health of the schoolteachers and other school personnel should be kept under careful observation to ensure that they do not transmit infection to the children. For example, schoolteachers should be routinely screened for tuberculosis and food handlers for enteric infections.

(6) *Nutrition*
The school health programme should include some mechanism for the promotion of adequate diet for schoolchildren. The programme should be designed to ensure that each child is adequately nourished and, where specific defects are noted, to provide some means of supplementation. The programme would include some health education of parents through group activities such as the Parent-Teacher Associations, or individually in cases of special problems. It may be useful to have a school meal programme; this can provide a valuable demonstration of good balanced diets, but the school meal can also be specifically designed to supplement the child's diet at home in such a way as to make up any major specific nutritional deficiencies. Practical instruction in nutrition can include the growing of food crops in the school garden and mother-craft and cookery classes especially for the girls.

(7) *Special Surveys*
Special epidemiological surveys can be conducted to investigate specific health problems. It can also be used as part of the assessment of health needs and evaluation of the school health programme.

Operation of the School Health Programme
The detailed organisation of the school health programme varies from one country to the other. In the more developed countries, the school health services employ numerous doctors, dentists, nurses, psychologists, speech therapists and other skilled personnel. In most developing countries, such elaborate schemes are not in operation. The objective in each country should be to exploit the available resources and co-ordinate them into a national school health programme.

The following services are usually provided in school health programmes:
    (*a*) *Medical inspection*
    (*b*) *Screening tests for defects*
    (*c*) *Clinics*—(i) Minor ailments, (ii) Consultation; (iii) Special clinics, e.g. orthopaedic, ophthalmological, ear, nose and throat and child guidance
    (*d*) *Dental services*—Preventive and therapeutic.

Co-ordination of the School Health Programme
The health care of the child at school requires the co-ordinated efforts of parents, teachers, school health personnel, family physicians and local health authorities. Each has an important role to perform; skilled dovetailing of these various units will provide the most effective school health programme. Since there are overlapping functions in several areas, it is important to avoid unnecessary duplication of effort especially where resources are scarce. Even where resources are lavish, it is essential to prevent avoidable conflict and friction.

The provision of a safe healthy environment is the responsibility of the school authorities. They are also responsible for health education and physical education at school. The personnel of the school health programme are responsible for the medical inspection of the children; in some places they also undertake treatment but in other countries any defect or illness is treated by the family physician. The school health personnel are also responsible for the control of communicable diseases, although again they or the family physician may be responsible for immunisation of the children. In developing countries, many of these functions are performed by medical auxiliaries who are working under the supervision of doctors.

Assessment and Evaluation
Evaluation of the school health programme depends in the first instance on a careful definition of the objectives of the programme.

First, there should be an assessment of the work load of the various units: the number of medical inspections, the number of cases treated at the clinics, the number of children immunised, the number of school meals served, etc. The health status of the children can be assessed from an analysis of the data gathered at the medical inspections, from sickness records and from special surveys. The data generated in the operation of the school health service should be compiled and analysed. Such information as the distribution of the heights and weights of the children, the haemoglobin level, and the frequency of dental caries can provide valuable assessment of the health of the children and the effectiveness of the school health programme.

Chapter Eleven

Environmental Health

The objective of environmental sanitation is to create and maintain
conditions in the environment that will promote health and prevent
diseases. Man's external environment contains elements which are
essential for life and for the maintenance of good health. In addition,
the environment contains potential hazards. Man has a wide range of
tolerance of environmental conditions because of his ability to adapt.
Such biological adaptation has its limits, and the breakdown of
adaptation represents the onset of disease. For example, the human
being can tolerate wide fluctuations in environmental temperature; he
has various mechanisms (sweating, shivering) for coping with these
changes. If however the heat stress is excessive, then adaptive mechanisms break down and disease results may be in the form of heat stroke.
Health can therefore be viewed as successful adaptation to the environment, whereas disease represents a breakdown of adaptation.

The breakdown of adaptation can be prevented by:

(*a*) increasing the host's ability to withstand stresses in the environment, e.g. by good nutrition

(*b*) reducing the hazardous and hostile elements in the environment.

Environmental Sanitation

This is the process of taming the environment so that it no longer
constitutes a hazard to man. In particular, environmental sanitation
deals with:

(1) Provision of a safe and adequate supply of water
(2) Disposal of wastes
(3) Safeguarding of food
(4) Provision of good housing
(5) Control of insect vectors and other pests
(6) Control of animal reservoirs of infection
(7) Air hygiene and prevention of atmospheric pollution
(8) Elimination of other hazards—noise, radiation, etc.

Many of these problems in environmental sanitation are dealt with
by public health engineers, technicians and other non-medical personnel
rather than by the physician. The doctor is therefore not usually required to know in detail how the various appliances are constructed

and maintained. Nevertheless, he should be familiar with the basic principles involved. This would enable him to give informed support to his environmental health team and for simple projects, guidance to the health auxiliaries.

Water Supplies
Each community needs a safe and adequate supply of water.

Uses of Water
(a) *Domestic*—(i) drinking and cooking, (ii) personal hygiene—for washing the body and clothes, (iii) environmental sanitation—for washing utensils, floors and for the disposal of wastes, (iv) temperature control—for heating and cooling, (v) gardening.

(b) *Industrial and agricultural.*

Sources of Water
These include: (*a*) rain water, (*b*) surface water—streams, rivers, ponds, lakes and sea, (*c*) underground water—wells, bore holes and springs.

(a) *Rain water*
Rain water is pure but it may pick up impurities from the atmosphere, roofs, roof gutterings and storage tank.

(b) *Surface water*
This source is easily polluted by direct contamination by human beings and animals, or indirectly when rain washes faeces and other pollutants from the banks into the streams and rivers. Surface water must, therefore, be purified before use.

(c) *Underground water*
(1) *Wells*—These may be:
  (*a*) Shallow wells—the water is collected above the first impervious layer. Shallow wells are liable to pollution by seepage from surface water.
  (*b*) Deep wells—water is drawn below the first impervious layer.

Protection of wells. (i) The wells should be situated at least 100 feet (preferably uphill) from any potential source of pollution, e.g. pit latrine. (ii) There should be a watertight lining for at least 10 feet from the surface. (iii) There should be a parapet about 2 feet high surrounded by a concrete apron to drain the waste water away. (iv) There must be a watertight cover. (v) Water should be drawn preferably by a pump, or at least through a permanent bucket which is anchored to the well.

(2) *Springs*
The water from a natural spring may be quite pure. It can be protected

by building a concrete dam so that the water accumulates in reservoir and is drawn through pipes.

Whatever its source, the supply of water should be:

(a) *Adequate*—A minimum of 5 to 10 gallons per person per day is required. The requirement is much higher in modern industrial urban areas (40 to 100 gallons per person per day, or more).
(b) *Safe*—It should be free from chemical and biological hazards.
(c) *Acceptable*—It should be acceptable in terms of its taste, colour and softness.

Diseases associated with Water

The water-related diseases can be broadly classified into five epidemiological groups:

Group I   Water-borne infections, e.g. cholera, typhoid, infective hepatitis.
Group II   Water-shortage diseases, e.g. skin infections, trachoma.
Group III   Water-impounding diseases, e.g. schistosomiasis, guinea-worm.
Group IV   Water-arthropod diseases, e.g. malaria, onchocerciasis.
Group V   Chemical constituents either excess or shortage, e.g. fluoride.

Purification of Water

The purification of water can be achieved by a combination of some of the following measures:

(a) *Protection of the source*

In particular, the source water should be protected from pollution from human faeces, a major source of pathogenic organisms and other human contact which could lead to contamination, e.g. with guinea-worm. Human beings and animals should be excluded from surface sources of water.

(b) *Storage*

Some of the human pathogens have a relatively short life in water, they may be absent from water that has been stored for a few days or longer. Cysts, e.g. *E. histolytica*, tend to survive for much longer periods.

(c) *Coagulation and sedimentation*

Addition of alum to water causes flocculation of the finely suspended matter; these larger particles settle more rapidly, leaving a clear supernatant.

(d) *Filtration*

Various devices are used for filtration: a thick linen cloth may remove large particles, including cyclops (intermediate host of guinea-worm), from the water: a sand filter consisting of sand and stones of graded size, with fine sand at the top and large stones at the bottom; simple domestic filter in which the water is filtered through a 'candle' filter which is made of fine clay. At best, filtration will remove bacteria, protozoal cysts and larger particles but viruses ('filterable viruses') will pass through the filter.

(e) *Disinfection*

Chlorination is the most widely used method of chemical disinfection of water. It may be used in the form of chlorine gas for large municipal schemes or as bleaching powder (chloride of lime), liquid bleach, or hypochlorite. Most vegetative forms of bacterial pathogens are killed by chlorination, but the cysts of *E. histolytica* may survive. *Super-chlorination* consists in the application of a dose of chlorine which considerably exceeds that required to disinfect the water. This method is often used in an emergency, e.g. during epidemics and after a suitable contact time the water is dechlorinated.

(f) *Boiling*

This is a reliable way of eliminating pathogens but it is impracticable on a large scale. It can be used in special circumstances, e.g. when there is sudden breakdown in treatment process of a municipal water supply. It is also advisable to boil all water to be used for feeding young infants.

Quality of Water

The quality of water is assessed by (*a*) physical, (*b*) microscopical, (*c*) chemical, and (*d*) bacteriological examination.

Chemical Properties of the Water

There should be no chemical constituent in quantities that could be a health hazard. Safety limits have been prescribed for some of the elements (Table 11.1).

TABLE 11.1

Safety levels of common elements in domestic water

	Maximum allowable concentrations in parts per million (i.e. mg/litre)
Lead (as Pb)	0·1
Arsenic (as As)	0·2
Selenium (as Se)	0·05
Chromium (as Cr hexavalent)	0·05
Cyanide (as CN)	0·01

With regard to fluoride, a high level (1·0 to 1·5 mg per litre) predisposes to dental and skeletal fluorosis; a low content (0·5 mg/litre) is associated with dental caries. Therefore, fluoride may be added to bring the concentration to about 1·0 mg/litre.

Biological Tests

Although pathogens such as *S. typhi* and *V. cholerae* can be isolated from water, the routine bacteriological examination of water concentrates on detecting evidence of faecal pollution of water. Coliform organisms are used as indicators of recent faecal pollution because these organisms are present in faeces in large numbers and they survive in water for relatively short periods. Faecal coli (*E. coli*) can be differentiated from other coliform organisms which occur in nature. A high coliform count ('presumptive coliform count') of 10 coliforms/100 ml or more is regarded as being suspicious or bad; and there should be no faecal coli.

Disposal of Wastes

The accumulation of waste products and their indiscriminate disposal represent a grave hazard to health. Systems of waste disposal are designed to eliminate these hazards. The broad objectives of a waste disposal system can thus be briefly summarised:

(a) *Eliminate hazards to man*
    (i) physical, e.g. broken bottles, empty cans
    (ii) chemical, e.g. poisonous chemicals in industrial wastes
    (iii) biological, e.g. the agents and vectors of disease harboured in wastes.

(b) *Prevent pollution of the natural environment*
The dumping of wastes on land, and the indiscriminate disposal into rivers and other surface waters, or into the air can cause destruction of the natural life.

(c) *Salvage of materials of economic value*
The following problems will be considered:
    (*a*) Disposal of sewage
    (*b*) Disposal of refuse
    (*c*) Disposal of industrial wastes.

Disposal of Sewage

Human excreta are an important source of pathogenic organisms, especially the causative agents of diarrhoeal diseases. In addition, faeces are attractive to flies and support the development of the larval stages ('maggots') of filth flies. Apart from these hazards, the indiscriminate disposal of faeces can constitute a grave nuisance from the offensive sight and smell.

The sanitary disposal of human excreta can be achieved only where there are adequate provisions in the community for the disposal of faeces and where the people have learnt to appreciate and use them. Ideally, there should be at least one latrine for each family, and the device should be kept clean and maintained in good working order. Public latrines are also required in markets and other places where people gather in large numbers.

Qualities of the Ideal Latrine

A good latrine must possess the following qualities:

(a) There should be no handling of fresh faeces
(b) There should be no contamination of surface soil
(c) There should be no contamination of surface water or underground water that may enter springs or wells
(d) The excreta should not be accessible to flies or animals
(e) There should be no unpleasant odours or unsightly conditions
(f) The method should be simple and inexpensive in construction and operation and in relation to the resources of the community
(g) The method should be acceptable in terms of the cultural beliefs of the community.

The common methods of sewage disposal are:

(a) Bucket latrine
(b) Trench latrine
(c) Pit-hole latrine
(d) Bore-hole latrine
(e) Water-seal latrine of Cheugmai type
(f) Aqua privy
(g) Chemical closet
(h) Water-carried disposal methods—to sewage pits, septic tanks, sewage farms or oxidation ponds.

The use of bucket latrine should be discouraged as widely as possible. It often involves the handling of fresh faeces, flies and animals are attracted to and can often reach the faeces, and it tends to cause offensive odours. Where bucket latrines are in use, the single-bucket system should be replaced by the two-bucket system.

In the single-bucket system, the conservancy worker empties the bucket into a large pail or tank and returns the empty but dirty bucket to the latrine. In the two-bucket system, a fresh clean bucket is brought in to replace the dirty bucket; meanwhile the dirty bucket is removed to the depot, where it is emptied, washed and disinfected.

Various methods, such as pit latrines, septic tanks, oxidation ponds and such other methods, rely on the natural process of decomposition of faeces. Excreta, wherever deposited, decompose and ultimately become converted to an inodorous, inoffensive and stable product. In the process, many human pathogens are destroyed. Thus faeces are self-digesting and self-purifying.

The main actions of decomposition are to break down the complex organic compounds such as protein and urea into simpler and more stable forms; reduce the volume and mass (80 per cent of the decomposing material) by the production of such gases as methane, carbon dioxide, ammonia and nitrogen which are dissipated in the atmosphere, and by the production of soluble materials which leach away into the underlying soil. Pathogenic organisms are unable to survive the processes of decomposition or are attacked by the rich biological life of the decomposing mass. Bacteria play the major role in decomposition. The process may be entirely anaerobic, as it is in aqua privies, septic tanks, bottom of deep pits or entirely aerobic as in composting (see p. 279).

Disposal of Refuse

This refers to the storage, collection and disposal of solid wastes in a community. Refuse includes various organic materials such as leaves and food remnants, and inorganic objects such as bottles, tins, and a variety of discarded objects.

Poor refuse disposal attracts fly breeding and other insects, and affords food and shelter for rodents. It creates fire hazard and is a source of accidents through cuts and puncture wounds from sharp objects.

(a) *Storage of Refuse*

This involves provision of a sufficient number of containers to hold the volume of refuse produced between collections; the selection of an approved type of container; the placement of containers where they will provide maximum convenience for the user and easy access to the collection crew; and the maintenance of the containers and their surroundings in a sanitary condition. The dustbin or garbage-can should be watertight and provided with a tight-fitting lid. It should be rust resistant; structurally sound; easily filled, emptied and cleaned, and finished with side handles. The bins should rest on a concrete slab, the sweepings from which should be put in the bin and not cleared off on to the adjacent ground.

(b) *Collection of Refuse*

Where a community has no collection service, conditions are generally favourable for high fly and rat populations. Even where service is available, a careless collection employee may spill refuse on the premises or street. Rough handling may damage the container rim so that the lid may not fit properly, thereby making the refuse accessible to flies and rats.

Collection of refuse should be frequent, systematic and reliable, and bin points maintained by Government or Municipal Cleansing Services. Great improvements in collection by specially constructed vehicles have been developed in recent years.

Where combined refuse collection is practised, this service should be provided daily or at least twice a week. This practice will favour sanitary storage and will contribute to an environment adverse to flies, mosquitoes and rats. Collection crews must be properly trained.

(c) *Disposal of Refuse*

In any system the final disposal of refuse must be considered first, since it has an important influence on both storage and collection. Regardless of how diligently the householder attempts to control flies in his premises, he stands little chance when a nearby dump is a prolific breeding ground.

The methods of refuse disposal commonly used are:

(1) *Dumping in the sea or river.* This method is used in coastal cities and riverine towns, it results in littering of shore-lines with refuse and becomes a health as well as an accident hazard. It is also a deterrent to the tourist trade.

(2) *Open dumping.* This is cheap, it requires little planning and is therefore unfortunately too frequently found in tropical communities. It provides ideal breeding places for rats, flies and mosquitoes. Every effort should be made to eliminate this health menace and to replace it with sanitary and practical methods of disposal.

(3) *Burning.* Low-temperature burning of combustible refuse is frequently used. Generally speaking, burning using oil drums and cages or open burning are unsatisfactory and surroundings are frequently littered with cans and broken bottles that constitute an accident hazard to children playing in the area. The smoke and odours contribute to air pollution and it is a fire risk. Moreover, half-burnt refuse can afford breeding places for flies and provide food for rats.

(4) *Composting.* This is a process in which under suitable environmental conditions aerobic micro-organisms, principally thermophilic, break down organic matter to a fairly stable humus. Composting requires frequent turning, and two main methods are used: (*a*) Refuse without nightsoil, e.g. Trengganu method and (*b*) Refuse with nightsoil, e.g. Calcutta and Indore methods. The details of these various methods are available in standard textbooks of hygiene and sanitation.

(5) *Controlled tipping.* This is an effective and proven method for the hygienic disposal of refuse and can be used wherever sufficient and suitable land is available. Basically it consists of four steps: (i) depositing refuse in a planned control manner, (ii) spreading and compacting it in layers to reduce its volume, (iii) covering the material with a layer

of earth, and (iv) compacting the earth cover. The initial investment is low and health hazards, fire and nuisance are eliminated.

(6) *Incineration*. The newer incineration plants have reduced atmospheric pollution and by this method the volume of material for ultimate disposal is greatly reduced.

The final choice of method to be used for the sanitary disposal of refuse will naturally vary from rural to city areas; it will depend on the population density, the availability of land and other facilities at one's disposal.

(d) *Salvaging*

Some of the materials in refuse can be sorted and used. Thus, paper, rags, metal containers, bottles and similar objects can be salvaged.

Industrial Wastes

Modern industrial processes produce chemical wastes which are potential hazards to man and other living things. Although each special problem cannot be examined in detail, some general principles can provide useful guide-lines.

Ideally the design of the plant should include a satisfactory means of disposal of the waste products. This may involve some processing of the effluent before it is ultimately discharged into a stream; it may require storage and final disposal by burying of solid wastes; or it may include a subsidiary process which can salvage and consume some of the waste products of the primary process.

In particular, the disposal of crude effluent into a stream should be strongly discouraged. Similarly solid wastes, such as slag heaps from mines, should not be indiscriminately dumped on land; nor should noxious fumes be blown from chimneys to cause atmospheric pollution.

Housing

The provision of good housing is an important aspect of environmental health. It represents:

(*a*) A significant part of man's environment
(*b*) Shelter from the elements
(*c*) Workshop: the kitchen for the housewife, the playroom for the children; the toolshed for the adult males.
(*d*) Home: the residence of the family, where this social institution carries out some of its major functions.

Good housing should minimise physical and biological hazards in the environment and should promote the health of the inhabitants. Good housing should eliminate or minimise the following hazards:

(a) *Biological*

The risk of the transmission of communicable diseases should be minimised. Poor ventilation and overcrowding, for example, predispose to the spread of respiratory infections. Good water supply, adequate facilities for washing utensils and other sanitary devices, good storage for food and well-designed kitchens, will help to minimise the spread of gastro-intestinal infections.

(b) *Physical*

Injury from falls, burns, electric shock, poisoning and similar physical hazards can be controlled by good design of homes to include appropriate safety devices. The maintenance of an equable temperature in the house, by heating in winter and cooling in the hot summer is also conducive to good health. The physical hazards include atmospheric pollution from smoky wood fires, excessive noise and poor lighting.

(c) *Social*

The home should be designed so that the family can function effectively in terms of its cultural background. This implies the required level of privacy for adults and a suitable setting for bringing up children.

The World Health Organisation has defined in some detail the requirements of a healthy residential environment (WHO Tech. Report Series No. 225, 1961).

The basic aspects of housing relate to the proper siting and construction of a residence which provides fundamental physiological, psychological and sanitary requirements. Types of housing in the tropics depend on the climatic environment and hence are quite different in arid zones, in savannahs, in upland jungle, in cold dry or humid high plateaux, in marshlands, in high mountain steppes and in tropical rain forest.

In many parts of the rural tropics, traditional huts are often small, ill-ventilated and lighted only through the door opening, with a smoky fireplace inside and without real furniture. Men, fowls, small and large animals may cohabit and lack of sanitation and safe water supply are all too obvious. Many model rural villages have, however, been started all over the tropical world with appropriate government help.

Housing for plantation, mining and industrial workers has been provided in many areas by employees and standards have been variable. Often government authorities have had to regulate the minimum standards including size, floor and air space, ventilation, cooking, storage, sanitary facilities and water supplies. Inspired by good management rather than by humanity or justice, industrial and agricultural companies in the tropics have learned much about the physical, biological, psychological, technical and economic problems involved in housing their employees.

K

For the rapid urbanising populations of the tropics provision of adequate low-cost housing is a primary responsibility of government and municipal authorities. Standards should be such that they can be made enforceable in a low income community and relate to local climate and cultural conditions.

Food Hygiene

The chief aim of food hygiene is to prevent the contamination of foodstuffs at all stages of their production, i.e. collection, preparation, manufacture, transportation, storage and sale. Sometimes, despite all precautions, organisms may contaminate food, in these instances adequate refrigeration may prevent multiplication of the organisms to a level sufficient to cause clinical symptoms.

The measures to be taken to maintain high standards of catering whether in the home or in the community at large will include:

  (i) the control of primary sources of food, e.g. avoidance of use of human manure as a fertiliser
  (ii) inspection of relevant premises, e.g. abattoirs
  (iii) supervision of foodhandlers, e.g. carriers
  (iv) health education
  (v) laboratory examination of foodstuffs, e.g. precooked meats
  (vi) legislation.

Disinfection

The aim of disinfection is to kill noxious organisms and there are several ways of achieving this, namely by: (i) heat, (ii) desiccation, (iii) sunlight, (iv) chemical agents, (v) filtration, (vi) aerosols, and (vii) irradiation.

The destruction of the bacteria in the discharges and excreta of a patient suffering from an infectious disease, e.g. typhoid fever, and on articles in contact with him is known as 'current disinfection'. The cleansing of a room which has been occupied by a patient suffering from an infectious disease, e.g. cholera, is known as 'terminal disinfection'.

(1) *Heat*

Heat kills bacteria and spores by coagulating their protein, moist heat is more efficient than dry heat. Thus boiling water will kill bacteria in a few minutes (5-10) and most spores in about half an hour. Pasteurisation destroys bacteria in milk without spoiling it. Steam is also an efficient method of disinfection. Burning ideally gets rid of infected fomites which are of no further use and hot air may also be used to kill bacteria although its penetrative powers are poor.

(2) *Desiccation*
Only delicate organisms, e.g. the meningococcus are killed when allowed to dry and this form of disinfection is therefore of limited value.

(3) *Sunlight*
Sunlight, especially ultraviolet rays, are lethal to many bacteria and ultraviolet light is sometimes used for the sterilisation of air.

(4) *Chemical Agents*
Chemical disinfectants, e.g. iodine, chlorine, hydrogen peroxide, alcohol, phenol and cresols (lysol), actively kill bacteria and are widely used for disinfection in a large variety of circumstances. 'Detergent' types of antiseptics are increasingly being utilised.

(5) *Filtration*
See page 274.

(6) *Aerosols*
In these days of automation aerosols are becoming extremely popular especially for the sterilisation of air, the disinfectant, e.g. sodium hypochlorite or propylene glycol being spread in a very fine spray.

(7) *Irradiation*
Gamma irradiation (cobalt-60 as source) has been used to sterilise food and thus eliminate *Salmonellae* and other bacteria. Similarly several medical appliances, e.g. catheters, disposal syringes, etc., are being radiation-sterilised.

Further Reading
Ross Institute Bulletin No. 10: *Small Water Supplies.*
Ross Institute Bulletin No. 8: *Rural Sanitation in the Tropics.*
Ross Institute Bulletin No. 5: *The Housefly and its Control.*
WHO Tech. Rep. Series. No. 484: *Solid Wastes Disposal and Control.*

Chapter Twelve

Health Education

The impulse to enlighten people in matters relating to health, hygiene and disease has been with the medical profession for many years. So has the desire of the people to learn about the body, its function and dysfunction. Between 1762 and 1835, several doctors working as individuals and as groups made several attempts to produce written material about health for the general public, or for special groups. Every such publication was quickly bought up by the public, and in many instances several editions in many languages were also produced. All of these sought to explain and give advice about health and diseases, based on the general principle that information and demonstrations of how to better conditions would, in the course of time, be adequate to improve them. From these beginnings 'Health Education' has moved from the campaigns of the middle and late nineteenth century, through the intensified educational activities of the early years of this century to the present situation.

The term 'health education' was first used at a conference in 1919. It very quickly became widely accepted and adopted and the process gained recognition as a special field of endeavour in public health. But, although it has gained steadily in importance, a universally accepted definition of health education has not been found. This gives rise to a situation in which the expression can mean, and does mean, different things to different persons, and even different things to the same person at different times.

When a health worker successfully imparts information, in such a way that the recipient is motivated to use that information for the promotion, protection, maintenance or restoration of his, his family's or his community's health, health education is a **tool**.

When a public health education department examines a situation and prepares guide-lines, approaches and materials for others which enhance their effectiveness; or when the work of the department in general or in specific projects is evaluated, health education becomes a **service**.

When teachers and education authorities provide effective health teaching for their pupils, or the community evolves an organised approach to the study and the solution of health problems, health education is a **process**.

If we accept health education as the translation of what is known about health into desirable individual and community behaviour patterns, through the education process, it becomes a **concept** as well.

Health education is an involved undertaking which is influenced and determined by attitudes, beliefs, tradition and education, and by the wants and the needs of the teacher and pupils. It is influenced by situation and by everything that affects the human animal. It is not the simple exercise of telling it loudly, telling it clearly and telling it often that it is sometimes believed to be. It seeks to bring about change in people, change in their knowledge, their attitudes and habits, to help them relate in the most effective way to their total (physical, mental, biological and social) environment.

Scope and Opportunities for Health Education

As Pierre Delore wrote in 1953: 'Over and above each technical act, there is a corresponding educational function which doubles the value of the act, prolongs it, increases its efficacy and endows it with real value'.

The opportunities offered to a doctor for health education are only limited by his ability to recognise them.

In countries which for want of a better designation are called developing, perpetuating the dichotomy between curative and preventive medicine offers no demonstrable advantages. With limited manpower resources and the preponderance of preventable diseases, the objectives of all medical practice must be to provide prevention at the classical five levels of *Health Promotion*, namely, (i) *Specific Protection*, (ii) *Early Diagnosis*, (iii) *Prompt Treatment*, (iv) *Disability Limitation* and (v) *Rehabilitation*. At each of these levels health education has specific functions:

(*a*) Most effective health promotion can centre around education about nutrition, care of the body with intelligent use of exercise and rest and the provision of a safe environment.

(*b*) Competent health education will enhance the chances of immunisation being accepted and special measures being taken to avoid particular diseases. Thus specific protection is provided.

(*c*) Teaching the public self-examination, the value of periodical medical examination and early manifestations of specific diseases will lead to early diagnoses and prompt treatment.

(*d*) Education about early mobility, or about immobility where indicated, and correction of traditional erroneous beliefs, can help to limit disability.

(*e*) Re-education and supportive educational measures for the handicapped facilitate his rehabilitation.

Overall, health education can increase the efficiency of health services by ensuring that they are indeed needed and wanted, and by helping the community to understand, accept and use those that are available in the most effective way.

The physician, in his recurring contacts with patients, has valuable opportunities for health education and he must recognise and utilise them. He occupies a position of high credibility and trust which make his pronouncements well received. But often no education takes place and the opportunity for health promotion is lost. Learning is a cumulative process which does not take place in a vacuum. One thing learned may facilitate the learning of a new thing as easily as it may prevent the learning of something else. The right knowledge and the correct practice in health has usually to displace, at least in part, what a person already believes and practises. Failure of the educational effort is certain, if it is not realised how vital it is to be aware of the current health beliefs and practices of the person or group one wishes to teach.

Methods of Health Education

Methods of communication are not to be confused with methods of health education. Communication is a process by which thoughts, ideas, wishes, intent and such are transmitted from one source (person, groups, things), referred to as the sender, to another source, referred to as the receiver. It is the basis of all human interrelationship without which education in any form cannot take place. It is thus an integral part of health education, but it is not the whole of health education.

The significant difference between health education and other types of education lies in the simple but important fact that, in other forms of education, the person to be educated is usually desirous of acquiring the education. He has a clear-cut objective in view which provides him with the drive towards the knowledge, the attitude or the skill to be acquired or learned. In health education, often the drive is with the educator who believes he can see a need in the person or group to be educated.

Every known method of education, conventional as well as unconventional, is applicable to health education. The validity of any one method, at any one time, depends on many factors. What is to be taught, why it is to be taught, when it is to be taught, where it is to be taught, who is to be taught, and the skill and competence of the teacher are the deciding factors of how it is to be taught.

Cicero (106-50 B.C.) once said, '. . . often, the opinion of those who teach is an obstacle to those who wish to learn'. This is a truism in the field of health education as in any other field. The health worker believes that health education consists of pouring accurate, simple, understandable information about health and disease into receptive and appreciative containers—his target or client. He thinks that if he says something with enough emphasis and intensity it must, somehow, penetrate, be understood and be accepted. He is disappointed and frustrated when this does not happen. He is not aware of the fact that the clients are human beings who know about themselves, know what they want and what they value. To them health is not as important as it seems to be to the health worker. Cause and effect relationships as regards illness are not fully accepted, clearly understood or sharply defined. The mother may be forgiven for her scepticism if she finds it difficult to believe that her baby is sick because she gave it unboiled water to drink when her neighbour's baby who drank the same water, at about the same time, is not sick; that her baby's diarrhoea and vomiting could have been caused by the same flies with which she has lived all her life, and which did not make her baby sick 2 weeks or 2 years ago. What appears so patently clear and straightforward, to a doctor or a nurse, the direct relationship between germs and disease, is not necessarily clear, or straightforward to uneducated persons whose values, beliefs and understanding do not equip them to encompass the concepts involved.

The most common method of communication employed by health personnel in health education is teaching. The emphasis should really be on learning. The doctor's preoccupation should be with how he can help his client(s) to learn, more than on how he can teach. The most effective methods, therefore, will be those that facilitate the learning process. Approaches which take into consideration the background, the social and cultural values of those it is desired to influence, and which are not limited to 'telling', have a better chance of succeeding. The doctor will have to learn to listen to and use the psychologist, the anthropologist and the sociologist as his most valuable associates if he wishes his health education efforts to bear fruit.

Components of Health Education

Communication forms the bulwark of health education. Thoughts, ideas, concepts and facts have to be transmitted in such a way that the fascination of the various forms of communications traps many into making communication an end, instead of the means that it is. All methods of communication are valid for health education, and provided they are used in appropriate situations, and used with skill, all methods have some effectiveness. Subtle methods, for example patients' clubs, fathers' societies and convalescence groups, have exceptional value in enhancing communication between members by providing a forum for discussion, amongst peers, in relatively relaxed atmosphere. As important as knowing, and being able to use the accepted channels of communication, is the ability to identify barriers to communication when they arise.

One such barrier is the tendency of the physician to 'talk down' to those he considers socially inferior to him. Planning to ensure that the educational aspects of health programmes are fully considered and integrated into the programme is an essential component of health education. Within this area the following must be included:

(i) determining the objectives to be attained by the programme
(ii) identifying, assessing and mobilising the resources available
(iii) involving those who will operate the programme in its planning
(iv) arranging the timing of the programme, and its educational aspects in relation to other services and programmes being carried out simultaneously
(v) selecting and testing various communication media
(vi) building in a method of evaluation to measure the extent to which objectives are attained.

The personnel who will occupy key positions in health education will depend on the basic programme for which the health education is planned. The doctor, the nurse, the sanitarian, the midwife; each has leadership roles in different types of programmes. And their selection and preparation can determine the success of the programme. Health education is a co-operative undertaking in which several health workers, of different disciplines and at different levels, participate. They combine to plan the programme and to operate it, each contributing according to his capability.

Activities in health education are principally of two kinds:

(*a*) A constant on-going health educational activity in which every member of the health team participates. Every contact with the target, in whatever situation presents itself, provides opportunities for health education, and every subsequent contact reinforces the teaching. Health education is not the primary purpose; it is one of the means by which the health team hope to improve child care, the sanitation of the area, or the control of a prevalent communicable disease.

(*b*) A component of a specific programme or activity. For example, an immunisation campaign, or a campaign to improve the nutrition in a particular area. Health education activities, usually precede the specific programme. They are used to prepare the community and increase the effectiveness of the basic programme.

The health educator includes amongst his responsibilities:

(i) co-ordination of the efforts of all those who work in the health field, including those of voluntary agencies
(ii) provision and development of communication and audio-visual material, especially those designed to meet special needs

(iii) contribution to the training of other workers, especially in areas relating to communication and health education

(iv) evaluation of health education activities, other programme activities and the overall activities of the organisation.

Evaluation

When the objectives of a health education programme have been decided they should be broken down into the specific intervening actions, steps and processes that will lead to the desired goals. Once this is done, it becomes relatively easy to devise ways to measure the extent to which the objectives are attained and to set the criteria for deciding whether the programme is succeeding or failing. It is for this reason that evaluation has such tremendous import for health education.

Evaluation has been defined as 'the art of the practicable'. In this connection, it is our way of finding out whether a programme, or an activity within the programme is valuable. It also discovers for us if there is lack of value in any portions of the programme. Thus, the prime purpose of evaluation should be to assist in determining the effective and ineffective aspects of a programme; the reasons for success or failure; and the factors that facilitate or inhibit achievement of health education objectives.

Health education is a valuable tool for helping people, singly and in groups, to improve their health status. But like every other tool, its effectiveness depends on the skill of the user.

Further Reading

DERRYBERRY, M. (1960). Health education—its objectives and methods. *Health Education Monthly*, No. **8**.

DOWELL, LINUS J. (1966). A study of selected health education implications. *Research Quarterly*, Vol. **37**, No. **1**.

GRIFFITHS, W. (1955). The learning process. *Bulletin of the National Tuberculosis Association*, **69-70**.

HOPPER, J. M. H. (1960). The value of various forms of publicity. *International Journal of Health Education*, Vol. **3**, No. **3**.

MASLOW, ABRAHAM (1966). *The Psychology of Science*. New York: Harper & Row.

PATTERSON, R. S. & ROBERTS, B. J. (1951). Community Health Education in Action. In *Nature and Scope of Health Education*, ed. C. V. Mosby, pp. 17-28. St Louis.

PAUL, BENJAMIN (1955). *Health. Culture of Community*. Russell Page Foundation.

ROBERTS, BERYL J. (1962). Concepts and methods of evaluation in health education. *International Journal of Health Education*, Vol. 5, No. 2.

STEUART, GUY W. (1969). Planning evaluation in health education. *International Journal of Health Studies*, Vol. 12, No. 2.

Chapter Thirteen

Other Aspects of Public Health

In this chapter the following subjects will be briefly dealt with: (1) International Health, (2) Social Welfare, (3) Sources of International Aid, (4) Public Health Laws, (5) Genetics and Health, (6) Mental Health and (7) Occupation and Health.

(1) International Health

The International Health Regulations are intended to ensure the maximum security against the international spread of disease with the minimum interference of world traffic. Recent experience has shown that these regulations do not constitute a sufficient safeguard against the introduction of the quarantinable diseases:

    (i) Smallpox (including *variola minor*)
    (ii) Cholera
    (iii) Yellow fever
    (iv) Plague.

The jet aeroplane has made a nonsense of incubation periods, and 'epidemiological surveillance' of selected diseases of international importance will have to be strengthened within the national health services of individual nations. In addition to the diseases mentioned above, poliomyelitis, influenza and malaria should also be covered. Surveillance means the epidemiological study of a disease as a dynamic process involving the ecology of the infectious agent, the host, the reservoirs, the vectors and the role of the environment (see p. 25).

Most countries have a Quarantine and Epidemiology Branch at the Ministry of Health which deals with

    (i) Port health
    (ii) Airport health
    (iii) Quarantine stations or hospitals and
    (iv) Vaccination.

The aim of such a division is to guard against the import and export of diseases, thus keeping the indigenous population reservoir as small as possible and *honestly* notifying w ho of the latest situation in the country irrespective of the local consequences. Unfortunately experience with cholera has shown that certain countries react most unfavourably to this concept. Although all points of entry into a country must be controlled, e.g. sea, air, road or rail, sea and airports present special problems.

TABLE 13.1

Vaccination certificate requirements for international travel*

VACCINE	Minimal period before travel	Duration of validity†
Smallpox (a) Primary (b) Re-vaccination	8 days after *successful* vaccination Same day	3 years, starting 8 days after vaccination 3 years, starting on day of vaccination
Yellow fever	10 days	10 years, starting 10 days after one injection of vaccine
Cholera	6 days	6 months, starting 6 days after one injection of vaccine

* Vaccination requirements vary from country to country and travellers are advised to check the requirements in the areas they propose to visit. This information is usually available through Embassies or High Commissions and travel agencies. A booklet, 'Vaccination Certificate Requirements for International Travel' is available from WHO.

† One injection of cholera or yellow fever vaccine given before the end of the validity of the certificate render the certificate valid for a further period of 6 months or 10 years respectively, starting on the day of injection. Travellers are advised that if the re-vaccination is recorded on a *new* certificate they should retain the old certificate for 6 days in the case of cholera, and 10 days for yellow fever, until the new certificate is valid by itself.

Seaports

When a ship is infected, e.g. with a case of smallpox, the following action has to be taken:

 (i) isolation of case
 (ii) re-vaccination of passengers and crew
 (iii) isolation of close contacts (14 days)
 (iv) surveillance of other contacts (14 days)
 (v) disinfection of patient's cabin, etc. (not whole ship)
 (vi) international notification.

All passengers should have their vaccination certificates checked and those without valid certificates require vaccination and surveillance. Yellow fever and pneumonic plague suspects must be isolated. At quarantine stations and hospitals compulsory re-vaccination takes place as well as group isolation and medical surveillance.

Sanitary examination of ships, especially water, toilets, kitchen and food storage compartments should be carried out and the deratisation certificate examined. When a ship flies the 'Q' flag, no one is permitted to board or leave the ship before the Port Health Officer.

Airports
Airport health services are rapidly being developed all over the world:
  (i) to perform vaccination and inoculation of passengers and crews when necessary
  (ii) to examine suspected passengers
  (iii) to place passengers under surveillance when necessary
  (iv) to inspect aircraft coming from yellow fever infected areas for the presence of *Aëdes* and to carry out disinsectisation if necessary
  (v) to vaccinate and inoculate all personnel in the airport who come in contact with aircraft coming from infected ports
  (vi) to inspect and see that the airport precincts are kept in a satisfactory state including the airport restaurant and flight kitchen
  (vii) to supervise the control of *Aëdes* and other mosquitoes within the control zone of the airport perimeter
  (viii) to maintain and run the casualty clearing station in case of air disaster
  (ix) to provide out-patient treatment facilities for cases of minor illnesses (for passengers and airport staff)
  (x) to take samples of toilet wastes from planes and to send the specimens for bacteriological examination to ascertain whether adequate disinfection is being carried out
  (xi) to take periodic samples of food and potable water that are supplied to the aircraft to ascertain whether these are fit for human consumption and that they have not been contaminated by bacteria or chemical substances.

Conclusion
The attitude towards the International Sanitary Regulations should be one where the security afforded to countries takes priority over the facilitation of travel. The infection status of neighbouring countries should be especially well known. Certain recent global trends in the spread of the quarantine diseases are very disturbing. The most notable has been the spread of El Tor cholera since 1961 across Asia, to southern Europe and the Middle East and now to Africa south of the Sahara, for the first time in history (Fig. 4.2). A number of outbreaks have taken place in many countries free of epidemic diseases as a result of the rapid development of international air travel, and the frequency with which travellers move about and change planes. A reappraisal of the existing International Sanitary Regulations and their function is overdue.

(2) Social Welfare

Departments of social welfare in the tropics provide a variable range of welfare services for the community. In some countries, e.g. Singapore, a very wide range is available while in some other countries, e.g. those of tropical Africa, social welfare services barely exist. The aim is basically to provide welfare and protection to needy children and young persons; to women and young girls with particular reference to brothels and to provide probation and aftercare services for young offenders, endeavouring to place them in employment whenever possible.

Public assistance schemes provide financial assistance to the aged, the chronic sick, the physically and mentally handicapped, the widows and orphans and the unemployed. Institutional care is provided for special cases.

Voluntary organisations have played and continue to play an important role in welfare work in the state. In some tropical countries the only welfare work available, e.g. care of handicapped children, is that provided by major voluntary organisations.

(3) Sources of International Aid

Major sources of world aid include:

- (i) World Health Organisation (WHO)
- (ii) United Nations International Children's Emergency Fund (UNICEF)
- (iii) International Labour Organisation (ILO)
- (iv) Food and Agriculture Organisation (FAO)
- (v) United Nations Educational, Scientific and Cultural Organisation (UNESCO)
- (vi) United States Agency for International Development (USAID)
- (vii) Colombo Plan.

The Regional Offices of the World Health Organisation are situated in the following cities:

(1) Western Pacific Region	(WPRO)	Manila
(2) South-Eastern Asian Region	(SEARO)	New Delhi
(3) Eastern Mediterranean Region	(EMRO)	Alexandria
(4) African Region	(AFRO)	Brazzaville
(5) European Region	(ERO)	Copenhagen
(6) American Region	(PAHO)*	Washington

The main functions of the World Health Organisation are given on page 319. In addition, WHO produces a manual of the international statistical classification of diseases, injuries and causes of death; as well as an international pharmacopoeia. It is responsible for the biological

* The Pan-American Health Organisation serves as the regional organisation for the Americas.

standardisation of drugs, sera and vaccines. It produces several publications: e.g. *World Health*, which is a popular monthly for lay people; *WHO Chronicle*, which gives brief accounts of conferences, field activities and meetings of expert committees and is also produced monthly; *WHO Bulletin*, which publishes scientific papers monthly; *Technical Report Series*, which gives the recommendations of expert committees. It also publishes a series of monographs on a wide variety of subjects of public health importance.

South Pacific Commission

The purpose of the Commission is to encourage and strengthen international co-operation in promoting the health, economic, social welfare and advancement of the peoples in the South Pacific region. The headquarters is in Noumea, New Caledonia. The health section of the Commission plays an advisory and consultative role to seventeen territories spread over a vast area with an estimated population of three million inhabitants.

International Red Cross (Red Crescent) Society

Its origin is associated with Henri Dunant in 1859 following the battle of Solferino, Northern Italy. It was instrumental in formulating the First Geneva Convention in 1864 which afforded protection to the wounded and those caring for them, and to provide medical supplies. Subsequent conventions in 1929 extended this protection to prisoners of war and civilians.

The League of Red Cross Societies, to which National Societies became affiliated, was set up in 1919.

The Red Cross is now a powerful well-organised International Health Agency active in both peace and war conditions. Programmes vary from country to country but invariably include First Aid, Home Nursing, Disaster Relief, etc. Children can join the Junior Red Cross.

Rockefeller Foundation

The huge funds accumulated by the Rockefeller family over the last 100 years are devoted to supporting a variety of medical and non-medical research and service programmes in many parts of the world. Fellowships for study and travel are also available. Recently more emphasis is being placed on agriculture and population control than on health.

(4) **Public Health Laws**

Public health laws are enacted in order to protect and promote individual and community health. The enaction of these laws is very variable and is dependent on the legal system of individual countries. The application and enforcement of these laws is a function of health officers, public health inspectors and the medical officers of health, who are given certain special powers for the purpose. The number of public health laws varies from country to country and they aim at covering such topics as:

    (i) registration of births and deaths
    (ii) quarantine and prevention of disease
    (iii) sales of food and drugs
    (iv) destruction of disease-bearing insects
    (v) registration of medical personnel
    (vi) registration of schools
    (vii) environmental health.

Under the above laws the health officers are given power to entry into premises and to take such action as they might deem necessary to prevent the propagation of disease.

(5) Genetics and Health

In recent years interest in genetics has been greatly stimulated in the tropics and subtropics by the discovery that high gene frequencies for some genetic traits are maintained by providing a protection to the carrier against falciparum malaria. The haemoglobin genetic markers vary in importance from one area to the other, thus while haemoglobin S is the most important abnormal haemoglobin in Africa, it is superseded by haemoglobin E and thalassaemia in South-East Asia. Many other examples of the interplay between genetic factors and health are available.

Glucose-6-phosphate dehydrogenase (G-6-Pd) deficiency, so common in many areas of the tropics, renders its bearer vulnerable to haemolytic anaemia on exposure to primaquine, the fava beans and other agents.

Some individuals inactivate isonicotinic acid hydrazide (isoniazid) rapidly. In these, antituberculous therapy with isoniazid is less satisfactory than in those patients in whom the drug is inactivated more slowly. On the other hand, the 'slow inactivator' is probably more likely to display toxic reactions, such as neuropathy.

It is known that a relatively high proportion of Africans lack demonstrable haptoglobins and it is reasonable to postulate that such persons are favoured by selection, but the search for such an advantage has yet to begin.

There is overwhelming evidence that patients with carcinoma of the stomach have a higher incidence of group A, and patients with peptic ulcer a high incidence of group O, than control populations from the same area.

The spread of insects resistant to DDT and other chemicals, of bacteria resistant to drugs, and of malaria parasites resistant to chloroquine are dramatic examples of changes in the genetic composition of natural populations of organisms in response to powerful selective forces.

When subjects heterozygous for two genes, e.g. (AS) are favoured by selection over both homozygotes (AA and SS), the situation is referred to as 'polymorphism'. One of the best examples of this is in fact provided by the sickle-cell gene which has remained common in parts of the world (especially in Africa), despite the fact homozygotes develop a severe anaemia from which most die in childhood. The hypothesis that the heterozygote enjoys a selective advantage against the lethal effects of *P. falciparum* malaria is now accepted and various facts confirm its veracity:

(i) The sickle-cell gene is found in its highest incidence in areas where *P. falciparum* malaria is, or was until recently, endemic

(ii) In areas of stable malaria, high *P. falciparum* densities are significantly less commonly found in children with the sickle-cell trait (AS) than in normal children (AA)

(iii) Post-mortem studies have revealed that death from cerebral malaria does not occur in the S heterozygote (AS)

(iv) There is evidence that the prevalence of the sickle-cell trait in a population increases with advancing years, which is suggestive of differential survival with a greater loss of normal genes

(v) It has been found that mothers with the sickle-cell trait had a slightly higher fertility and lower stillbirth rate, and that the birth weights of their children tended to be slightly higher than those of non-sickling mothers. This could be attributed to partial protection against *P. falciparum* malaria, as in pregnancy there is evidence that there is some lowering of immunity to this infection.

The mechanism whereby the sickle-cell haemoglobin partially protects the bearer from the severe effects of *P. falciparum* malaria is obscure. The red cell assumes the sickle shape when the oxygen tension is lowered, so it would appear reasonable to postulate that the utilisation of oxygen by the malarial parasite might enhance this effect, with consequent disposal of the young parasite and cell by the reticuloendothelial system. Maturation of the parasite would thereby be prevented. However, on estimating the incidence of gametocytes of *P. falciparum* in sicklers and non-sicklers no significant differences have been found, which implies that maturation can occur. It has also been suggested that the parasite might not be able to metabolise S as well as normal adult haemoglobin. It has been shown also that sickling children in Nigeria have significantly higher γ-globulin levels than non-sickling children which may imply that the trait enhances the antibody response against the malarial parasite.

Haemoglobin C and Malaria

The C gene occurs in its highest incidence in an area of Africa where malaria is stable. Unfortunately it also occurs in an area where the S gene is found in high incidence. The incidence of the S gene would appear to vary inversely with the incidence of C, in Northern Ghana being 12 to 18, Southern Ghana 18 to 12 and in Western Nigeria 24 to 6 per cent, the total incidence of S and C remaining very roughly constant at 30 per cent in these areas.

Pure haemoglobin-C disease (CC) causes little disability, but double heterozygosity of S and C frequently occurs and death from SC disease is not uncommon, especially in pregnancy. The C gene is therefore at a disadvantage, although the selection is much smaller than in the case of the S gene, where procreation by homozygotes (SS) is rare.

It has been suggested that, just as in the case of S haemoglobin, C may protect the bearer from the severe effects of *P. falciparum* malaria, thus offsetting the loss of C genes in SC disease. In this connection it has also been suggested that if this were so, C might have evolved from S mutation, a less harmful gene being substituted for a more lethal. It is, however, considered that, as the abnormality in both S and C haemoglobins is in the sixth position of the β chain, where the amino-acid residue glutamic acid is substituted by valine and lysine residues respectively, it is most likely that haemoglobins C and S arose as independent mutations from haemoglobin A, the mutation A to C being comparatively recent. All evidence to date points to the fact that the presence of C haemoglobin confers no partial protection against malaria.

Haemoglobin F and Malaria

It has been suggested that the presence of the 'F gene' might partially protect the bearer against the effects of *P. falciparum* malaria. An analysis of the results of various observers who have examined infants living in malarious districts of Africa reveals a comparatively low level of malaria infection in infants under 3 months of age. An apparent relationship was found in Gambian infants between the disappearance of foetal haemoglobin and the onset of malaria infection, but no definite evidence exists that haemoglobin F protects against the lethal effects of *P. falciparum*.

Haemoglobin E and Malaria

The few series of children so far investigated have failed to show any protection of haemoglobin-E heterozygotes against malaria. It has also been posited that increased iron absorption in the E-trait carrier might confer an advantage, but there is no evidence that the trait carrier does absorb more iron.

Thalassaemia and Malaria
Since the β thalassaemia gene is often lethal when homozygous, the heterozygote frequencies of 20 per cent found in some places must be explained by heterozygous advantages, and once again it has been suggested that malaria was involved. The evidence to date is inconclusive.

G-6-PD and Malaria
Confirmation of the malaria-protection hypothesis has been sought in various ways: gene-frequency-distribution studies in populations living in areas of different malarial endemicity; malaria-parasite-density surveys in G-6-PD normal and deficient children; induced-falciparum malaria in human volunteers; and G-6-PD deficiency among patients with severe clinical falciparum malaria. The results of recent studies have provided evidence that G-6-PD deficiency offers a selective advantage to the carrier against potentially lethal malaria infection.

Rh-negative Gene and Malaria
A most interesting hypothesis has been put forward about the possible selection against the Rh-negative gene by malaria. The incidence of the Rh gene is generally low in areas in which malaria is or was endemic. It was suggested that a population subject to a heavily malarious environment might be superior antibody producers owing to selection by elimination of poor antibody producers. If this were so, erythroblastosis foetalis should be more intense in malarious areas, and Rh-negative genes should be selectively eliminated if the frequency of the gene is or was below 0·50. Hence Rh-negative mothers in a malarious area should show a higher incidence of sensitisation to an Rh-positive foetus than their counterparts in northern areas. In Ibadan, Nigeria, over 400 Rh-negative pregnant multiparae were studied and, apart from some who had had previous transfusions of Rh-positive blood, the evidence of those sensitised by pregnancy was only 2·5 per cent—a lower incidence than the figures recorded from Europe and elsewhere. This evidence does not, therefore, substantiate the above hypothesis.

Human genetics is one of the elements that can be used in the planning of co-ordinated attacks on disease, since it can sometimes differentiate individuals who are susceptible from those who are not.

Genetic factors often determine *group susceptibility* or resistance to disease, e.g. the racial immunity to vivax malaria of West African Negroes; alternatively *individual susceptibility* can be a reflection of genetic factors, e.g. twins are sometimes more liable to certain morbid conditions. In addition, immune deficiencies whether cellular or humoral, e.g. agammaglobulinaemia, are consequent on genetic factors, while genetic failure may be responsible for altered patterns of disease, e.g. defective cellular immunity in lepromatous leprosy.

Population genetic studies are a recent important expansion of the field of genetics and the knowledge thus acquired can be of practical value in preventive medicine, in the form commonly referred to as genetic counselling. This is particularly important in the situation as it is at present in Africa, where sickle-cell anaemia has an incidence of nearly 2 per cent in some countries and may be responsible for a childhood mortality of approximately 5 per 1000.

(6) Mental Health

Throughout the world there is an increasing awareness of mental illness as a significant cause of morbidity. This awareness has increased with the steady decline of morbidity due to nutritional disorders, communicable diseases and other forms of physical illness. There is also a better understanding of certain behavioural and social problems which had previously not been properly recognised as manifestations of mental illness. The role of the community both in the prevention of mental illness and the care of the mentally sick has now been widely recognised and it is regarded as the only appropriate basis for the development of mental health programmes.

Various forms of mental illness are encountered:

(a) *Sub-normal intelligence*
Arrested or incomplete development of the mind.

(b) *Psychoses*
These include the manic-depressive psychoses and schizophrenia, and a variety of organic psychoses which are related to demonstrable lesions of the brain.

(c) *Psychoneuroses and psychosomatic disorders*

(d) *Behavioural disorders*
These include maladjustment in childhood, juvenile delinquency, absenteeism, etc.

(e) *Psychopathic disorders*
These present as irresponsible, often aggressive antisocial acts, repeated in spite of appeals, warnings and sanctions.

Objectives of Mental Health Programme
The main objective of a mental health programme is to ensure for each individual optimal development of his mental abilities and a satisfactory emotional adjustment to his community and environment. Thus, the programme will include the promotion of mental health, the prevention of mental illness and the care of the mentally sick.

Promotion of Mental Health
The positive aspect of the mental health programme involves the design and creation of social and environmental situations in which mental health will grow and flourish. The factors which promote mental

health are both physical and socio-cultural. The physical aspect includes the promotion of the general physical fitness of the individual and the control of environmental stresses such as excessive noise. The socio-cultural factors include the consolidation of family life, the control of economic stresses, and the resolution of conflicts within the society.

The Prevention of Mental Illness

The prevention of mental illness is to some extent limited because the aetiology of some of these disorders is not known. A number of underlying causes, predisposing or precipitating factors have been identified. The main aetiological groups are:

- (*a*) Genetic factors
- (*b*) Organic brain damage
- (*c*) Socio-cultural factors
- (*d*) Idiopathic group.

(a) *Genetic factors*

There has been a tendency to exaggerate the role of genetic factors in the aetiology of mental illness. The familial occurrence of certain forms of mental illness may be determined by social and environmental factors rather than by genetic factors. Thus, mental illness in the child of alcoholic parents may have resulted from the stresses of an unsuitable home background rather than from genetic inheritance. There are, however, some clear examples of mental subnormality resulting from genetic factors, e.g. Down's syndrome, which is determined by a demonstrable chromosomal abnormality. More subtle genetic factors which are manifested in the form of personality types, response to stresses and other behavioural patterns are recognised but are difficult to quantify. The role of genetic factors in the aetiology of the major psychoses (manic-depressive psychoses and schizophrenics) has not been clearly defined.

(b) *Organic brain damage and degenerative lesions*

Organic brain damages may result from:

- (i) *Trauma*—including birth trauma
- (ii) *Infections*—e.g. meningitis, syphilis, trypanosomiasis, kuru, and other forms of encephalitis, acute febrile illness, hyperpyrexia.
- (iii) *Malnutrition*—e.g. vitamin deficiency—pellagra, beri-beri, Korsakov's psychosis; protein-malnutrition—clinical and experimental studies suggest that severe protein malnutrition in childhood may result in permanent mental retardation.
- (iv) *Toxins*—alcohol, opiates and other habit forming drugs, amphetamines, cannabis, lysergic acid.
- (v) *Degenerative lesions*—senility, specific degenerative diseases, e.g. Sydenham's chorea, changes secondary to arteriosclerosis.

The increasing human life span has brought the problems of old age into greater prominence.

(c) *Socio-cultural factors*

The social environment of the individual plays a prominent role in determining the state of his mental health. Social stresses can often be identified as initiating and precipitating factors of acute mental illness. This association is most prominent in relation to behavioural problems in childhood which often reflect emotional problems within the family.

Although patterns of non-organic psychoses are similar in many communities, the manifestations are conditioned by cultural factors. Thus, the recognition of mental illness depends on a careful evaluation of the norms, beliefs and customs within the particular culture. Thus, for example, a man who would not touch a particular object because he believes that it is inhabited by evil spirits may in one culture, be manifesting signs of acute mental illness, but in another culture, may be showing no more than reasonable caution.

(d) *Idiopathic group*

Within this group are various psychotic and psycho-neurotic illnesses, psychopathic personality, problems and behavioural disorders. It seems likely that in most cases, each condition is not the result of a single aetiological agent, rather the occurrence of disease is determined by a chain or a web of interrelated factors—a genetic predisposition, facilitating and inhibitory social, cultural and environmental factors, and the existence of various precipitating factors.

The Elements of a Community Mental Health Programme

The basic ingredient of a community health programme is community concern for the patients and their families, and community acceptance of its responsibility for the prevention and care of mental illness. It has been rightly said that 'Community care is possible only in a community which cares'. Community health education is therefore vital to the success of these programmes and it should be directed to the following objectives.

(i) *Eradication of superstitious fears and prejudices*

Traditional attitudes to mental illness include superstitious fears that the ill patients are possessed by devils and evil spirits. Even in modern societies there are many social attitudes to mental illness which are unfounded and illogical. These attitudes result in painful social stigma against the mentally ill and permanent prejudices against those who have fully recovered. Successful treatment and social rehabilitation of patients will be much enhanced by a tolerant and understanding attitude within the community.

(ii) *Dissemination of knowledge of the manifestations of mental illness*
It is particularly important that the early signs of mental illness be
recognised so that remedial action can be promptly taken. The early
signs may be misinterpreted by relatives, friends and society as merely
anti-social behaviour calling for punishment rather than treatment.
The community should be taught that 'a person who is troublesome,
may be a person in trouble'.

(iii) *Participation of the community in the care and rehabilitation
     of the mentally sick*
The attitude in many communities is to seek custodial care for the
mentally ill, where the patients can be isolated for indefinitely long
periods. The modern concept is to treat the patients as far as possible
within the community, thereby minimising the effects of the illness on
the patient and his family, and also facilitating his social rehabilitation.

Patterns of Care

The prevention and curative services take many forms. Facilities are
required for out-patient and in-patient care, follow-up services and
general mental health promotion in the community.

Out-patient care within the community would include psychiatric
out-patient clinics, a variety of special clinics (child guidance, counselling) and day hospitals. The advantages of the day hospital are
that it:

(*a*) conserves limited in-patient hospital resources for patients who
     require them
(*b*) exploits the social dynamic forces of the community in the care
     of the mentally ill
(*c*) avoids the disturbing effects of the unfamiliar and artificial en-
     vironment of the hospital
(*d*) assists in the rehabilitation of the patient in his home, family and
     job.

The mental health problems of the community are stratified in terms
of age and other social features. The mental health programme would
include measures to prevent mental illness which are appropriate at
each age-group:

(a) *Pre-natal*—to provide good ante-natal care and delivery services
        to ensure normal foetal development
     to prevent congenital infections (e.g. syphilis)
     to avoid intrapartum trauma.
(b) *Infancy*—to provide emotional security within the family circle
     to care for abandoned children and children without families
     to prevent malnutrition, communicable and other diseases.

(c) *School age*—to provide a balanced programme of work and play
    to avoid excessive fatigue—physical and mental
    to encourage positive use of leisure hours
    to establish satisfactory social adjustment inside and outside the
        family.
(d) *Adolescence*—to prevent, identify and deal with emotional prob-
    lems at puberty by health education including sex-education.
(e) *Young adult*—to assist adjustment of working life, especially where
    rural/urban, agrarian/industrial transfers are involved.
(f) *Adults*—to provide counselling service for family life and con-
    sultant service for resolving conflicts in relation to self, family
    and community.
(g) *Old-age*—to provide substitute systems of care where traditional
    extended family systems are breaking down
    to re-phrase the leadership roles of the elderly where they have
        been deprived of their traditional position of authority, e.g.
        provide ritual functions in the commuity.

It is clear from these examples that a successful mental care programme cannot be operated solely by professional psychiatrists and
other specialist personnel, but it must include all medical and health
workers, voluntary agencies and other community resources.

(7) Occupation and Health

The health problems of workers in developing countries are more
complex than those of industrialised nations because of the high
prevalence of epidemic and endemic diseases in most areas of the tropics.
Modern concepts of occupational health embrace all types of employment including mercantile and commercial enterprises, service trades,
utilities, forestry and agriculture. The distinction between environmental, occupational and industrial health is academic in the context of
many tropical families where the husband may work in a factory while
the wife and children cultivate a plot for food.

Agriculture and Health

Although industrialisation is the common path for the achievement of
the fullest use of each nation's natural resources, the economy of many
tropical countries is still basically agricultural and agricultural workers
constitute a high proportion of the working population.

All forms of activities connected with growing, harvesting and
primary processing of crops; with breeding, raising and caring of
animals; and with tending of gardens and nurseries is agriculture.

Accidents take a large toll of life or result in permanent and disabling
injuries. They may be associated with farm machinery or inadequate
housekeeping around farms.

Infections and parasitic diseases can be contracted directly or indirectly during the course of an agricultural occupation (Table 13.2). The use of pesticides, insecticides and other chemicals has greatly increased in developing countries resulting in acute or chronic poisoning from compounds ranging from the toxic organo-phosphorus compounds,

TABLE 13.2
Some occupational diseases of agriculture (After WHO 1962)*

	A. Principally contracted through an agricultural occupation	B. Occasionally contracted through an agricultural occupation	C. Questionably contracted through an agricultural occupation
VIRAL	Tick-borne encephalitis Tick-borne haemorrhagic fever	Psittacosis Rabies Mosquito-borne encephalitis Mosquito-borne haemorrhagic fever	Mosquito-borne fever Tick-borne fever Cowpox Foot and mouth disease African tick-borne fever
RICKETTSIAL	Q fever	Scrub typhus	
BACTERIAL	Anthrax—Brucellosis Leptospirosis Tetanus Bovine tuberculosis Tularaemia	Plague Human tuberculosis	
PARASITIC	Ancylostomiasis Schistosomiasis	Hydatid disease Malaria	Filariasis Leishmaniasis Onchocerciasis
FUNGAL			Actinomycosis Blastomycosis— South American Histoplasmosis

* Joint ILO/WHO Committee on Occupational Health (WHO 1962).

nitrated and chlorinated phenols to DDT. Besides communicable disease and exposure to chemicals, the extremes of *climatic conditions* such as temperature, humidity and solar radiation impose additional stresses upon the tropical worker.

Thus the health problems of agricultural workers are numerous and complex and methods for their prevention must be developed taking into consideration the differing conditions of every country.

Industry and Health

Most tropical countries are committed to industrialisation: it is the pace at which this is occurring which differs. Mass labour migration from rural to industrial areas immediately introduces enormous problems in housing and one is only too familiar with the growth of insanitary slums around industrial complexes, which adversely affects the physical, mental and social well-being of the worker and his family.

Many small factories and workshops have been built where *dangerous chemicals* are being handled in a very indiscriminate and careless fashion. Lead acid battery makers and repairers are a particularly vulnerable group. In these little, often neglected workshops, a variety of occupations are going on—making; grinding; welding; cutting; moulding and painting various things.

In addition to chemicals, *heat* and *poor ventilation* are serious hazards in hot weather leading to heat cramps, heat exhaustion and fatigue resulting not only in low and faulty production but also in an increasing risk of accident.

Compressed-air illness in divers and caisson workers on the many dams and bridges that are constantly being built in the tropics must be borne in mind.

With the expansion in mining and the utilisation of mineral wealth all types of *pneumoconiosis, silicosis* and *asbestosis* are on the increase in the tropics, as are the vegetable-dust diseases. *Byssinosis*, due to cotton dust, has been reported in cotton mills as well as in ginneries in Egypt, the Sudan and other tropical countries where this product is grown and exported, while respiratory diseases due to exposure to mouldy sugar cane (bagassosis), mouldy hay (farmer's lung), wool, gum acacia, ricinus, etc., are on the increase.

Accidents in factories are a major hazard, especially among the agrarian population coming into contact with industrial machinery for the first time. The danger of *cancer* in the chemical, asbestos, rubber and other industries must be borne in mind.

Thus a number of very important industrial hazards already exist in the tropics and they are likely to increase in magnitude and complexity.

Labour Legislation

Legislation covering health, safety and welfare of workers is now operative in many tropical countries and will become universal before long. Without such labour laws progress in occupational health is virtually impossible. They should cover occupational diseases, worker's compensation, medical examination, protection of women workers, protection of young persons, radiation protection and labour inspection. These labour laws must be adequately enforced and are essential prerequisites to any effective occupational health programme.

Occupational Health Programmes

The type of occupational health programme needed will vary from country to country and a constant reappraisal of the situation is required as the degree of industrialisation increases and trained personnel become available. Many countries in Africa, for example, are developing occupational health units within the Ministry of Labour, and these usually have a staff consisting of a medical specialist with a diploma in industrial health, a qualified occupational hygienist and a registered nurse trained in industrial and occupational medicine.

Private occupational health services are sometimes provided by big industrial enterprises in the tropics undertaking total medical care for employees and dependants.

In other areas, group occupational health services are being organised by industry itself, providing membership to companies and firms of all sizes, employing as many as 3000 employees to small enterprises employing as few as 10 workers.

Where public and private services are deficient, such a group occupational health service is welcomed by industry and fulfils a dire need.

Certain basic concepts are essential for the organisation of occupational health programmes. Management has to be convinced that the benefits of the programme justify the costs involved. The co-operation of management is also essential to ensure a high attendance rate for preventive programmes.

The collaboration of trade unions, shop-stewards, worksite committees and the individual workers sometimes is the determining factor as to whether a programme will succeed or fail. Such co-operation can only be forthcoming if the medical staff succeed in convincing labour that they are neither the tools or spies of management.

In worksites where most of the workers are non-residential, it is essential to obtain whenever possible the co-operation of general practitioners who may be able to help to complete immunisation courses and give information about employees suffering from communicable diseases. Vaccination programmes should be carried out at the worksite and planned to avoid clashing with particularly busy periods. An occupational health doctor must be familiar with the disease patterns in the community outside the worksite, and the whole socio-economic setting of the worker must be appreciated.

In developing and industrialising countries, health patterns are changing so rapidly that one cannot be content to sit back after devising a preventive programme, however well planned and ably executed. New priorities may have to be established in the face of some of these changes.

Summary

The essential principles of prevention of the occupational diseases can be listed as follows:

(1) Sanitation and hygiene of factories:
  (*a*) Cleanliness of factories
  (*b*) Avoidance of overcrowding
  (*c*) Adequate heating, ventilation and lighting
  (*d*) Adequate sanitary facilities
  (*e*) Protection against inhalation of dust fumes, e.g. by use of respirators
  (*f*) Protection of eyes when applicable, e.g. by suitable goggles or effective screens
  (*g*) Food hygiene in canteens.
(2) Monitoring of the environment (e.g. radiation) and of the individual (e.g. lead workers)
(3) Substitution of noxious substances or processes whenever possible
(4) Limiting exposure to hazardous processes to the minimum of persons
(5) Pre-employment examination
(6) Notification of specified occupational diseases
(7) Health education and training
(8) Accident prevention, e.g. by adequate protection of machinery
(9) Rehabilitation.

Further Reading

International Health Regulations (1969). 1st annotated edn. 1971. WHO, Geneva.

Vaccination Certificate Requirements for International Travel. 1971. WHO, Geneva.

International Sanitary Regulations, 3rd annotated edn. 1966. WHO, Geneva.

Health and Safety at Work, ed. W. O. Phoon. 1971. National Safety First Council and Singapore Medical Association.

Health in Industry, by R. C. Browne. 1961. London: Edward Arnold Ltd.

Chapter Fourteen

The Organisation of Health Services

Introduction

Health activities aim at maintaining a way of life, an active continuing attitude of mind and code of conduct and behaviour which enables individual members, as well as the community as a whole, to adjust continuously to the changing circumstances of the environment in order to maintain general well-being.

There are examples from the earliest times of how communities tried to induce their members to lead healthy lives and to take steps to regain lost health. The books of Leviticus and Deuteronomy contain references to prohibition of the use of unclean animals for food; to methods of examination, diagnosis, treatment and prevention of the spread of leprosy and other skin diseases; to injunctions for the safe disposal of human excrement as a protection against certain diseases, etc. The kind and location of house in which people live, the food they eat, the work they do, even their thoughts and feelings directly influence their health for good or ill. Measures which the individual takes for the specific purpose of influencing his own health, or the health of relatives and dependants, are usually sporadic measures related to particular episodes of sickness or disability. When a community takes steps to improve health it is due to one or a combination of two or three main motives:

(1) The fear of epidemic disease and its devastating effect on all and sundry irrespective of social class
(2) The fact that those whose health are protected and whose diseases are treated adequately live longer and produce more towards family or national economic development
(3) Out of altruistic compassion for others, particularly the poor and those afflicted with disease and disability.

Every community has evolved some form of organised effort for the purpose of preventing and treating disease and disability. The differences in extent, sophistication and effectiveness between the organised efforts which different communities have evolved for this purpose reflect and express the differences in sophistication and social and economic development between the respective communities.

However, health-promoting and disease-controlling activities will not produce significant growth in a country's economy by themselves alone. Effective activities have to be undertaken in other fields such as agriculture, education, social and industrial development. Such national economic activities strive towards an ample production and equitable distribution of wealth, to ensure the well-being of the people of the country under constantly changing human and environmental conditions. Obvious economic advantages can be derived from specific health measures which favour agricultural and industrial production. Similarly certain agricultural policies can have a very beneficial effect on the nutritional status of the population; and economic development is essential for rapidly increasing the provision of institutions and the training of personnel for the delivery of better health services. Therefore, the basic and most important objective and function of health workers should be to try and alter the attitudes, beliefs and behaviour of people among whom they work in order to encourage the adoption of more effective social, economic and medical measures for promoting health and for preventing and coping with sickness, disability and injury, and improving the health situation.

The Nature and Scope of Health Services

In most parts of the tropical world today health services are more concerned with the study of diseases and how to cure them than with the study of health and how to promote and maintain it. This is due to the historical development of scientific medicine in Europe and America, and the influence which these advanced countries have had, and continue to exercise, over tropical countries which are still poor and underdeveloped. Development took place much more rapidly in the purely biological sciences than in the social and allied sciences of health promotion and protection. This led to the creation of a sharp distinction between these sciences and between their respective services. More intellectual effort and money was and continues to be devoted to the diagnosis and cure of disease and injury in the individual patient than to the promotion of health and prevention of disease in the individual and community, or to the diagnosis and treatment of disease, injury and the attendant social disruption, on a community basis. The result is that 'curative' and 'preventive' medicine tend to be conceived, planned and organised as separate disciplines. In advanced countries the disadvantages of this arrangement are obvious enough in the irritation, frustration and loss of time caused by fragmentation of services; the rising costs of medical care and the utilisation of doctors who might otherwise have been available for, and some of whom have actually come from, the underdeveloped countries. In tropical countries where the important operative factors are poverty and low levels of social and economic development, rather than geography and climate, the results are more serious and unfavourable to progress.

Health services were defined almost fifty years ago as being designed to prevent disease and accidents, promote physical, social and mental health, efficiency and happiness and prolong useful life; through organised community effort for the sanitation of the environment, the control of diseases and education in personal hygiene. Their role includes organising medical and nursing services for the early diagnosis and adequate treatment of diseases, and developing good social standards to ensure the health and longevity of members of the community. This means that the organisation and administration of the entire range of services which are usually described and provided separately as curative, preventive, public health, etc., should be much more closely related to each other especially at the community level. They should be integrated wherever possible, and certainly always co-ordinated. They include all those services which provide for promotion of health, happiness and efficiency by teaching healthy living and by providing adequate housing, nutrition, etc. These are the community services which prevent illness by vaccination and other forms of immunisation, by the control of water, food, animals and insects and refuse collection and disposal, and by the control of atmospheric pollution. The curative services include the detection of diseases and abnormality, adequate treatment, rehabilitation and after care, including remedies for social factors which lead to delayed recovery or increased disability.

Adequate Health Services imply more than the mere provision of medical and health institutions, facilities and technical staff to perform the functions listed above. Their effectiveness depends on their being available and readily accessible to most members of the community in forms which people are able to understand, accept and utilise. It depends also on the ability and willingness of doctors, nurses and other health workers to give explanation and advice and to render service based on an understanding of the attitude of the people among whom they work towards the prevailing diseases, deficiencies and unfavourable conditions of their environment.

Existing Patterns of Organisation

The patterns of health services which exist vary between different groups of countries and in different parts of the same country, depending on the level of social and economic development. Certain features are however characteristic of the underdeveloped countries, many of which are in the tropics. The services are grossly inadequate to meet the needs of the vast majority of the population. They tend to be concentrated mainly in urban areas, but even in these areas they only provide an adequate service for a small proportion of the community. They tend to be based on institutions which provide treatment for specific diseases or groups of diseases. Usually curative and preventive services are strictly separated with regard to personnel and buildings. In those areas where an attempt is made to combine the provision of curative and preventive services within the same building, as a rule, separate personnel are used for each service.

A considerable proportion of the population still rely wholly or in part on unscientific medical care, including household and folk remedies and the ministrations of herbalists, medicine men and soothsayers. People resort to such unscientific methods and healers either because scientific services in dispensaries, clinics, hospitals and by medical practitioners are not readily available, are too expensive, or have not been accepted as being relevant to the particular illness. Often both scientific and unscientific methods and remedies are used at the same time. Usually this section of the community also suffers from a lack of basic social services like good housing, water supply, refuse disposal, educational and recreational facilities, because of poverty. Some of them may be protected by vaccination or other forms of immunisation from certain communicable diseases like smallpox. They may have had prophylactic mass treatment against diseases; they may have had their homes sprayed with insecticide to destroy malaria-carrying mosquitoes; or may have had samples of their blood taken in malaria or sleeping-sickness surveys. If they are in urban or semi-urban areas, a few are likely to have had chest X-ray examinations and/or BCG vaccination; some scientific care during pregnancy and/or delivery, in infancy, during school attendance and in relation to their employment in large government, agricultural or industrial undertakings; and to have heard radio programmes or seen film shows on health.

In some territories almost all the health work in rural areas is done by centrally or regionally based mobile field units although there is a steady increase in the provision of dispensaries, clinics and health centres. Such work is organised in response to epidemics of specific diseases, the particular interest of research workers and organisations. In more developed countries rural areas are divided into health districts under the control of district medical officers. They are responsible for the total health care of the population, but they spend most of their time in purely curative work in their base hospital or clinic, and in the outlying clinics and dispensaries which they visit at intervals. When they exist, preventive services like the control of refuse disposal, water supply, food insect-vectors and smallpox vaccination are left almost entirely to sanitarians. Usually the doctors, dispensers, nurses and mobile field unit workers are employed by the central national government, while the auxiliary nurses, dispensary attendants, sanitary orderlies and overseers are local or district council employees.

A few towns have local authority health services with responsibility for environmental health control, care of pregnant women and children, the control of communicable diseases and the collection and registration of vital statistics, but in most of them the doctors, nurses and sanitarians are employees of the central, regional or provincial government. These services are usually quite distinct from the hospitals and clinics with the result that the impression is created that they are in competition with each other for the allocation of funds and personnel. Usually hospitals and clinics are run by the central and sometimes by the local government, foreign missionary or aid-giving organisations, commercial or industrial companies or the military service. They vary from modern teaching hospitals, large general hospitals with or without specialist units, special hospitals, to medium sized, cottage or small rural hospitals and what are merely clinics or dispensaries with a few beds.

In capital cities there is a Director of Medical or Health Services responsible directly or through a lay administrator to a Minister of Health or of Health and Social Welfare for the administration of the health services of the entire country. His immediate assistants are usually senior doctors responsible for hospitals and curative services, laboratory services; preventive services or mobile health units; senior nurses and pharmacists; and senior administrative staff responsible for management, personnel, stores and finance. This represents the central health administration. The larger and/or more developed tropical countries have state, provincial or similar administrative organisations, which cannot readily be considered as intermediate level health administrations in many cases because they are either practically autonomous with no real control direction, supervision or feed back; or they are merely outposts of the central administration with no delegated functions and responsibilities: and with little or no relationship with other units of administration like education, public works, agriculture, public utilities, social welfare, etc., at a comparable level.

Guiding Principles for organising Health Services
The first and most important principle for the organisation of health services in poor underdeveloped areas is that the government should assume responsibility for ensuring that the best arrangements possible are made, within the of limits available technical, human and financial resources, for the protection, promotion and maintenance of the personal and communal health of all members of the population. These arrangements should be based on the nature and extent of the existing and foreseen health problems, and should involve non-governmental, private and commercial agencies. Whatever services exist at present will give better results if they are planned and organised in a more satisfactory manner. Special attention should be given to the establishment of priorities, to adapting existing services along modern lines, and to the training of, and duties performed by, various levels of health

L

personnel. Considerable benefits can be derived from developing a certain amount of uniformity in organisation and practice and inter-territorial health co-operation and co-ordination, particularly in the control of communicable diseases, the alleviation of malnutrition and the training of personnel. Doctors must assume more general administrative and organisational responsibility for their work and for the work of the staff under their supervision. They must give greater consideration to the cost of the services which they render and to the ways in which community health services are financed.

The central health organisation should be headed by a national health ministry including a national health planning body to formulate the country's health policy within the framework of its national socio-economic plan. The ministry should have statutory responsibilities for co-ordination of existing facilities; for education and registration of members of the medical, nursing and allied professions, for giving grants-in-aid, specific grants, technical assistance, or providing emergency or supporting service to the provinces or regions; and for evaluation and research. Medical and nursing schools should play a vital role in planning and providing health services. Health services should be organised to serve communities—a community being defined as a grouping of individuals in a geographically demarked area and dependent on each other for the achievement of common political, economic and social goals. Thus a national health service should serve the entire nation. It should be in relation to regional or provincial health services, which should be related in turn to local district health services serving their respective areas. Every attempt should be made to preserve the same pattern of subdivision into local districts, provinces or regions as is used in the political and administrative field, without sacrificing efficiency. This facilitates joint consultation, planning, operation and evaluation of those services within other fields.

Much confusion arises in the consideration of health service organisations because the various categories of staff and types of institutions do not subserve the same functions in different countries. Attempts which have been made in a number of tropical countries to plan health organisations on the basis of the ratio of doctors to population, nurses to population and beds to population, have not taken account of the fact that institutions subserve widely different functions even when they go by the same name. The distribution of doctors, nurses and institutions is often very arbitrary. Another source of confusion is the fact that to many people the concept of a basic health service is limited to a network of peripheral health units established to perform a narrowly selected group of functions by personnel based almost exclusively in the units themselves. A basic health service should include intermediate and central health units and administrations, hospitals and health departments, right on to the central ministry. Its 'basicness' lies in its being simple, effective, integrated, comprehensive, available and readily accessible, free or at nominal cost to the vast majority of the population, in respect of their most important and pressing health needs and problems. In fact in poor underdeveloped tropical countries the most that can be hoped for in the foreseeable future is the development of such a health service. It is therefore superfluous to use the word 'basic' in this context.

The Local Health Organisation

Each local community should ensure effective planning of health objectives and services based on the existing needs, problems and available human, material and financial resources. Such a local community could consist of a village or group of villages; one or more towns and their surrounding villages; or a municipal city or its constituent districts or municipal wards. Its health services should aim at providing facilities for the following activities, to an extent which will vary with the particular locality, and should make use of one or more multipurpose health units, clinics or centres, staffed by governmental, non-governmental, professional, auxiliary and lay personnel as required and as available.

(1) *Recording of births, deaths, and certain diseases*

Simple but accurate records for use locally, returns of which are made to the intermediate level of organisation on a routine basis; or directly to the intermediate and central level in the case of notifiable infectious diseases or a sudden or unusual outbreak or disaster.

(2) *Family health*

Antenatal and postnatal care including family planning. Arrangements for childbirth in a clinic, centre or at home. Family health protection in and out of school and at work. Home visiting, immunisation and promotion of sound nutrition and emotional development. Diagnosis and out-patient treatment of diseases and injuries. There should be facilities for referring cases of serious or complicated illness requiring hospitalisation, consultation or investigation, to an intermediate or central service level; for obtaining the services of more competent staff from such levels; for exchange of staff between levels and for regular supervision by staff from those levels.

(3) *Environmental health*

Control of environmental sanitation as described in Chapter 11.

(4) *Health education and community development*

In the normal course of their work all health personnel should help people to understand that diseases have a natural history which is often closely related to the physical and social environment. They should try and impart the necessary knowledge and skills to enable people to do the best they can in promoting their own health and well-being, and in dealing with minor ailments and disabilities. They should help them to accept the principles of scientific medicine and to make full and proper use of available health services.

The Provincial or Intermediate Health Organisation

The natural referral points from outlying health units are district or provincial hospitals. They have consultant services, facilities for conducting surgical and other operations and a wide variety of laboratory and other clinical investigations and supporting services should exist. They should have facilities for transporting patients and staff on consultative or supervisory visits; for storage and distribution of medicines and equipment and for the in-service training of staff. A hospital already provides certain features of a comprehensive service for the individual patient. It promotes his health and recovery by giving adequate housing, food and water supply in healthy surroundings. Diseases and injuries are diagnosed and treated, thus preventing the development of more serious diseases and complications.

It should be possible to make the hospital serve the health promotion and disease prevention, personal and social welfare needs of the population of the geographical area in which it is situated. In this way it would become the seat of the district or provincial health organisation. Its various units would become more co-ordinated. They would provide the staff and organisation necessary for giving direction and supervision to the integrated work which goes on in local health units. At present there is hardly any such support, supervision and stimulus for continuing in-service training of staff and improvement of service. It should provide epidemiological intelligence and analysis of records from local health units, co-ordination of their health, social welfare and community development programmes, and liaison with other government and non-governmental services. Separate provincial or district health units may already exist, or it may not be considered practicable or desirable to build such units as part of or close to hospitals. But even in such cases much of the desired effect can be obtained if the different units co-ordinate their work to an increasing extent.

Central Health Organisation

The main functions of the central health administration should be planning, establishment of standards, evaluation, provision of advisory services, technical assistance and transport to intermediate and local levels, budgetary provision for the national services, collection and analysis of health statistics, liaison with other government ministries and with commercial, industrial and non-governmental agencies, procurement, storage and distribution of equipment, supplies and drugs, epidemiological surveillance and control activities, staff recruitment and training, central laboratory services and environmental and occupational health supporting services.

One of the problems of national health administrations is that of ensuring a multi-purpose and integrated organisational approach at its intermediate and central levels. At the consumer level in the local district service, it is clear that a multi-purpose worker is essential to provide health care. There it can be seen that a multi-purpose health unit is valid and practicable. But immediately beyond that level there is an ever-increasing range of specialisation between health and health-related disciplines, between different health disciplines, and even within individual health disciplines. This specialisation tends to become more marked in more sophisticated services. There is no comparable increasing expertise in, and responsibility for, providing multi-disciplined and integrated service which is needed at these higher and more sophisticated levels. The supervision and direction of multi-purpose auxiliary workers is to a large extent carried out by single-purpose professionals. There should be more emphasis on the development of the multi-purpose approach at higher levels of organisation. One can almost say that a specialist is one whose work benefits fewer and fewer people directly. Therein lies much of the difficulty in providing total health coverage of the population.

Financing Health Services

Lack of funds is one of the important limiting factors in improving the health situation in tropical countries. Already many governments allocate up to 10 per cent of their total expenditure on medical and health services, and it is unlikely that this proportion will be increased under prevailing conditions of underdevelopment. On the other hand, the cost of such services continues to increase because of increase in the size of the population; increase in medical knowledge and in the cost of its application; and increase in awareness of the benefits of scientific medicine. In addition to the funds spent by government, non-governmental and commercial agencies, there is a considerable amount of individual private expenditure by the public for medical care and attention, both scientific and unscientific, and in particular for the purchase of medicines.

A significant feature of health services expenditure in tropical underdeveloped countries is that those members of the public who are wealthier, better educated, better motivated towards healthful living and indeed healthier, make more use of and derive greater benefit from the free or highly subsidised government or non-government health services. There it is essential that health services should be planned and organised to make more efficient use of the limited available financial resources for the benefit of the greatest number of people. Centrally made laws should provide for a health organisation, outline its work and allocate funds to carry out its work. At both intermediate and local levels of administration there should be the possibility of making health rules and regulations and of allocating funds for specific health purposes. This should be in addition to funds provided, and powers delegated, by the central authority.

In some countries consideration has been given to schemes for a contributory health insurance; to making commercial and industrial firms responsible for providing medical care and health promotion and disease prevention services for their employees.

International Health Organisations

The idea of co-operation of different groups, clans and nations for their common good is not a new one. What is new is faith in fundamental human rights, and the dignity and worth of the human person, in the equal rights of men and women, of nations large and small, to enjoy better standards of health, happiness and freedom. Expression is being given in the United Nations and its related agencies, to this concept. The guiding principles which underlie the activities of the World Health Organisation, other members of the United Nations and related agencies and the technical health assistance given by advanced countries to tropical underdeveloped countries are as follows:

Health is an important element in the social and economic circumstances which determine and guide most human activities, at the local, national and international level; therefore it is essential to co-ordinate activities in the health field with other economic and social development activities to ensure balanced national development.

Careful planning is essential for the orderly development of an efficient central health administration, and the provision of adequate basic health services, as an integral part of national economic and social development.

It is imperative that assisted countries should have as rapidly as possible their own cadres of trained staff in all fields of health; this is the only real and lasting solution to their health problems.

Priority is given to specific requests for technical aid from governments according to the following criteria:

(i) The probability of achieving successful, useful and permanent results.

(ii) The relative importance of the problem in the whole health programme of the requesting country.

(iii) The ability of the country to provide the services required as measured by the availability of trained personnel and means of training personnel.

(iv) The financial and administrative ability of the country to absorb the requested assistance, taking into account all the health projects planned and in operation, as well as assistance in other forms which might overload the country's operating capacity.

(v) Reasonable assurance of satisfactory working relationships with the government throughout the programme.

(vi) Reasonable assurance that the project will be continued, and particularly that the government will provide adequate personnel and financial support for their continuation.

(vii) Balanced expenditure among the various health sectors.

(viii) Equitable distribution of funds among the countries in the region.

(ix) The strengthening of basic health services needed to assist economic and social development.

The main purpose of the work programme of WHO may be briefly described as:

(i) The strengthening of national health services.

(ii) The education of professional, technical and auxiliary staff in medicine and allied fields

(iii) Measures against the communicable, and certain non-communicable diseases and against adverse environmental and nutritional factors.

(iv) The provision of assistance in matters of international health interest.

(v) Medical research.

(vi) The co-ordination of health with other economic and social activities.

General Further Reading

Davey & Lightbody's *Control of Disease in the Tropics*, 4th ed. 1971, ed. T. H. Davey and T. Wilson. London: H. K. Lewis & Co. Ltd.

Control of Communicable Diseases in Man, ed. A. S. Benenson, 11th ed. 1970. American Public Health Association, Washington D.C. 20036.

Epidemiologic Methods. 5th Printing 1972. B. MacMahon, T. F. Pugh, J. Ipsen. Boston: Little, Brown & Co.

Index